Supporting Women for Labour and Birth

This new edition provides an up-to-date and thoughtful guide to supporting women in labour, looking at a range of approaches that promote a safe and positive experience of birth for women and their families.

Across the world, support in labour has been shown to reduce obstetric interventions and improve outcomes for women and babies. Written by two highly experienced midwifery authors, this text draws on a wide range of cutting-edge research on this topic, identifying how evidence can be applied to everyday practice. Narratives from women and practitioners, including midwives, doulas, childbirth educators and students, are used to illustrate a range of situations where the quality of support is central to the quality of experiences and outcomes. *Supporting Women for Labour and Birth* encourages readers to reflect on their experiences and examine evidence provided by both research and the experiences of women and practitioners in order to explore how this might be incorporated into their practice.

The only book to deal directly with the practical and emotional issues associated with labour support, this is an ideal text for student midwives and an important reference for practising midwives, doulas and other childbirth practitioners.

Nicky Leap is an Adjunct Professor of Midwifery at the University of Technology Sydney, and at the Molly Wardaguga Research Centre, Charles Darwin University, Alice Springs. Nicky divides her time between living in Bristol (UK) and the Blue Mountains (Australia).

Billie Hunter is Professor of Midwifery at Cardiff University, UK. She holds an Honorary Chair at the University of Surrey, UK and is an Adjunct Professor of Midwifery at the University of Technology Sydney, Australia. Billie is also the Director of a World Health Organization Collaborating Centre for Midwifery Development at Cardiff University, which contributes to global efforts to strengthen midwifery and midwifery education.

Supporting Women for Labour and Birth

A Thoughtful Guide

SECOND EDITION

Nicky Leap and Billie Hunter

Routledge
Taylor & Francis Group

LONDON AND NEW YORK

First published 2022
by Routledge
4 Park Square, Milton Park, Abingdon, Oxon, OX14 4RN

and by Routledge
52 Vanderbilt Avenue, New York, NY 10017

Routledge is an imprint of the Taylor & Francis Group, an informa business

First edition published by Routledge 2016

British Library Cataloguing-in-Publication Data
A catalogue record for this book is available from the British Library

Library of Congress Cataloging-in-Publication Data
A catalog record for this book has been requested

ISBN: 978-0-367-55232-9 (hbk)
ISBN: 978-0-367-55233-6 (pbk)
ISBN: 978-1-003-09252-0 (ebk)

DOI: 10.4324/9781003092520

Typeset in Times New Roman
by Apex CoVantage, LLC

We dedicate this book to our friend and mentor, Andrea Robertson, who died suddenly while we were bringing the first edition of this book to fruition. A childbirth educator and birth activist for over 40 years, Andrea raised awareness about the need for woman centred maternity care in many countries. Thousands of midwives across the world attended Andrea's workshops, learnt from her publications and used the extensive teaching aids, equipment and resources that she made accessible through her company, Birth International.

Andrea gave us much encouragement and a wealth of resources to draw on in the writing of this book: not least, permission to use her line drawings of support in labour. Her vision and determination to make the world a better place, starting with birth, will continue to inspire us:

> I believe that the health and wellbeing of our planet and our very lives depend on caring, empathetic people taking responsibility and working together for the betterment of all. This process has its roots in birth, and midwives have a major role to play at this pivotal time. We humans need to achieve better birth outcomes as a demonstration of our commitment to the future. We must reduce intervention and pay more attention to protecting nature's intricate system for the survival of our species. A generous dose of love and compassion for our fellow beings, especially women striving to do their best in labour, would be one place to start.
>
> (Andrea Robertson, *The Midwife Companion: The Art of Support During Birth*. Sydney: Birth International, 2007, p.ix)

Contents

Figures

Tables

Foreword to 1st edition

It is always an honour to be asked to write a Foreword to a book, but to be asked to write a Foreword to a book by Nicky Leap and Billie Hunter is to be tasked with a quest. With a quest you gain more than you ever give, and indeed I have.

There have been, there are and there will be many great midwives who make the world a better place for childbearing women, but to 'sit at the feet' of Nicky Leap and Billie Hunter, as I felt I was doing reading this book, is to truly understand the meaning of wisdom. As I read this book I found my midwife heart overflowing with hope and excitement, and I was reminded of Ina May Gaskin's words, 'If a woman doesn't look like a goddess in labour then someone isn't treating her right'.* As midwives, we have the amazing privilege of being a part of a woman's transformation into a goddess.

Just recently I was caring for a woman having a long and challenging labour. As I watched her sway with the contractions, her skin glisten with sweat, caught like diamond drops in the soft, dappled light, I thought this must be what a goddess looks like. Love swirled in that room, eyes were misted with awe, hands touched with love, cool cloths were swept along her face and neck, and warm towels and hands were pressed against her back, moving in time with her labour dance. There was so much love in that room – enough to make you feel drunk on it. Once again, as I have seen many times before as a midwife, I saw the fingers of our limited human existence pierce that thin veil into 'other worlds'. There are not many times in life that humans get to experience this connection to the universe at such a profound level. I often wonder why it is that we rob so many women of this possibility. Without love, support and trust, the goddess cannot shine.

I remember another lovely woman I cared for saying to me recently about her first birth in hospital, 'yes they touched me, but it was a functional touch. I don't want a functional touch when I give birth.' When women are in labour, pretence is stripped bare and imposters are exposed with brutal clarity. Nicky and Billie give us the tools and understanding in this beautiful book to be truly present as midwives and to go beyond being 'functional' to being the co-creators of goddesses. Now that is something I want to put on my resumé!

This book begins with a lovely dedication to the wonderful Andrea Robertson, who sadly left this world recently. However, she left this world with a beautiful legacy that lives on today and shines through the pages of this book. The book is divided into nine chapters that midwives will find so useful for informing their practice. I think the most refreshing thing about this book is all the activities and reflections throughout it. This is not a 'sit back and be filled up with information' sort of book; it is one that will challenge you and make you think and grow as a midwife.

Helping women to work with pain and fear sits at the heart of the book. Pain and fear both challenge women giving birth and indeed the midwives who care for them. Being able to work with pain and women's fear (and, I would add, health providers' fear, too) is the fulcrum that normal labour and birth pivot on. Sometimes it takes only a word or a dispassionate look to take birth in a totally new direction. 'Who' we are and 'how' we are with women is of more importance than 'where' we are and 'what' we are doing as midwives. The emotional aspects of labour support are key to midwives being able to work with women and be truly present for them, and this is dealt with beautifully in the book. The book ends appropriately with 'midwifing the midwife' and the importance of looking after each other and ourselves.

If every midwife absorbed the lessons in this book, then most women we care for would be able to join with Debra Adelaide to say the following:

> So far it was his [her son's] and my greatest achievement. Together we had written the complete works of Beethoven, scaled the Himalayas, flown to the moon and back, then around the earth several times for good measure. Nothing I had ever done was as clever, as beautiful, as pure or as perfect as this. Now I knew how God felt after the sixth day of creation. Why he had done it. I was a god. I was a goddess. I was God. I had commanded creation, said 'Fiat Lux', and witnessed life in all its glory. Had I also blasphemed?
>
> (Adelaide, 1996, p.216)

Support during labour and birth does not and cannot start when contractions commence. Support must be threaded through the fabric of every midwife/woman encounter; it sits in every expression we use, it rests on every word we utter and it is passed to women by the way we touch them. Women can smell our fear and pick up on our doubts and, if we don't do the work we need to ourselves, we will never be able to be truly present for them.

I want to end my Foreword with this wonderful quote from Anna Maria Dell'oso. For me this sums up the need for support, the experience of support and the impact of support, and it captures so well the essence of this beautiful and timely book.

> Being with someone, murmuring along with their heartbeat, breathing with them is a lost art. The true midwives of birth and death, those who keep vigil at the bedposts are rare. They are people whose eyes are accustomed to darkness and light, who stand waiting by night and by dawn, holding cloaks and soft wrappings at the cross-roads and gateways; they stand at the threshold, at the breaking of the paths, watching the lights, rain and the winds, welcoming and farewelling our journeying souls. The price of such people is above rubies. No machines that go ping can stand in their place. Yet so often that is all we have. Thank God it doesn't happen to me.
>
> (Dell'oso, 1989, p.201)

by Hannah Dahlen

Note

* For Ina May Gaskin quote, see: www.azquotes.com/author/37677-Ina_May_Gaskin

References

Adelaide, D. (1996). Desiring the unknown. In Adelaide, D. (ed.), *Mother Love* (pp.211–225). Australia: Random House.

Dell'oso, A.M. (1989). *Cats Cradles and Chamomile Tea*. Australia: Random House.

Foreword to 2nd edition

It is an absolute honour and joy to be asked by Nicky Leap and Billie Hunter to write this Foreword. I feel humbled, and somewhat inadequate, as I admire and have been fortunate to learn from these wonderful, inspirational midwives.

As a midwife for over 30 years and working in academia for the last nine years, I was completely blown away by the first edition of this book. So much so that I recommended it as pre-course reading to all new student midwives, and we use the book throughout the Bachelor of Midwifery (Hons) programme. The sensitive, insightful analysis of support that women, pregnant people and families need and deserve during labour is presented in a way that makes you think afresh. The stories bring the book to life and the reflections and resources are invaluable. This revised 2nd edition further challenges us all to be thoughtful, as well as providing an invaluable resource for education.

Nicky and Billie have highlighted the importance of cultural safety in this edition, and now is the time that we, as midwives, must lead in calling out racism, unconscious bias and intersectional inequalities, so that support for labour and birth is equitable, respectful and accessible for all.

I write this Foreword during the unimaginable Covid-19 pandemic when families face unprecedented challenges across the globe. More than ever now, women need kind, caring, supportive, compassionate midwives who can walk with them on their childbirth journey; providing safe, effective care and sharing clear, accurate evidence to support them to choose the right path for themselves and their families.

Midwives and student midwives are also challenged during this pandemic, with reconfiguration of maternity services and academic learning moved to online virtual provision. Nicky and Billie make reference, in the introduction, to the transformative opportunities that the pandemic offers, which are outlined in the paper I co-authored with Mary Renfrew and colleagues (Renfrew *et al.*, 2021). The subtitle of that paper is 'I have never learnt as much in my life, as quickly, ever', and this 2nd edition of *Supporting Women for Labour and Birth* provides thought-provoking learning and renewal for all midwives. This is especially pertinent as we recover and rebuild after the pandemic, and seek to provide sensitive support, both for women and families, and for each other as midwives.

This book is such a great resource for student midwives. The Reflective Activities are really valuable as they can be utilised in a variety of ways: individual or in groups, face-to-face or virtual. They serve to scaffold student learning and add to rich discussions of women's experiences during labour and birth. Asynchronous sessions are a vital part of virtual learning and the thought-provoking activities promote self-awareness, mindfulness and examination of resilience as well as the development of compassion. Blended learning pedagogies will continue following the pandemic, and this excellent resource can support student midwives' education in a creative way.

This book is a labour of love by Nicky and Billie, two amazing, kind, supportive, erudite midwives and academics who continue to inspire the current and future generations of midwives and women.

Midwives and student midwives – let this book be your guide and your constant reference point as you provide compassionate and sensitive support for labour and birth. It will make you think, it will challenge your thinking, make you smile, bring tears, give you encouragement and guidance, refreshment and learning. And always remember the words of the Dalai Lama, 'Be kind whenever possible. It is always possible.'

by Grace Thomas FRCM
Reader in Midwifery
Lead Midwife for Education/Professional Head and Deputy Director,
WHO Collaborating Centre for Midwifery Development
School of Healthcare Sciences
College of Biomedical and Life Sciences
Cardiff University

Reference

Renfrew, M.J., Bradshaw, G., Burnett, A., Byrom, A., Entwistle, F., King, K., . . . Thomas, G. (2021). Sustaining quality education and practice learning in a pandemic and beyond: 'I have never learnt as much in my life, as quickly, ever'. *Midwifery, 94*, 102915.

Acknowledgements

Acknowledgements from the 1st edition

For both us, this 'thoughtful guide' represents ideas and experiences gained across several decades of supporting women for labour and birth. We first and foremost acknowledge all the women and families from whom we have learnt so much.

This book is rich with stories from women about their experiences of labour and birth support, and from midwives, childbirth educators and birth supporters who describe providing that support. Special thanks are due to the thoughtful individuals who told us their stories and gave us permission to share them with readers: Gina Augarde, Marleen De Rijk, Jaclyn Hill-Smith, Meg Hitchick, Margaretha Huese, Jo Hunter, Sue Kildea, Annie Lester, Rachael Lockey, Jane McMurtrie, Andrea Robertson, Jilly Rosser, Ruth Sanders, Rachel Smith, Angela Thompson, Jen Watkins, Jacqui Wood, Annie Yates and Katie Yiannouzis.

Many of the ideas that are shared throughout the book reflect the contributions of people who have contributed to research that we have been involved in. We have used both published and unpublished data in quotations that reflect their wisdom and experiences. We are deeply grateful for their generosity.

Nicky's Master's thesis, *A midwifery perspective on pain in labour*, was influenced by several midwives whose thoughtful approach to practice enabled the development of the 'working with pain' theory: Alice Coyle, Jill Demilew, Valerie Fray, Jo Naylor, Becky Reed, Julie Rochford, Beatrijs Smulders, Helen Stapleton, Holliday Tyson, Marleen De Rijk and Cathy Walton. Their knowledge and their insights are shared throughout this book.

We have also quoted extensively from the research that Nicky was involved in with Jane Sandall and colleagues at the Health and Social Care Research Division of King's College, London: *Supporting women to have a normal birth: Development and field testing of a learning package for maternity staff* (funded by a grant from the National Service Framework for Children, Young People and Maternity Services Research Initiative, Department of Health, England). The experiences and ideas of women, their partners, midwives, obstetricians, birth supporters and childbirth educators make significant contributions to this book – their words bring to life the theory of how we support women for labour and birth.

Nicky and Billie acknowledge the influence of their colleagues at the University of Technology, Sydney. In particular, Caroline Homer and Maralyn Foureur have led cutting-edge interdisciplinary research into multiple aspects of midwifery education and practice; this has stimulated our thinking about interactive learning and the way we have approached writing the Reflective Activities in this book.

Billie's PhD thesis, *Emotion work in midwifery*, laid the foundation for developing her understanding of the emotional work of midwives. She would like to thank all those who participated in this ethnographic study, as well as the Iolanthe Midwifery Trust for awarding her a Research Fellowship to partly fund the research. Billie's understanding of how emotions affect the support that midwives provide continues to evolve. Two further studies have contributed to this understanding: *A policy ethnography of the All Wales clinical pathway for normal labour* (funded by The Health Foundation) and *Investigating resilience in midwifery* (funded by the Royal College of Midwives). Billie is indebted to those who supported and participated in these projects, as well as colleagues and students in the Universities of Swansea and Cardiff and in the Welsh University Health Boards, with whom she has discussed these ideas over many years. Particular thanks are due to: Laura Goodwin, Marie Lewis, Myfanwy (Van) McAteer, Jeremy Segrott, Grace Thomas and Lucie Warren.

We were thrilled when Professor Hannah Dahlen agreed to write the Foreword to the 1st edition, and even more thrilled when we read what she had written. Thank you, Hannah, for articulating so clearly and strongly the importance of providing excellent support during labour and birth.

Dr Leissa Roberts generously allowed us to use the Coping with Labor Algorithm © profiled in Chapter 7 and positively engaged with us in providing suggestions for the activity that we devised to practise using the algorithm.

In the chapter on communication we drew heavily on the wisdom and insights of Dr Allan Cyna, who continues to inspire midwives and others to think about the power of language and suggestion. In particular, we thank him for giving us permission to profile the LAURS of communication and other concepts from the *Handbook of Communication in Anaesthesia and Critical Care. A Practical Guide to Exploring the Art.*

Nicola Beauman from Persephone Press gave us permission and encouragement to include a passage from *The Squire*, written in the 1930s by Enid Bagnold – an extraordinary semi-biographical novel about the emotions around pregnancy and childbirth that we recommend to our readers.

Rhea Dempsey's dynamic and profound book, *Birth with Confidence: Savvy Choices for Normal Birth*, has stimulated a lot of our thinking around how we engage with women and their supporters in preparation for labour and birth. We thank her for her inspiring work and for giving us permission to reproduce her diagram about Pain Attitudes.

Before her sudden death in April 2015, Andrea Robertson gave us permission to use the line drawings that so beautifully illustrate how women can best be supported in labour. Andrea gave us a lot of encouragement around the writing of this book. Her inspiration continues, and we think she would have liked it that we gave her the first and last word in the Dedication and Epilogue.

Thank you to Nicky's son, Reuben Turkie, for help with digitalising some of the line drawings and to her daughter, Hester Lean, for her diligent assistance with proofreading.

The approach taken to writing this 'thoughtful guide' has meant that we have sought the support and advice of many respected colleagues and friends in our efforts to create a useful and stimulating book. We would like to thank them all for their knowledge, generosity and overall enthusiasm for our project. In particular, the following people have provided us with additional resources and expert advice: Pauline Armstrong, Jenny Browne, Sarah Davies, Deborah Davis, Jude Davis, Ruth Deery, Soo Downe, Nadine Edwards, Jenny Fenwick, Marilyn Foureur, Jenny Gamble, Kathryn Gutteridge, Athena Hammond, Caroline Homer, Mervi Jokinen, Inga Karlsdottir, Eleanor Kelly, Holly Kennedy, Mavis Kirkham, Sue Kruske, Amali Lokugamage, Rosemary Mander, Jackie Moulla, Mary Newburn, Janet O'Sullivan, Lesley Page, Jane Raymond, Mary Ross-Davie, Denis Walsh, Cathy Walton and Lucie Warren.

The book has taken several years to grow from our initial ideas to publication. We thank Louisa Vahtrick and Grace McInnes, our editors at Routledge, for their patience and confidence in our approach. Our thanks also to Sheila Garrard for her diligent attention to detail in copyediting our manuscript.

Finally, we would like to thank our partners, Pat Brodie and Nick Wells, who have supported us during the book's long gestation. They have always believed in the potential value of the book and have steadfastly continued to provide us with nourishment, time and space to write whenever we could, never-ending beverages and encouraging words just when we needed them. Special thanks are due to the wonderful Pat Brodie whose eagle eye and clever attention to detail contributed to the many draft chapters. She has brought her midwifery support skills of perceptive and thoughtful comment, reassurance and encouragement to the editing process – indeed, the very support skills that we describe throughout this book. The final birth of this book is due in no small part to her skilful midwifing.

Addendum: Additional acknowledgements for the 2nd edition

Returning to our 'thoughtful guide' almost five years on, we are very aware that the book is needed now more than ever, and that all of our previous thanks and acknowledgements remain relevant. We would like to thank our editor Grace McInnes for taking the initiative in commissioning a 2nd edition and for her encouragement and enthusiasm as we've been writing. We would also like to thank the anonymous reviewers of the book proposal for the 2nd edition; their suggestions were invaluable in alerting us to gaps in the 1st edition, and areas where new evidence was available.

Grace Thomas has written an insightful Foreword to this 2nd edition. Drawing on her extensive experience in midwifery education and practice, Grace has captured the essence of what we hope this book offers in terms of encouraging thoughtful approaches to supporting women for labour and birth. Thank you, Grace, for articulating the importance of questioning our individual values, attitudes and experiences in order to engage with the politics of maternity care and provide culturally safe, woman centred care.

During the years since we wrote the 1st edition of this book, a number of midwifery leaders in different countries have engaged with us in thoughtful discussions; these midwives have reinforced our belief in the potential of research and collective action to convince others of the need for systems change and midwifery continuity of care. Their publications are peppered throughout this book, identifying the importance of being proactive in the promotion of positive experiences of birth for women, their families and society.

We would like to thank everyone whose thinking and research has influenced the changes and additions that we have made in this 2nd edition of our book. Whilst it is impossible to name everyone, there are a few who deserve to be singled out. Both Sheena Byrom and Deborah Fox have been generous in suggesting resources; they have both been a mine of information and a 'sounding board' for exploring critical issues related to education and practice.

Nicky would like to acknowledge her midwifery sisters in the team at the University of Technology Sydney, who continue to influence her thinking as well as offering encouraging feedback about how they have used the 1st edition for teaching and learning purposes.

A number of people have entrusted Nicky with their inspiring practice stories in recent years. Special mention is due to midwifery friends in the Blue Mountains, Australia, who attend women who choose to give birth at home: Jo Hunter, Lucretia McCarthy and Jacqui Wood, you are an absolute inspiration. Student midwives have shared some very different personal stories of their experiences in institutions with soaring intervention rates, particularly during the Covid-19 pandemic. A special mention is due to Bronie Condon who exemplifies how inspiring the next generation of midwives is.

Since the publication of the 1st edition, Billie has conducted research into the sources of stress and burnout in midwifery and how stress and burnout impact on midwives' experiences. This research has enhanced her understanding of the emotional wellbeing of midwives and how this affects the care they give to women, which is reflected throughout this edition. Attending to the emotional wellbeing of midwives has become even more important during the Covid-19 pandemic. Billie would like to thank her collaborators Josie Henley, Joanne Cull, Mary Sidebotham, Jenny Fenwick and Eleanor Cramer for their insights and stimulating conversations.

Billie would also like to thank the midwifery students (present and past, undergraduate and postgraduate) at Cardiff University, as well as her colleagues in the midwifery education team, for their enthusiastic responses to the 1st edition, and for being such engaged 'guinea pigs' for the reflective activities.

Finally, we both want to pay tribute to Nicky's wife Pat Brodie and her daughter Hettie Lean for their eagle-eyed critical reading of numerous drafts, especially when we could no longer see the wood for the trees. You have both been such stalwart supporters – a very big thank-you. Pat did a final, meticulous proofread of the manuscript and has been the source of many 'thoughtful' suggestions and 'words of encouragement'.

Prologue

In this prologue, we set the scene for the rest of the book by providing a brief historical overview of how women have been supported in labour over the centuries. This is just a whistle-stop tour; we have focused on some key areas that are relevant to supporting women today, rather than the history of childbirth and midwifery per se.

Pre-twentieth century support in labour: women with women

It is common throughout the world for women to support each other when they give birth and in the weeks following birth. This was certainly true in the past; for example, historian Adrian Wilson (1990) describes how, in seventeenth-century England, childbirth was very much a social event. Pregnant women would invite female friends, relatives and neighbours to be present during labour and birth, and it was considered a great honour to be included. The women would bring baskets of food and beverages, which would sustain them all through the woman's labour and after the birth. Wilson proposes that the word 'God-sip' or 'gossip' comes from this gathering of women surrounding the new mother, telling stories and sipping mead.

Figure 0.1 Support for childbearing women in sixteenth-century Germany

Source: Woodcut from: *The Expert Midwife or An Excellent and Most Necessary Treatise on the Generation and Birth of Man*. Jacob Rueff, 1637.

An influential sixteenth-century German textbook, *The Expert Midwife*, written by doctor Jacob Rueff (Dunn, 2001), provides interesting insights into the physical and emotional care given by the midwife and the woman's supporters. Rueff describes how, once the labouring woman was seated on her birth chair ready to birth, 'the midwife shall place one woman behind her back which may gently hold the labouring woman, taking her by both the armes. . . . But let her place other two [women] by her sides, which may both with good words encourage and comfort the labouring woman' (Rueff, cited in Dunn, 2001, F222).

There are similar descriptions of midwives and local women working together in the memoirs of the Dutch (Frisian) midwife, Catharina Schrader, who attended over 4,000 births between 1693 and 1740 (Marland, 1987). Her fascinating diary gives unique insights into her practice, including how she combined physical support and skill with psychological support to achieve a positive outcome for mother and baby. In this example, Catharina describes how she attended a birth where it was feared that both the mother and baby would die:

> When I came there her husband and friends were weeping a great deal. I examined the case, suspected that I had a chance to deliver [her]. The woman was very worn out. I laid her in a warm bed, gave her a cup of caudle, also gave her something in it; sent the neighbours home, so that they would let her rest a bit. An hour after her strength awakened again somewhat. And I had the neighbours fetched again. . . . The friends and neighbours were very surprised. The mother and child were in a very good state.
>
> (Memoirs of Catharina Schrader, in Marland, 1987, pp.63–64)

Figure 0.2 Woman on a birth chair with her midwife and birth supporters

Source: Woodcut from: *The Expert Midwife or An Excellent and Most Necessary Treatise on the Generation and Birth of Man.* Jacob Rueff, 1637.

In this account, there is a strong sense of Catharina's attention to the woman's need for warmth, rest and nourishment as well as the needs of her birth companions. Caring and empathy are implicit in her words.

The involvement of local women as essential birth supporters, working with the midwife, can be seen in other historical accounts, such as the eighteenth-century diary of the North American midwife, Martha Ballard. Martha attended nearly 1,000 births in rural Maine, and her diary is meticulously explained by historian Laurel Thatcher Ulrich (1990). Ulrich describes how Martha considered women's labours and births to be divided into three stages but that, unlike today, these were *social* rather than physiological stages: 'each marked by the summons and arrival of attendants – first the midwife, then the neighbourhood circle of women, finally the afternurse. Parturition ended when the mother returned to her kitchen' (Ulrich, 1990, p.183).

It is clear from Martha's diary entries that she was often present in the family home for several days before the birth, probably because of the long distances she needed to travel on foot between families. She supported women in the lead-up to established labour by taking part in everyday domestic activities: 'I helpt Mrs. Lithgow make Cake and Pies & knit on my Stockin' (Ulrich, 1990 p.183). By the following day Martha writes that she has finished her knitting and that the baby was born that evening! Such accounts give a strong impression of the importance of the midwife's presence and attention to the woman she was caring for, a point we shall return to later in this book.

Early twentieth-century support in labour: professional midwifery care

By the first half of the twentieth century, support in labour in the United Kingdom (UK) was increasingly provided by trained midwives. When writing our oral history of midwifery and childbirth in pre-National Health Service (NHS) Britain – *The Midwife's Tale* (Leap and Hunter, 2013) – we were told many stories about midwifery care that described this support. For example, district midwife Elizabeth C. lived and worked for many years in Battersea, where she was known as 'Aunty Betty'. She described her empathic approach to supporting women:

> I think there's a lot in being a personal friend to the person having the baby. You want a bit of sympathy and someone you can talk to just then. Not someone telling you, 'Now shut up. Stop making a noise.' I used to say, 'Shout if you want to dear, I won't take any notice.'
>
> (p.63)

In these midwives' stories there were vivid descriptions of the practicalities of providing labour support, at a time when most births took place at home and pharmacological pain relief was rarely used. For example, Esther S. described the value of water immersion and massage for helping women to cope with long or difficult labours:

> I might give her another hot bath. I think that helps – you can't really quicken it up I don't think. . . . Nature is its only best way, but you can aid. I used to rub her back because the contractions there were more severe with a posterior position. They get more backache with the posteriors, don't they; very, very, painful, I believe, from what they say.
>
> (p.160)

Esther also described the importance of women being mobile during labour:

> We kept them moving around in labour, never went to bed until the last minute. . . .
> Nature needs you to move. You let them have the freedom of what she's wanted. You got
> as tired as they were; you walked miles when you had deliveries.
>
> (p.162)

Midwives like Esther knew how necessary it was for midwives to give emotional support
and reassurance to women, especially those having long labours:

> And well, I just have to keep on trying to encourage her and tell her that some people do
> have slower labours – to see if you could put her mind at ease as well.
>
> (p.161)

As we will see in the following chapters, the importance of upright positions, moving around,
labouring in water and encouragement has now been formally recognised. Supported by a
robust research evidence base, these approaches to supporting the normal physiology of
labour and birth are central to the UK National Institute for Health and Care Excellence
intrapartum guidelines for healthy women and babies (NICE, 2014) and professional guidelines for supporting women in labour, such as those published by the UK Royal College of
Midwives (RCM, 2018).

The importance of caregiver attitude and the value of continuity of care for women's experiences are now also supported by high-level research evidence (Bohren *et al.*, 2019; Sandall *et al.*, 2016). Many of the midwives whom we interviewed emphasised the importance
of the relationship between the midwife and the woman, as a means of offering effective
emotional support. 'Knowing the midwife' (that is continuity of care) was seen as important.
Elizabeth C. told us:

> I'm sure it's really important to know the person who's going to look after you in labour.
> I've never had a baby, of course, but I'm sure it's very comforting to have someone that
> you know and that knows you and sort of knows your temperament, knows what you
> can take and what you can't. And having a home back up, too. Knowing the midwife, it's
> better than dope or something because it's a normal thing, you see.
>
> (Leap and Hunter, 2013, p.164)

The attitude of the midwife was thought to be critical by the midwives we interviewed. The
important attributes identified were kindness, friendliness, empathy, sympathy and patience:

Esther S: Practical, down-to-earth knowledge is important, but it's having the right attitude
that's so important, too. You have to be their friend. If you can befriend a mother
and get her on a level with you, there's an understanding and you're both far better off. I think the midwife in her own mind should remember that the mother is
important to her. She, the midwife, is not the most important person. She isn't.
The mother is the most important person.

Elsie K: Kindness for one thing. You have to be in sympathy with the woman. And
patience and love of the job.

(p.183)

Women's memories of care provided in labour

Decades after they have given birth, women have vivid memories of the kind and unkind things that people said to them in labour. We were very moved by the vivid recollections and strong emotions expressed by the elderly women we interviewed. All could recall the exact words of midwives and doctors when they were in labour some 70 years earlier. There were many positive stories. Sissy had four babies in the 1930s in Deptford, south-east London, attended by the much-loved community midwife Elsie Walkerdine. She told us:

> Having a baby with Nurse Walkerdine, I can't express it. It was marvellous, just marvellous. She was an angel through and through. If you needed bed clothes, that nurse found them. In them days, you often relied on neighbours if you never had nothing. And Nurse Walkerdine always found things for you. She'd say, 'We'll see if we can find you some bits.'
>
> (Leap and Hunter, 2013, p.184)

In conclusion, over the centuries, women have sought support from other women when they are in labour: friends, neighbours and midwives. What matters to women is that this support is encouraging, compassionate and kind. As we shall explore, there is now a wealth of evidence that confirms the importance of such support for women during labour and birth.

References

Bohren, M.A., Berger, B.O., Munthe-Kaas, H., Tunçalp, Ö . . . (2019). Perceptions and experiences of labour companionship: a qualitative evidence synthesis. *Cochrane Database of Systematic Reviews*, Issue 3. Art. No.: CD012449 doi:10.1002/14651858.CD012449.pub2.

Dunn, P.M. (2001). Jacob Rueff (1500–1558) of Zurich and 'The Expert Midwife'. *Archives of Disease in Childhood. Fetal and Neonatal Edition, 85,* F222–224.

Leap, N. and Hunter, B. (2013). *The Midwife's Tale: An Oral History from Handywoman to Professional Midwife*, 2nd edn. Barnsley: Pen & Sword.

Marland, H. (ed.). (1987). *'Mother and Child Were Saved': The Memoirs (1693–1740) of the Frisian Midwife Catharina Schrader*. Amsterdam: Rodopi.

NICE (2014). Intrapartum care: care of healthy women and their babies during childbirth. Clinical guideline 190. National Collaborating Centre for Women's and Children's Health UK. Commissioned by the National Institute for Health and Care Excellence (NICE): www.nice.org.uk/guidance/cg190.

RCM. (2018) *Midwifery care in labour guidance for all women in all settings. RCM Midwifery Blue Top Guidance. No. 1*. London: Royal College of Midwives. https://www.rcm.org.uk/media/2539/professionals-blue-top-guidance.pdf.

Sandall, J., Soltani, H., Gates, S., Shennan, A. and Devane, D. (2016). Midwife-led continuity models versus other models of care for childbearing women. *Cochrane Database of Systematic Reviews*, Issue 4. Art. No.: CD004667. doi:10.1002/14651858.CD004667.pub5.

Ulrich, L.T. (1990). *A Midwife's Tale: The Life of Martha Ballard, Based on Her Diary 1785–1812*. New York: Vintage Books.

Wilson, A. (1990). The ceremony of childbirth and its interpretation. In V. Fildes (ed.), *Women as Mothers in Pre-Industrial England* (pp.68–107).

Introduction to the 2nd edition

What does a woman need from those who care for her when she gives birth? Evidence from research and from the personal experiences of women and their birth attendants shows that *support* is the most important ingredient: support that is respectful, sensitive, empathic and finely tuned to an individual woman's needs. Whoever she is, wherever she is giving birth, whatever labour and birth she has, a pregnant woman will need support as she approaches and experiences birth and new motherhood. In this book we explore how best that support can be provided.

As we write this 2nd edition, the Covid-19 pandemic continues to challenge the way that maternity care can be safely provided worldwide. Compassionate sensitive support has never been more important. Given the changing profile of the pandemic and the rapidly growing Covid-19-related literature and knowledge, we have not focused on these issues in any depth, recognising that all involved in maternity care during a pandemic will be fully versed in how to access key resources and ever-changing sources of information.

The pandemic has also affected the way that midwifery education can be provided worldwide, with many programmes being moved online. We hope that this book will be a valuable resource, as many of the activities can be easily adapted for online teaching and learning. We have made the decision not to convert our activities into online resources. Educators have rapidly become skilful at adapting to distance teaching and blended learning, so we have left the Reflective Activities in this book open to enable a variety of approaches to be used. We trust this will offer an opportunity to adapt and create bespoke materials that will suit the needs of students. We encourage educators to use our Reflective Activities creatively, for example with students collaborating online in small groups before, during and after online classes, using breakout rooms, and multimedia programmes and resources to share ideas and present to each other. We recommend enhancing student participation by linking reflective activities to assignments.

We also recommend reading the paper by Mary Renfrew and colleagues (Renfrew *et al.*, 2021) which takes an Appreciative Inquiry approach using case studies to investigate strategies for midwifery education during and after a pandemic. Focusing on the positive learning opportunities that the pandemic has offered, the authors sound this hopeful note: 'The pandemic provides an opportunity for student midwives to be re-imagined as essential members of midwifery teams and not 'just students'. Transformative actions identified include whole-system working, tackling longstanding problems including racism, poverty, prejudice, and systemic discrimination, and keeping students at the heart of the education system' (Renfrew *et al.*, 2021, p.1). We hope that this book will play a part in contributing to these 'transformative actions' (Renfrew *et al.*, 2021, p.1).

DOI: 10.4324/9781003092520-1

Why is this book needed?

The initial impetus for writing this book was prompted by worldwide debates amongst maternity care professionals and in the media about the quality of maternity services. As we write the 2nd edition, these debates and concerns have not gone away. Women continue to report feeling unhappy with the level of emotional support they receive; they describe being frightened of labour pain and childbirth, despite widespread use of pharmacological pain relief. This is particularly worrying as we now have strong research evidence demonstrating the global importance of continuous support in labour, which is associated with improved outcomes and positive experiences for women and their supporters (Bohren *et al.*, 2017). We also now have robust evidence which demonstrates that, for women across the world, what matters most during childbirth is 'giving birth to a healthy baby in a clinically and psychologically safe environment with practical and emotional support from birth companions, and competent, reassuring, kind clinical staff' (Downe *et al.*, 2018, p.1).

High levels of epidural use mean that students increasingly lack experience of supporting women through an unmedicated labour and often have little opportunity to develop skills in providing practical and emotional support during childbirth. In our experience, students are often bemoaning a lack of role models and asking for information about how best to support women in labour. Students (and qualified midwives) also encounter a plethora of dilemmas around 'informed choice' and epidurals, fears of litigation and how to support women who are not confident about their bodies and abilities.

In this book we address these issues and consider a range of situations where midwives provide support. This includes where women labour with and without pharmacological 'pain relief', and how we support healthy pregnant women having a normal birth as well as those who experience the challenges of complicated labours and intrapartum loss.

When we talk about 'supporting women', it is a given that we also mean that we shall be supporting the people whom the woman has chosen to support her in labour, often referred to as 'birth supporters' or 'birth companions'. This is usually her partner and may also include family members and close friends. For some women, this also includes a 'doula' or lay birth supporter who she has asked to be there, specifically to help and guide her through the challenges of labour.

It is important to note that this book is not a manual for performing the clinical tasks associated with labour or for identifying the properties and ways of administering pharmacological 'pain relief'. These topics are covered in the well-known midwifery textbooks and other contemporary texts (see, for example, Bayes and de-Vitry Smith, 2018; Chapman and Charles, 2017; Johnson and Taylor, 2016).

What approach does this book take?

We continue to call this book a 'thoughtful guide'. It is not a book that provides all the answers. Instead, we have created a text that will encourage readers to explore their practice and reflect on their experiences. We believe that, before learning about the practicalities of providing labour support, we have to consider how our attitudes, values and ways of communicating might all impact on the experiences of women and their supporters.

It is also a thoughtful guide in that we encourage readers to examine a wide range of evidence sources and explore how the insights gained could be incorporated into their practice. We have drawn on updated research evidence as well as sources of practice-based evidence, using stories and testimony from women and midwives to illustrate a range of ideas and practices. In using this broad definition of evidence, we have been influenced by the original explanation of evidence-based medicine proposed by David Sackett in 1996. This explanation focused not only on research evidence, but also included clinical experience and expertise and patient preference as equally important forms of evidence. This notion of evidence-informed practice is embedded in Lesley Page's widely used '5 Steps of Evidence-Based Midwifery':

1   Finding out what is important to the woman and her family
2   Using information from the clinical examination
3   Seeking and assessing evidence to inform decisions
4   Talking it through
5   Reflection on outcomes, feelings and consequences

(Page, 2000, p.9.)

We have also been influenced by a study of practitioners' 'mindlines' undertaken by John Gabbay and Andree Le May (2011), which showed how healthcare professionals draw on a wide range of sources when making clinical decisions. Their ethnographic studies showed that practitioners created personal and group mindlines, webs of knowledge which incorporated: personal experiences; the experiences of colleagues and communities of practice; training; research evidence; information from professional bodies; and recognition of the significance of local context. The concept of mindlines allows us to explore tacit knowledge as well as the interactions and relationships that we have with others as we create, enact and share knowledge (Wieringa and Greenhalgh, 2015).

The stories and testimony that we have included give insights into some midwifery mindlines. They show the various forms of knowledge that midwives draw on when providing support to women. As Mavis Kirkham has discussed, stories are valuable sources of midwifery knowledge (Kirkham, 1997). From our experience, we think that there is a culture of learning from storytelling in midwifery. This was borne out in Hannah Williams's (2003) study of midwifery conversations at the desk in a midwife-led birth centre in the UK. Whenever a midwife described what was going on in the room where she was caring for a woman, a colleague would respond by sharing a story about a similar situation they had been in. Williams suggested that, 'I had a woman once who . . .' is the midwifery equivalent of 'Once upon a time . . .'. We hope that the narratives in this book will 'bring to life' the experiences of women and those who provide support in labour, and also provide real-life examples of the theories of labour support that we discuss.

In the interest of contributing to knowledge development using an approach that embraces the concept of mindlines, throughout the book we have placed boxes identifying key research evidence (Research Briefing), Recommended Resources and Reflective Activities.

Research Briefing boxes

These provide an overview of relevant research, with recommendations for further reading. At times we have selected key research papers and discussed these in more detail. We have also included book chapters and books in these Research Briefing boxes as we think these are particularly important for the in-depth exploration of concepts related to our practice.

All Research Briefings have been updated to ensure that they reflect the evidence base; however, they are not meant to be comprehensive literature reviews on any one topic and you will see that we have included references that are more than five years old. We make no apology for this. There are many groundbreaking texts that continue to enhance theory development and stimulate our thinking. In our commitment to language awareness we avoid using the word 'seminal' when referring to these important texts, honouring Sheila Kitzinger's (2015) suggestion that we use instead 'ovular' in order to avoid the sexist roots of language and Sara Wickham's (2017) proposal that 'germinal' might be a better alternative, since it encompasses both egg and sperm!

Recommended Resources

We encourage you to 'think outside the box' when exploring these resources. They include different forms of media, some of which are only available online.

Reflective Activities

Throughout the chapters, there are boxes identifying interactive Reflective Activities. These have been designed to be thought provoking and to stimulate reflection and learning. We hope that they will encourage readers to interrogate the research evidence and consider testimonies from women, midwives and others in light of their own experiences and ideas.

The activities can be adapted for students to undertake alone, in pairs or groups, and they could form the basis of classroom, workshop or online activities. We have deliberately not attached learning outcomes to them and hope that you will adapt them for different situations and contexts.

In suggesting these activities we have drawn on theory from a number of disciplines which has shown how rehearsing improves practice and that what you think, model or pretend will ultimately become part of the way you behave (Gould, 2008). We have also been mindful of the potential for further developing skills related to emotional intelligence, self-awareness and resilience through the sharing of ideas and stories (Patterson and Begley, 2011).

Postscripts

Each chapter ends with a postscript, usually a longer account, which exemplifies or challenges our thinking about what has been discussed in the chapter. These can also be used for learning activities and reflection.

The language that we have chosen to use

Throughout the book we refer to the woman who is in labour or giving birth as 'the woman' and the person accompanying her as her 'partner'. We have chosen the term 'partner' or 'those who support women' purposefully, so that this can include male or female birth supporters such as the woman's partner, significant others (mothers, friends, other relatives), as well as doulas or other lay supporters/companions and students (midwifery or medical). This is not in any way meant to undermine the importance of including 'fathers' in every aspect of support as identified in the Preparation for Birth and Beyond resource that we profile in Chapter 4 (Department of Health, 2011).

In Chapter 5 we have explored the concept and use of woman centred language. We have attempted to reflect this throughout the book. Thus, we tend to refer to the 'birthing unit'; we describe women 'giving birth' rather than delivering; and having a 'caesarean birth', rather than a caesarean section. After some deliberation we have chosen to use the terminology, 'healthy women and babies' and birth with or without 'complications'. Depending on the context, we also use the terminology that others have used, so at times we talk about 'straight-forward labour and birth', 'uncomplicated labour' and 'normal birth'.

For ease of understanding and, given that the majority of midwives are women, we have chosen to use 'she' for midwife rather than the cumbersome she/he. This is not meant in any way to deny the role played by male midwives in providing labour support.

We have chosen to use the words 'woman' and 'women' and see 'woman centred care' as an important philosophical concept underpinning midwifery practice. In so doing, we do not mean to exclude people having babies who do not identify as women. In Chapter 1, we have touched on the importance of using inclusive language when a person's gender may not necessarily denote their role, identity, or language preferences (Allen, 2019; Darwin and Greenfield, 2019; Greenfield, 2017).

Addressing diversity

Since the 1st edition, there has been increasing awareness that people accessing maternity care have inequalities in their experiences and outcomes, and that it is essential for all involved in the planning, implementation and evaluation of maternity services to address how the social determinants of health impact on access to services and the health of childbearing women and their families. Socioeconomic inequalities continue to have devastating effects on the health of women and children living in disadvantaged circumstances in Western countries like the UK (Marmot *et al.*, 2020) and Australia (Australian Institute of Health and Welfare, 2020)

The concerns and experiences of women of colour have been particularly highlighted in the UK because of the continuing, greatly increased chance of negative outcomes for them and their babies (Draper *et al.*, 2020; Knight *et al.*, 2020). These concerns have gained the prominence they deserve in 2020, partly because of the spotlight on endemic racism shone by the Black Lives Matter movement in the aftermath of the shocking murder of George Floyd, and also because of the evidence that Covid-19 poses signifi-cantly greater health risks for the Black, Asian and minority ethnic (BAME) community (Aldridge *et al.*, 2020). We hope that our revisions in this book reflect the importance of cultural safety and the dangers posed by ethnocentricity in maternity care. We also hope that this new edition pays proper attention to the need for care providers to be alert to racism in all its insidious forms (such as unconscious bias, institutional racism) and to understand how this contributes to inequalities in women's experiences and outcomes (Cross-Sudworth, 2007; Durey, 2010; Horn, 2020; Lokugamage and Meredith, 2020; Macedo *et al.*, 2019; Wren Serbin and Donnelly, 2016). We acknowledge that, as two white women, we are writing this book from a position of privilege, but we hope that we've been able to use this privilege to highlight these crucial concerns.

Although the book focuses mainly on maternity care in high income countries, many of the issues we discuss have relevance globally, especially the need for all women to receive respectful and supportive care wherever they live. Important international resources have been noted in the briefings, and it should be possible to adapt some reflective activities to suit a range of settings. It is worth noting that this book was used in 2018 in Zimbabwe as a core text for 'Respectful Maternity Care/Woman Centred Care' workshops with midwives and obstetricians. These workshops were successful with positive evaluations; the workshop materials have since been developed into a Training in Respectful Maternal Care: Supporting Mothers During Labour and Birth Toolkit.

Sources of evidence

We have referenced a large body of published evidence from different disciplines; you will find reference lists at the end of each chapter We have also drawn on published and unpublished material from studies that we have personally been involved in over the years, where the data still have relevance for contemporary practice.

In preparation for writing this book, we carried out interviews with women, their partners, midwives and other health professionals. These took the form of informal discussions that were focused on informing our writing. People told us their stories and shared their ideas with the specific purpose of contributing and gave permission for us to use their testimony.

A timely book

The time has never been more right for this book. We now have a strong research evidence base demonstrating the importance of labour support for optimising women's wellbeing and the wellbeing of their babies. We know more than ever about what works and what doesn't work in terms of supporting women and have better insights from hormonal physiology about why that might be (Buckley, 2015). The imperative to promote physiological birth is being articulated through new insights from microbiology and epigenetics; increasingly, we are cautioned to think about the iatrogenic side effects and human costs of increasing rates of caesarean section and other interventions in childbirth (Dahlen *et al.*, 2014).

We also now have strong research evidence, in the form of the Lancet Series on Midwifery, which demonstrates the significant impact which midwifery care can have on maternal and newborn outcomes. The papers in the series highlight the importance of the midwifery values of respect, communication and individualised care, as well as midwifery's distinguishing philosophy of 'optimising biological, psychological, social and cultural processes; strengthening women's capabilities; expectant management, and using interventions only when indicated' (Renfrew *et al.*, 2014, p.12). The Quality Framework for Maternal and Newborn Care developed in this series incorporates these values and philosophy and has had a global impact: for example, it is embedded in the World Health Organization (2019) *Framework for Action: Strengthening Quality Midwifery Education for Universal Health Coverage 2030* and forms the foundation of the UK Nursing and Midwifery Council Standards for Midwifery (NMC, 2019).

There is also new evidence about what women want from childbirth (Downe *et al.*, 2018; Olza *et al.*, 2018), which emphasises the importance that women place on feeling psychologically safe and receiving support from skilled and caring staff. This evidence also indicates that most women hope for a physiological labour and birth, but if interventions are needed, they want to be actively involved in any decisions so that their sense of control is optimised (Downe *et al.*, 2018).

Despite this increased knowledge, however, since we wrote the 1st edition global caesarean births and induction rates have continued to rise, soaring in some places to unprecedented heights. These increases, which frequently have no clinical justification, have implications for the long-term wellbeing of women and their babies, as well as financial consequences (Miller *et al.*, 2016).

Our responses to these challenges require a sophisticated exploration of the culture, relationships and practices that surround childbirth. This textbook will enable readers to grapple with some of these issues and to consider the far-reaching impact that our efforts to promote a positive experience of birth may have on childbearing women's lives.

These are not new concerns. For the past 50 years, concerns about trends in maternity care that de-humanise the birth process have been highlighted by birth activists. While we were writing this book many of those notable authors and campaigners have died: for example, Mary Cronk, Murray Enkin, Doris Haire, Sheila Kitzinger, Elizabeth Noble, Andrea Robertson, Marsden Wagner. . . . These pioneers have made a huge contribution by challenging those working in maternity care to focus on the needs and experiences of women and their families, rather than those of the professionals. Many of their concerns have not gone away and there is much work left to do if we are to contribute to making women's experiences of labour and birth as positive as they can possibly be.

Key recommended texts to stimulate thinking

Byrom, S. and Downe, S. (eds). (2015). *The Roar Behind the Silence: Why Kindness, Compassion and Respect Matter in Maternity Care*. London: Pinter & Martin.

Catling, C., Cummins, A. and Hogan, R. (2016). *Stories in Midwifery: Reflection, Inquiry, Action*. Chatswood, NSW: Elsevier Australia.

Chapman, V. and Charles, C. (eds). (2017). *The Midwife's Labour and Birth Handbook*, 4th edn. Chichester: John Wiley & Sons Ltd.

Downe, S. and Byrom, S. (eds). (2019). *Squaring the Circle: Normal Birth Research, Theory and Practice in a Technological Age*. London: Pinter & Martin.

Newnham, E., McKellar, L. and Pincombe, J. (2018). *Towards the Humanisation of Birth: A Study of Epidural Analgesia and Hospital Birth Culture*. London: Palgrave Macmillan.

Page, L. and McCandlish, R. (eds). (2006). *The New Midwifery. Science and Sensitivity in Practice*, 2nd edn. Edinburgh: Churchill Livingstone/Elsevier.

Simkin, P., Ancheta, R. and Hanson, L. (2017). *The Labor Progress Handbook: Early Interventions to Prevent and Treat Dystocia*, 4th edn. Chichester: Wiley-Blackwell.

Simkin, P. with Rohs, K. (2018). *The Birth Partner: A Complete Guide to Childbirth for Dads, Doulas, and All Other Labor Companions*, 5th edn. Boston, MA: Harvard Common Press.

Walsh, D. (2012). *Evidence and Skills for Normal Labour and Birth*, 2nd edn. London: Routledge.

Walsh, D. and Downe, S. (eds). (2010). *Essential Midwifery Practice: Intrapartum Care*. Chichester: Wiley-Blackwell.

References

Aldridge, R.W., Lewer, D., Katikireddi, S.V., Mathur, R., Pathak, N., Burns, R., . . . Hayward, A. (2020). Black, Asian and Minority Ethnic groups in England are at increased risk of death from COVID-19: indirect standardisation of NHS mortality data. *Wellcome Open Research*, 5(88), published online: doi:2010.12688/wellcomeopenres.15922.12682.

Allen, J. (2019). Midwifery continuity of care for specific groups. In C. Homer, N. Leap, P. Brodie and J. Sandall (eds), *Midwifery Continuity of Care*, 2nd edn (pp.207–230). Australia: Elsevier.

Australian Institute of Health and Welfare. (2020). *Health across Socioeconomic Groups*. Canberra: Australian Government.

Bayes, S. and de-Vitry Smith, S-A. (2018). *Skills for Midwifery Practice Australian & New Zealand edition*, 1st edn. Sydney: Elsevier Australia.

Bohren, M.A., Hofmeyr, G.J., Sakala, C., Fukuzawa, R.K. and Cuthbert, A. (2017) Continuous support for women during childbirth. *Cochrane Database of Systematic Reviews*, Issue 7. Art. No.: CD003766. doi: 10.1002/14651858.CD003766.pub6.

Buckley, S.J. (2015). *Hormonal Physiology of Childbearing: Evidence and Implications for Women, Babies, and Maternity Care*. Washington, DC: Childbirth Connection Programs, National Partnership for Women and Families.

Byrom, S. and Downe, S. (eds). (2015). *The Roar Behind the Silence: Why Kindness, Compassion and Respect Matter in Maternity Care*. London: Pinter & Martin.

Catling, C., Cummins, A. and Hogan, R. (2016). *Stories in Midwifery: Reflection, Inquiry, Action*. Chatswood, NSW: Elsevier Australia.

Chapman, V. and Charles, C. (eds). (2018). *The Midwife's Labour and Birth Handbook, Fourth Edition*. Chichester: John Wiley & Sons.

Cross-Sudworth, F. (2007). Racism and discrimination in maternity services. *British Journal of Midwifery, 15*(*6*), 327–331.

Dahlen, H.G., Downe, S., Kennedy, H.P. and Foureur, M. (2014). Is society being reshaped on a microbiological and epigenetic level by the way women give birth? *Midwifery*, 1149–1151.

Darwin, Z. and Greenfield, M. (2019). Mothers and others: the invisibility of LGBTQ people in reproductive and infant psychology. *Journal of Reproductive and Infant Psychology, 37*(*4*), 341–343.

Department of Health (Producer). (2011). Preparation for Birth and Beyond: a resource pack for leaders of community groups and activities. www.gov.uk/government/uploads/system/uploads/attachment_data/file/215386/dh_134728.pdf.

Downe, S. and Byrom, S. (eds). (2019). *Squaring the Circle: Normal Birth Research, Theory and Practice in a Technological Age*. London: Pinter & Martin.

Downe, S., Finlayson, K., Oladapo, O, T., Bonet, M. and Gülmezoglu, A.M. (2018). What matters to women during childbirth: a systematic qualitative review. *PLoS ONE, 13*(*4*), e0194906.

Draper, E.S., Gallimore, I.D., Smith, L.K., Fenton, A.C., Kurinczuk, J.J., Smith, P.W., . . . on behalf of the MBRRACE-UK Collaboration. (2020). *MBRRACE-UK Perinatal Mortality Surveillance Report, UK Perinatal Deaths for Births from January to December 2018*. Leicester: The Infant Mortality and Morbidity Studies, Department of Health Sciences, University of Leicester.

Durey, A. (2010). Reducing racism in Aboriginal health care in Australia: where does cultural education fit? *Australian and New Zealand Journal of Public Health 34*, S87–S92.

Gabbay, J. and Le May, A. (2011). *Practice-based Evidence for Healthcare: Clinical Mindlines*. London: Routledge.

Gould, D. (2008). Taught to be kind. *British Journal of Midwifery, 16*(*7*), 430.

Greenfield, M. (2017). He's not the mother. *AIMS Journal, 29*(*2*). Available from: https://www.aims.org.uk/journal/item/hes-not-the-mother.

Horn, A. (2020). Racism matters: 'When people show you who they are, believe them': why Black women mistrust maternity services. *The Practising Midwife, 23*(*8*), 15–17.

Johnson, R. and Taylor, W. (2016). *Skills for Midwifery Practice*, 4th edn. London: Elsevier.

Kirkham, M. (1997). Stories and childbirth. In M.J. Kirkham and E.R. Perkins (eds), *Reflections on Midwifery* (pp.183–204). London: Bailliere Tindall.

Kitzinger, S. (2015). *A Passion for Birth. My Life: Anthropology, Family and Feminism*. London: Pinter & Martin.

Knight, M., Bunch, K., Tuffnell, D., Shakespeare, J., Kotnis, R., Kenyon, S., . . . (eds). (2020). *Saving Lives, Improving Mothers' Care – Lessons Learned to Inform Maternity Care from the UK and Ireland Confidential Enquiries into Maternal Deaths and Morbidity 2016–18*. Oxford: National Perinatal Epidemiology Unit, University of Oxford.

Lokugamage, A. and Meredith, A. (March 2020). Women from ethnic minorities face endemic structural racism when seeking and accessing healthcare. *BMJ Opinion (online)*. https://blogs.bmj.com/bmj/2020/03/05/women-from-ethnic-minorities-face-endemic-structural-racism-when-seeking-and-accessing-healthcare/.

Macedo, D.M., Smithers, L.G., Roberts, R.M. and Jamieson, L.M. (2019). Racism, stress, and sense of personal control among Aboriginal Australian pregnant women. *Australian Psychologist, 55*, 336–348.

Marmot, M., Allen, J., Boyce, T., Goldblatt, P. and Morrison, J. (2020). *Health Equity in England: The Marmot Review Ten Years On*. London: Institute of Health Equity.

Miller, S., Abalos, E., Chamillard, M., Ciapponi, A., Colaci, D., Comandé, D., . . . Althabe, F. (2016). Beyond too little, too late and too much, too soon: a pathway towards evidence-based, respectful maternity care worldwide. *Lancet, 388*, 2176–2192.

Newnham E., McKellar L. and Pincombe J. (2018) *Towards the Humanisation of Birth: A Study of Epidural Analgesia and Hospital Birth Culture*. London: Palgrave Macmillan.

NMC. (2019). Standards of proficiency for midwives. The Nursing and Midwifery Council, UK. Available at: https://www.nmc.org.uk/globalassets/sitedocuments/standards/standards-of-proficiency-for-midwives.pdf.

Olza, I., Leahy-Warren, P., Benyamini, Y., Kazmierczak, M., Karlsdottir, S.I., Spyridou, A., . . . Nieuwenhuijze, M.J. (2018). Women's psychological experiences of physiological childbirth: a metasynthesis. *BMJ Open Access, 8*, e020347.

Page, L. (ed.). (2000). *The New Midwifery: Science and Sensitivity in Practice*. Edinburgh: Churchill Livingstone.

Page, L. and McCandlish, R. (eds). (2006) *The New Midwifery: Science and Sensitivity in Practice*, 2nd edn. Edinburgh: Churchill Livingstone.

Patterson, D. and Begley, A.M. (2011). An exploration of the importance of emotional intelligence in midwifery. *Evidence Based Midwifery, 9*(2), 53–60.

Renfrew, M.J., Bradshaw, G., Burnett, A., Byrom, A., Entwistle, F., King, K., . . . Thomas, G. (2021). Sustaining quality education and practice learning in a pandemic and beyond: 'I have never learnt as much in my life, as quickly, ever'. *Midwifery, 94*, 102915.

Renfrew, M.J., McFadden, A., Bastos, M.H., Campbell, J., Channon, A.A., Cheung, N.F., . . . Declercq, E. (2014). Midwifery and quality care: findings from a new evidence-informed framework for maternal and newborn care. *Lancet, 384*, 1129–1145.

Sackett, D. (1996). Evidence based medicine: what it is and what it isn't. Editorial. *British Medical Journal, 312*, 71–72.

Simkin, P., Ancheta, R. and Hanson, L. (2017). *The Labor Progress Handbook: Early Interventions to Prevent and Treat Dystocia*, 4th edn. Chichester: Wiley-Blackwell.

Simkin, P. with Rohs, K. (2018). *The Birth Partner: A Complete Guide to Childbirth for Dads, Doulas, and All Other Labor Companions*, 5th edn. Boston, MA: Harvard Common Press.

Walsh, D. (2012). *Evidence and Skills for Normal Labour and Birth*, 2nd edn. London: Routledge.

Walsh, D. and Downe, S. (eds). (2010). *Essential Midwifery Practice: Intrapartum Care*. Chichester: Wiley-Blackwell.

Wickham, S. (2017). The language of birth: crossing the Ts and promoting positivity. *The Practising Midwife*, 20 January 2017 online supplement. Available at: https://www.sarawickham.com/articles-2/the-language-of-birth-crossing-the-ts-and-promoting-positivity/.

Wieringa, S. and Greenhalgh, T. (2015). 10 years of mindlines: a systematic review and commentary. *Implementation Science, 10*, 45.

Williams, H. (2003). Storied births: narrative and organizational culture in a midwife-led birth centre. Unpublished thesis completed as part of MSc in Advancing Midwifery Practice, Kings College London.

World Health Organization. (2019). *Framework for Action: Strengthening Quality Midwifery Education for Universal Health Coverage 2030*. Geneva: World Health Organization.

Wren Serbin, J. and Donnelly, E. (2016). The impact of racism and midwifery's lack of racial diversity: a literature review. *Journal of Midwifery and Women's Health, 61*(6), 694–706.

1   What do we mean by 'support' in labour?

Introduction

'Continuous support in labour' or 'one-to-one support in labour' are terms used to describe the recognised gold standard of a woman having someone alongside her, responding to her physical and emotional needs throughout whatever transpires during her labour. In this chapter we shall explore the features and value of support during labour, with reference to the experiences of women, and those who provide support, including: midwives, doulas and the woman's chosen labour supporters or birth companions. The importance of this support cannot be over-stated, as this childbirth educator and birth supporter notes:

> We've had all this emphasis on giving women choices – and that comes quite a way down the hierarchy of importance for me. Support is the most important thing, and with support comes encouragement. Just connecting with the woman and telling her, you know, demonstrating through your body language and also through murmuring comforting and encouraging words that she's doing really well.
>
> (Childbirth educator/birth supporter, Sandall *et al.*, 2010, unpublished data)

We recognise that you may be working in a situation where the culture and organisation of the birthing environment dictates that continuous support for women in labour is the exception rather than the rule. The concepts that we shall be discussing in this chapter are still relevant: however fragmented or fleeting your interactions are with a woman in labour, you can make a difference to her experience through the way you connect with her. We encourage you to remember the oft-quoted words of autobiographer, poet and Black activist Maya Angelou:

> I've learned that people will forget what you said, people will forget what you did, but people will never forget how you made them feel.
>
> (www.goodreads.com/author/quotes/3503.Maya_Angelou)

Conceptualising support in labour

Definitions of support in labour

Multiple definitions and meanings are attributed to support in labour; this can cause confusion about how studies are compared and how the concept of one-to-one support is translated into practice (Sosa *et al.*, 2012).

DOI: 10.4324/9781003092520-2

Box 1.1   Research Briefing: The concept of continuous support in labour

Sosa, G., Crozier, K. and Robinson, J. (2012). What is meant by one-to-one support in labour: analysing the concept. *Midwifery*, *28*, 451–457.

This paper provides an overview of evidence related to one-to-one support in labour and discusses the complexities associated with the myriad of ways that the concept has been interpreted and incorporated into policy and practice in different settings. The researchers suggest that translating evidence into practice is problematic when there is no unanimous agreement about the level of presence, who should provide it, when it should happen and what type of model of care should be applied.

The Cochrane systematic review, *Continuous Support for Women During Childbirth*, identifies beneficial elements of supportive care in labour that were identified in 26 randomised controlled trials from 17 different countries, involving 15,858 women:

> Research shows that women value and benefit from the presence of a support person during labour and childbirth. This support may include emotional support (continuous presence, reassurance and praise) and information about labour progress. It may also include advice about coping techniques, comfort measures (comforting touch, massage, warm baths/showers, encouraging mobility, promoting adequate fluid intake and output) and speaking up when needed on behalf of the woman.
>
> (Bohren *et al.*, 2017, p.3)

In an article designed to encourage American obstetric nurses to value their role in providing supportive care, Penny Simkin offers a broader definition, suggesting that supportive care can be defined as:

> non-medical care that is intended to ease a woman's anxiety, discomfort, loneliness and exhaustion, to help her draw on her own strengths and to ensure that her needs and wishes are known and respected. It includes physical comfort measures, emotional support, information and instruction, advocacy and support for the partner.
>
> (Simkin, 2002, p.721)

The tone of this definition reflects qualitative studies suggesting that, when women reflect on the support that they received during labour, emotional support – feeling cared for as an individual – tends to be rated more highly than competence or physical care (Lunda *et al.*, 2018). A 16-year-old woman reflecting on the birth of her first baby offers an example of this:

> I felt really close to them. They were like sisters to me, they were really close, just making me feel that I was fine.
>
> (Mother, Leap, 2007, unpublished data)

Rosemary Mander (2001) questions the value of separating out different definitions of midwifery support, suggesting that the boundaries are often blurred; instead she suggests that it is useful to think of midwifery relationships as having the potential to embrace the full complexity of the physiological and psychological impacts of emotional and practical support. This means placing the individual woman at the centre of care; thus support is directly related to the concepts of 'woman centred care' (Leap, 2009) and 'being with woman' as opposed to 'being with institution' (Brodie, 1996; Hunter, 2004).

Evidence for continuous support in labour

Updated versions of the Cochrane systematic review of continuous support for women during childbirth (Bohren *et al.*, 2017) continue to identify a reduction in: caesareans, instrumental births, the use of intrapartum analgesia and epidurals, and low Apgar scores. Women who have continuous support are more likely to have shorter labours and report a positive experience of labour and birth.

Box 1.2   Research Briefing: The Cochrane systematic review of continuous support for women during childbirth

Bohren, M.A., Hofmeyr, G.J., Sakala, C., Fukuzawa, R.K. and Cuthbert, A. (2017) Continuous support for women during childbirth. *Cochrane Database of Systematic Reviews*, Issue 7. Art. No.: CD003766. doi: 10.1002/14651858.CD003766.pub6.

The key text for studying high-level evidence about continuous support in labour, the Cochrane systematic review, can be accessed freely via the Internet. Apart from encouraging you to study the comprehensive description of studies and findings in this review, we recommend the Background, Discussion and Authors' Conclusion sections as these provide a wealth of information to inform discussion and practice.

Bohren, M.A., Berger, B.O., Munthe-Kaas, H., Tunçalp, Ö. *et al.* (2019). Perceptions and experiences of labour companionship: a qualitative evidence synthesis. *Cochrane Database of Systematic Reviews*, Issue 3. Art. No.: CD012449. doi: 10.1002/14651858. CD012449.pub2

This review complements the Cochrane systematic review of continuous support in labour in exploring the perceptions and experiences of women, partners, community members, healthcare providers, administrators and others regarding labour companionship, drawing on 52 qualitative studies. The review is a source of rich information about the features of support that women appreciate and factors that affect the successful implementation and sustainability of labour companionship in facilities.

Evidence-based guidelines: continuous support in labour

The evidence for the considerable benefits of continuous support in labour has informed a number of practice guidelines; for example, the World Health Organization recommends a companion of choice for all women throughout labour and childbirth (WHO, 2018, 2020). Evidence-informed guidelines published by the Royal College of Midwives in the form of 'Blue Top Guidance' include a section on supporting birth companions.

Box 1.3   Recommended Resource: Birth companions: Recommendations for practice

RCM. (2018). Birth companions. *Midwifery Care in Labour Guidance for All Women in All Settings. RCM Midwifery Blue Top Guidance.* No. 1. London: Royal College of Midwives, pp.23–24. https://www.rcm.org.uk/media/2539/professionals-blue-top-guidance.pdf.

This section of the guideline focuses on supporting birth companions from the woman's family and friends. Evidence is identified to inform recommendations and practice points, including the following considerations:

- Making companions feel welcome, valuing their contribution, and asking whether they would like to receive suggestions on the ways they can provide support
- Recognising that not all companions need to be directed to ways to physically support the birthing mother
- Making sure a member of staff is tasked with providing information and support to the birth companion if an emergency arises
- Avoiding using the word 'fathers' when speaking about groups of parents and asking women and their families how they want to be addressed; this is one aspect of providing inclusive and sensitive care for lesbian couples
- Welcoming doulas as part of the woman's birth support network

---

Factors affecting the implementation of continuous support in labour

The Cochrane review of perceptions and experiences of labour companionship (Bohren *et al.*, 2019) found that most maternity services did not appear to address the key features of continuous support in labour that are associated with improved outcomes and experiences for women (Bohren *et al.*, 2017). The authors suggest a range of institutional policies and practices that can inhibit the implementation of continuous support in labour, including the following factors:

- Health workers and women not recognising the benefits of companionship
- A lack of space and privacy in birth environments

- Failure to design or implement policies to promote companionship
- Fears of increased risks of infection
- Resistance and conflict due to a lack of understanding of how to work alongside companions

Similar findings were identified in a review of factors that affect the implementation of schemes to enable women to have a companion of their choice (Kabakian-Khasholian and Portela, 2017). Although healthcare providers thought that companions might be useful in facilities with midwifery and nursing shortages, negative attitudes were common. Concerns were expressed about: cross infection; crowding; the cultural preferences of the companion; interference with clinical decision making; and the companion interfering with activities in the labour ward.

Developing a vision for continuous support in labour for all women

As research evidence of improved outcomes associated with continuous support in labour grew throughout the twenty-first century, a familiar catch cry in midwifery circles has been: 'If one-to-one support in labour were a drug, it would be unethical not to give it to all women'.

In lamenting how hard it is to make changes happen in institutions and in our planning efforts, we often find ourselves focusing on barriers, rather than potential solutions or existing strengths. We have found that adopting an Appreciative Inquiry approach (Cooperrider *et al.*, 2000; Mohr and Magruder Watkins, 2002) is worth considering as an alternative to 'problem solving', especially when we find ourselves slipping into disgruntlement, or even despair, about all the problems associated with how difficult it is to change the culture and practices of contemporary maternity care.

Appreciative Inquiry enables people to reflect on 'what is' and 'what could be' in a four-stage process that promotes positive thinking: Discovery, Dream, Design and Destiny. You will find explanations of Appreciative Inquiry in many online resources as well as articles describing how it has been used in maternity care and midwifery education settings. See, for example, Dewar *et al.* (2020); Schmied *et al.* (2019); and Sidebotham *et al.* (2015).

The following activity provides an opportunity for you to use an Appreciative Inquiry approach to reflect on your experience of one-to-one support in labour within your local context and think about a vision for your service in the future.

**Box 1.4   Reflective Activity: Exploring local implementation of
one-to-one support in labour**

In preparation for this activity:
1   Familiarise yourself with the principles of an Appreciative Inquiry approach
2   Read the paper by Sosa, G., Crozier, K. and Robinson, J. (2012) in Box 1.1.

Particularly focus on the list of antecedents and defining attributes of one-to-one support in labour, which include the following factors:

*   Woman centred philosophy of care
*   Adequate midwifery staffing
*   Midwife (or birthing partner) motivated to be with woman
*   Ratio of one midwife (or birth partner) to one woman
*   Equal relationship
*   Continuous support
*   Presence, being with, being available.

(p.456)

In pairs or small groups:
1   Discuss how each of these factors relate to:

*   the way in which you see support for women being provided in your working environment
*   policy documents in your setting

2   Using an Appreciative Inquiry approach, develop a local context map identifying your vision of any changes or improvements that are needed. This should include how and when these should happen and who will be involved in making them happen. There are many online examples of visual context maps, but often the best method is to let the map evolve during the discussion, using large sheets of paper and Post-it (sticky) notes.
3   Share your context map with the larger group and discuss the value of engaging in this activity, including the use of an Appreciative Inquiry approach.

Identifying and measuring quality midwifery support in labour

Mary Ross-Davie and colleagues at the University of Stirling in Scotland developed and tested a computer-based instrument (The Supportive Midwifery in Labour Instrument – SMILI) for systematically measuring the quality and quantity of midwifery support during labour (Ross-Davie et al., 2013). The study was carried out in four diverse NHS maternity units in Scotland and involved making comparisons between the researchers' observations of care provider behaviours in labour and women's views of the care they received. The instrument was found to be valid, reliable, feasible and usable. Importantly, it has the potential to be used in other settings.

Box 1.5   Research Briefing: Identifying and measuring quality support in labour

Ross-Davie, M.C. (2012). Measuring the quantity and quality of midwifery support of women during labour and childbirth: the development and testing of the Supportive Midwifery in Labour Instrument. University of Stirling, Scotland. This e-thesis can be accessed online: https://dspace.stir.ac.uk/handle/1893/9796.

Ross-Davie, M.C., Cheyne, H. and Niven, C. (2013). Measuring the quality and quantity of professional intrapartum support: testing a computerised systematic observation tool in the clinical setting. *BMC Pregnancy and Childbirth, 13*, 163.

Mary Ross-Davie's PhD study (2012) is a valuable resource that you can access freely via Stirling University, Scotland. Chapter 2 in her thesis provides a useful synthesis of literature related to women's views of labour support. This work contributed to the publication of a literature review identifying how far the nature of labour support shapes women's assessment of their birth experiences (Ross-Davie and Cheyne, 2014).

Box 1.6   Research Briefing: Support in labour – what do women want?

Ross-Davie, M.C. and Cheyne, H. (2014) Intrapartum support: what do women want: a literature review to identify how far the nature of labour support shapes women's assessment of their birth experiences. *Evidence Based Midwifery, 12(2)*, 52–58.

This paper provides a comprehensive overview of the key concepts and behaviours that women consider are central to the provision of high-quality intrapartum care. The researchers conclude that high-quality support promotes normal birth, reduces interventions and improves women's perceptions of their birth experiences. It also has the potential to promote a positive adaptation to motherhood and reduce the risk of post-traumatic stress disorder and other perinatal mental health problems.

Talking about support in labour with pregnant women and their supporters

In Chapter 4, we explore ways of engaging with pregnant women and their families in preparation for labour and birth. Exploring the myriad of ways that individual women might benefit from support in labour is a primary consideration in conversations and in any group sessions focussed on preparation for birth.

Box 1.7   Reflective Activity: Talking to women about support in labour

The *Cochrane Database of Systematic Reviews* provides 'Plain Language Summaries' for each review. These are easily accessible for those who want to access a quick impression of research findings and can be a useful resource for sharing with women and others who are unfamiliar with the reporting methods and language of systematic reviews.

Individually, in pairs or in small groups:

- After reading the Cochrane 'Plain Language Summary: Continuous Support for Women in Childbirth' (Bohren *et al.*, 2017), discuss how you might incorporate aspects of this summary into a discussion in an antenatal clinic when a pregnant woman says: 'I'm thinking of hiring a doula to support me in labour as I'd really like to have a normal birth. Do you think that's a good idea?'
- Write a script with fictional characters, paying attention to the language and communication skills that the midwife uses as she engages in an information-sharing discussion with the woman. Draw on the articles and reflective activities about language and suggestion in Chapter 5. This will help you think about how the midwife listens and responds to the woman as well as the potential impact of the language used in the discussion by both the midwife and the woman.

Supporting birth partners to support women in labour

A large survey conducted in England demonstrated the considerable sociodemographic variations in partner support and engagement; the authors of the study remind us not to assume that all women will be well supported by their male partners; some women will be more reliant on staff for support (Redshaw and Henderson, 2013). Undoubtedly, though, the majority of male partners want to be involved and welcome information about how to provide support (Poh *et al.*, 2014; Xue *et al.*, 2018). Since the majority of parents will search the Internet for advice about support in labour, we recommend the following activity:

Box 1.8   Reflective Activity: Advice about supporting women in labour – YouTube

Individually, in pairs or in small groups:

- Search YouTube using 'How to support women during labour'.
- After watching a selection of videos discuss how women and their birth supporters might feel and learn when looking for advice in this way.
- Write an annotated bibliography (a list of the videos with a short critique of each) to share with the whole group, identifying which ones you would recommend to women and their birth supporters.

Creating environments that enable companions to provide support

A meta-synthesis of fathers' experiences of their partners' labour and the birth of their babies highlighted that men often expressed overwhelming feelings of inadequacy in their ability to support their partner. Being well prepared and receiving support were essential elements of positive experiences and contributed to partners' ability to provide adequate support (Johansson *et al.*, 2015). The physical environment for labour and birth in institutions can have a profound effect on the experiences of supporters, enhancing or inhibiting their feelings of being needed and being able to engage in activities that are useful for the labouring woman (Davis Harte *et al.*, 2016).

Box 1.9   Reflective Activity: Creating environments that enable companions to provide support

Davis Harte, J., Sheehan, A., Stewart, S. and Foureur, M. (2016). Childbirth supporters' experiences in a built hospital birth environment: exploring inhibiting and facilitating factors in negotiating the supporter role. *Health Environment Research & Design Journal*, *9*, 135–161.

Individually, in pairs or in small groups:

*   After reading about the study by Davis Harte *et al.*, discuss how you felt when looking at the images in the paper.
*   How does the physical environment portrayed relate to your own experiences of working in institutions and supporting birth companions to provide support?
*   Design features that would facilitate supporters' roles are outlined in Table 4 of this article. How many of these are available and used in the birthing environment that you are familiar with?
*   How might you adapt the environment you work in to better facilitate positive experiences for a woman's chosen birth companions?

Providing culturally safe support and addressing racism

There is a wealth of childbirth literature identifying the importance of providing culturally safe and responsive care for pregnant women who are most likely to experience poor outcomes. This could be, for example, for Aboriginal women in Australia (Brown *et al.*, 2016; Kruske *et al.*, 2006; Macedo *et al.*, 2019), refugee and migrant women (Goodwin *et al.*, 2018; Higginbottom *et al.*, 2019; Rogers *et al.*, 2020) or asylum seekers (Frank *et al.*, 2021). However, providing culturally safe care is important for all women who are at risk of the effects of systemic racism (Cross-Sudworth, 2007; Horn, 2020; Lokugamage and Meredith, 2020; Wren Serbin and Donnelly, 2016).

In the UK, concerns about the fact that women from Black, Asian and minority ethnic (BAME) communities are more likely to die during pregnancy and after birth (Knight *et al.*, 2020) are prompting discussions about how to address the ways in which racial inequalities, racial discrimination and racism contribute to poor outcomes for BAME women and their babies. Citing the improved outcomes for women and babies cared for by the Albany Midwifery Practice (Homer *et al.*, 2017), the *NHS Long Term Plan* (NHS, 2019) proposes an NHS England target of 75 per cent of women in BAME communities receiving continuity of care from their midwife throughout pregnancy, labour and birth and the postnatal period by 2024.

Box 1.10   Recommended Resource: Racism Matters

Horn, A. (2020). Racism Matters: 'When People Show You Who They Are, Believe Them': Why Black women mistrust maternity services. *The Practising Midwife, 23*, Download from: https://www.all4maternity.com/racism-matters-when-people-show-you-who-they-are-believe-them-why-black-women-mistrust-maternity-services/.

This paper is the first in a series of articles published by *The Practising Midwife* entitled, 'Racism Matters'. Anna Horn, a Black American woman, UK maternity service user and equity advocate, offers insight into 'a deeper, systematic and historical precedent of racism and injustice as underlying contributor to health inequalities'. We recommend that you study all the papers in this series.

Supporting women from refugee and migrant backgrounds

The resources in Box 1.11 are examples of guidelines for responsive, culturally safe care for refugee and migrant women; they can all be downloaded from the Internet.

Box 1.11   Recommended Resources: Guidelines for culturally responsive care for refugee and migrant women

Migrant and Refugee Women's Health Partnership. (2019a). *Culturally Responsive Clinical Practice: Working with People from Migrant and Refugee Backgrounds*. Canberra: Migrant and Refugee Women's Health Partnership.

This resource provides a competency standards framework for clinicians, identifying optimal culturally responsive practices and communication when working with migrant and refugee women.

Migrant and Refugee Women's Health Partnership. (2019b). *Guide for Clinicians Working with Interpreters in Healthcare settings*. Canberra: Migrant and Women's Health Partnership.

A complementary resource to the competency standards framework, this document focuses specifically on effective communication and working with interpreters. It recommends relevant approaches and evidence-informed good practice points.

Vivilaki, V., Soltani, H. and van den Muijsenbergh, M. (eds). (2017). *Practice Guide for Perinatal Health Care of Migrant, Asylum-seeking & Refugee Women (D4.1)*. Co-funded by the Health Programme of the European Union: ORAMMA Operational Refugee and Migrant Maternal Approach.

This document provides evidence-informed guidelines for practice, emphasising the importance of effective communication, building trust and nurturing a friendly relationship with women, ensuring that women are listened to and that there is an efficient interdisciplinary team providing holistic woman centred care throughout all stages of pregnancy, birth and the postnatal period.

Supporting women who are asylum seekers

As identified in the review profiled in Box 1.12 women seeking asylum in high-income countries are likely to have different needs to refugee and migrant women, due to their insecure status.

Box 1.12   Research Briefing: Supporting women who are asylum seekers

Frank, G.D., Fox, D., Njue, C. and Dawson, A. (2021). The maternity experiences of women seeking asylum in high-income countries: a meta-ethnography. *Women and Birth.*

The review highlights the reasons why asylum seekers are at an increased risk of mental health issues and poor outcomes, including their tenuous visa situation, isolation, racism, discrimination, relocation, fear of deportation and sub-optimal maternity care. The importance of health professionals having education in the provision of culturally appropriate, respectful maternity care and supportive strategies for women seeking asylum is emphasised.

Supporting women around gender-based violence

The term gender-based violence (GBV) refers to any harmful acts directed at an individual based on their gender. It can include sexual, physical, mental and economic harm inflicted in public or in private, and includes threats of violence, coercion, manipulation and humiliation. Gender-based violence can take many forms, such as intimate partner violence, sexual violence, child marriage, female genital mutilation, grooming and trafficking. The UNHCR (2020) estimates that one in three women will experience sexual or physical violence in their lifetime and that, during displacement and times of crisis, the threat significantly increases for women and girls.

As we discuss in Chapter 6 in relation to supporting women who are in relationships involving intimate partner violence, where the midwife has not met the woman before or GBV only becomes obvious for the first time during labour, it is essential that the midwife finds time to initiate a discussion with the woman after she has given birth. This involves appropriate responses when a woman discloses GBV and knowledge of appropriate support and relevant agencies (Smith *et al.*, 2018). It also means having an empathetic and non-judgemental attitude and an awareness of how our own values and beliefs related to violence against women, including our prejudices and biases, might impact on the woman's experiences.

During labour, touch, vaginal examinations, pain, and feelings of powerlessness and fear can provoke disturbing memories of child sexual abuse for survivors. Naomi Waddell (2019) draws on literature to remind us that, for some survivors, becoming a mother and nurturing a baby can play a role in helping them reclaim their bodies and sexual identities. Midwives are in a unique position as health professionals to build trusting relationships and foster aspects of this potential for women to heal, particularly when they are able to provide continuity of care (Eustace *et al.*, 2016; Waddell, 2019).

Respecting diversity

Supporting families from LGBT communities

As highlighted earlier in the 'Blue Top' guidelines for midwifery care in labour produced by the Royal College of Midwives in the UK (RCM, 2018), it is important that we think carefully about using inclusive language. Many lesbian, gay, bisexual and transgender (LGBT) families do not conform to the model of two parents of two genders; there may be more than two parents with different roles and levels of involvement and a person's gender may not necessarily denote their role (Allen, 2019; Darwin and Greenfield, 2019; Greenfield, 2017).

Box 1.13   Recommended Resource: Inclusive language when working with LGBT families

Reproduced from: Allen, J. (2019). Midwifery continuity of care for specific groups. Chapter 10 in C. Homer, N. Leap, P. Brodie and J. Sandall (eds). *Midwifery Continuity of Care*, 2nd edn. Sydney: Elsevier Australia, p.218.

1   If you're not sure what pronoun a person wants to use, simply ask.
2   Use *names* instead of roles (e.g. 'mother' implies there is only one and that the person who is pregnant identifies as female).
3   Be aware of your assumptions and be open to alternative possibilities (e.g. there may be one mother, two mothers or no mother – one father, two fathers or no father).
4   Don't be afraid to ask questions, but first think about whether they're necessary.
5   Ask open questions (e.g. 'Who are the baby's parents?' 'Who gave birth?').
6   Avoid questions about why and how parents decided to conceive, who was to carry the child, and non-medically relevant details of transition.
7   Think about what it is you actually want to find out and then phrase your question accordingly.
8   Avoid repeated questions (i.e. record the answers to your questions).

Adapted from: Greenfield, M. (2017). He's not the mother. *AIMS Journal, 29(2)*, 7–9. https://www.aims.org.uk/journal/item/hes-not-the-mother.

Examining our own values and attitudes

Providing culturally safe and respectful care requires a careful examination of our values and attitudes and an understanding of the devastating effects of systemic racism on outcomes and experiences for women from BAME communities in the UK (Cross-Sudworth, 2007; Knight *et al.*, 2020; Lokugamage and Meredith, 2020) and Aboriginal women and families in Australia (Durey, 2010; Macedo *et al.*, 2019).

Box 1.14   Reflective Activities: Exploring the potential effect of our values and attitudes when supporting women in labour

The following activities can be used for personal reflection or discussion in pairs. They could also be adapted as workshop activities or written assignments.

1   Search the Internet for definitions of 'cultural safety.' Discuss what the principles of cultural safety mean to you as an individual and to your family. How might this affect how you support women and their families for labour and birth?
2   Tell (or write) a story about an occasion when you have felt put down or misunderstood by others. What was your role? What social group were you part of? What was the power relation between you and the other person/s? What is the relevance of your story to how you support women in labour?
3   The following words are associated with descriptions of identity:

Race	Ethnicity	Indigenous heritage
Sexual orientation	Gender	Religion
Body size/shape	Physical ability	Mental illness
Socioeconomic status	White privilege	Age

Choose one of these identities as you respond to each of the following questions. In your reflection/discussion, identify how this might affect how you support women in labour.

1   This is the identity I know most about.
2   This is the identity I know least about.
3   This is the identity I am most unsure about how to talk about.
4   This is the identity that I think most people judge me by.
5   This is the identity that is most important to me.

Continuous support in labour: a fundamental principle

> One thing I do tell partners: 'You don't have to worry about what you do; just being there is enough.' I always quote that Guatemalan study where just having another woman in the room, someone who the woman hadn't even met before, having that one person sitting there with them shortened their labours. So having the person you care about more than anyone else in the world there is going to make it even better! I like telling them that story.
>
> (Midwife, Leap, 2015, unpublished data)

The research that this midwife is referring to is the study carried out by Sosa *et al.* (1980) in the Social Security Hospital in Guatemala City. With an average of 60 births every two hours, no family member or support person was allowed to accompany labouring women. Forty women having their first babies, with uncomplicated labours, were recruited in labour. Half were allocated to standard care without a support person. Women in the intervention group had continuous support from an untrained 'lay' woman – someone they had not previously met – from admission to birth. The support they received was in the form of back rubbing, hand holding and friendly encouragement.

Mother–baby interaction with skin-to-skin contact was observed for 45 minutes for women in each group. The women who had had support in labour were much more likely to stroke, smile and talk to their baby. An unexpected finding was that they also had shorter labours. The research team repeated this study in the same hospital with larger numbers of women and again showed that women who had support had shorter labours; they also had fewer caesarean births and less augmentation of labour (Klaus *et al.*, 1986).

In spite of the highly context-specific nature of these studies, they became legendary. Large trials of continuous support in labour in other countries followed (Bohren *et al.*, 2017), yet the early studies in Guatemala are often the ones that are quoted anecdotally (hence the comment of the midwife cited earlier).

These studies were mainly carried out in countries where the alternative to continuous support was little or no support in labour. It is thus easy to comprehend how a supportive companion might ameliorate the fear, stress and loneliness for women who face labour in an unfamiliar environment without support, and how their presence might lead to a reduction in the stress hormones that are counterproductive to the neurobiology and physiology of labour (Mander, 2001).

Box 1.15   Recommended Resource: A critical look at trials of continuous support in labour

Mander, R. (2001). Chapter 5. Support in Labour. *Supportive Care and Midwifery*. Oxford: Blackwell Science.

Using a theoretical framework that allows for consideration of the training or professional education of those involved, the context of each study and the methods used, Rosemary Mander reviews the multiple studies in this area up to and including 2000. She presents a compelling critique of research undertaken and the emerging impression of: 'abysmal birthing environments being rendered less hostile by the endeavours of a kind-hearted woman companion' (Mander, 2001, p.111).

Doulas supporting women for labour and birth

The birth of the 'doula' movement

Members of the research team who carried out the early studies in Guatemala used the findings to highlight the value of a person they named a 'doula'– a Greek-derived term embodying the idea of 'mothering the mother.' Their book, *Mothering the Mother – How a Doula Can Help You Have a Shorter, Easier and Healthier Birth* (Klaus *et al.*, 1993) played a major role in the introduction of the doula as a new provider of services in maternity care in the USA.

For decades, randomised controlled trials have consistently shown that the presence and support of a trained doula reduces a woman's chance of having a caesarean section or forceps birth in institutionalised settings (Fortier and Godwin, 2015). It is therefore a logical choice for a woman who wants to avoid interventions to hire a doula, particularly if she is not confident about the level of support she can expect from her birth attendants in institutions that have high intervention rates.

Increasingly, across Northern America and, to a lesser extent, in other high-income countries, women can hire a trained, professional doula to go on the journey with them and support them through pregnancy, labour and birth, and new motherhood. For women who cannot afford the services of a doula, the case has been made for a low-cost alternative; labour support provided by a minimally trained female friend or relative, selected by the mother-to-be, also has the potential to enhance positive experiences of birth and new motherhood (Campbell *et al.*, 2006). This argument raises controversial issues about the professionalisation of doulas, their role and issues of equity of access to services.

> Before I was a midwife I was a doula. I worked mostly with women who had no support or women who were trying to negotiate something different within the system, like a vaginal breech birth. I also attended the births of a lot of lesbian mothers, who were not confident about how maternity staff would support them. It was very much a lay person role. I worry about the professionalisation of the doula – we had a woman come in the other day with her birth plan on the doula's very flashy headed notepaper and I thought, 'Who's birth plan is that?' And having to charge fees means that some women can't access a doula. But they do an important job; and of course they have to be paid for that. But sadly, I think they're filling the gap where midwives aren't providing continuity of care.
>
> (Midwife, Leap, 2015, unpublished data)

Box 1.16   Reflective Activity: The roles of the doula and the midwife in community-based continuity of care

In pairs or small groups:

1   In preparation for this activity, access two websites: one identifying services offered by doulas and another identifying the services offered by midwives working in a community-based, midwifery continuity of care service (in your local area, if available).

2   Make a list of the services offered by both the doulas and the midwives and discuss:
   - What are the differences and similarities in the services offered?
   - What are the cost implications (if any) for women?
   - How might a pregnant woman and her partner feel when accessing these websites?
   - How do the roles of the doula and the midwife correspond with the traditional role of women supporting women in labour outlined in the Prologue to this book?

Working with doulas to provide support for women

Box 1.17   Research Briefing: Doulas and midwives – conflict or collaboration?

Stevens, J., Dahlen, H., Peters, K. and Jackson, D. (2011). Midwives' and doulas' perspectives of the role of the doula in Australia: a qualitative study. *Midwifery, 27,* 509–516.

The potential for doulas to take over the midwife's role of continuity of care, continuous care in labour, advocacy, protecting normal birth and being part of the community was seen in this study as being driven by 'broken maternity systems' that are failing women. The benefits of doula care for women are outlined. Some of the areas where conflict between doulas and health professionals can arise are explored with recommendations for how these might be addressed and collaboration improved in order to optimise the provision of quality services for women.

We have probably all encountered concerns about doulas 'filling the gap' where maternity systems prevent midwives from providing woman centred continuity of care (Lundgren, 2010; Stevens *et al.*, 2011). Over time, the blurring of roles can split into two, resulting in situations where student midwives conceptualise continuous support in labour as 'doula' skills, separate from the more familiar midwifery tasks associated with providing care in labour (Thorstensson *et al.*, 2008).

The role of the doula: working alongside maternity care staff

In many high-income countries women turn to doulas where they are unable to access midwifery continuity of care. Doulas offer an opportunity to build a trusting relationship with women and their chosen birth companions and guarantee to be there to offer support during labour, however that may eventuate. Many doulas also visit women at home after they have had their babies and help women tap into local friendship networks and online resources. Ample time is spent during pregnancy exploring the woman's hopes and discussing evidence to support any potential choices she may make. As this experienced doula explains, from her perspective the emphasis should not be speaking on behalf of the woman and her partner, but rather on supporting them to have useful interactions with staff:

> In labour it's all about the information sharing that you've done with the woman previously, the conversations that you've had with the couple beforehand. If a doula is appearing obstructive to the staff, that's not a good situation for anyone. I teach doulas and I tell them that we are not the woman's advocate. That's not our role. We're going in to support the woman but we're not the one who should be saying, 'She wants that, she doesn't want that.' Rather than me as a doula directing it back to the doctor saying, 'She doesn't want an episiotomy,' I would say to the woman, 'They want to cut an episiotomy now' as another reminder for them to be the voice. I always try to put it back to them. I just remind them of the things we've discussed previously.
>
> (Doula, Leap unpublished data, 2020)

Midwives and doulas: avoiding assumptions and stereotypes

> In any profession there are some who excel and some who are a bit of a worry. I've met some doulas who think that they have to fight for the woman and they're almost antagonistic towards you – they make assumptions that you're not on the same wavelength when it comes to supporting women. But when I've worked with what I'd call 'good' doulas, they're there completely for the woman and they take good care of her in a nurturing way. They support the partner to support her too, often steadying them. Mind you I think that's our role too.
>
> (Midwife, Leap, 2015, unpublished data)

Georgina Sosa and colleagues (2012) identify the lack of studies on continuous support in labour in countries where midwives are the main providers of labour care (including in women's homes and midwifery-led units). They make the argument that there is insufficient evidence to conclude that doulas, rather than midwives, should be the primary carer providing one-to-one support in labour in all settings.

Approaches to supporting women for labour and birth

The art of supporting women for labour and birth is fostered by the relationships between the woman and those who will be close to her as she journeys through pregnancy, birth and new motherhood. Midwives who are able to be alongside a woman on this journey are ideally placed to engage with the woman in working out what sort of support she might need along the way (Homer *et al.*, 2019). At any stage of our interactions with women, though, including if we are not providing midwifery continuity of care, we can be there for women in a way that makes a difference. The skill lies in knowing when this means simply reinforcing women's confidence in their capabilities to find a way through any given situation or stepping in and offering more 'hands-on' support.

> When it was getting near the end of my labour, I was on all fours and I felt her just lightly put her hands on my back for a few seconds. I knew it was her. It was like an orb of light. That was enough. It gave me all the energy I needed to finish.
>
> (New mother, Leap, 2020, unpublished data)

In labour, such approaches are akin to the philosophies of midwifery care that have been described as:

- 'the less we do the more we give' (Leap, 2010)
- 'the art of doing "nothing" well' (Kennedy, 2000)
- 'presence' (Kennedy *et al.*, 2010)
- 'guardianship' (Fahy *et al.*, 2008)
- being an 'anchored companion' (Lundgren and Dahlberg, 2002)

Anecdotally, it seems that these concepts have often been misinterpreted as, 'letting the woman get on with it on her own'. On the contrary, this way of supporting women requires: 'maintaining concentration, sensitivity, energy and unobtrusive assistance' (Robertson, 2007, p. x);

it involves the quiet support of being an 'anchored companion' (Lundgren and Dahlberg, 2002) and creating a safe space in which a woman can labour, where her individual needs for intimacy, respect and patience can be addressed (Kennedy and Shannon, 2004; Kennedy *et al.*, 2010).

> No one told me to breathe, no one told me to do anything. They just watched the way I was doing it. And I could make a noise without someone feeling like they had to fix my problem. They just kind of heard it. And that was perfect for me in my labour. And of course, everybody's going to need different things in labour but for me what was most important was having calm people, keeping a safe space and trusting that I knew what I was doing.
>
> (Mother, Leap, 2015, unpublished data)

The concept of presence

In the concept analysis of one-to-one support that we explored earlier in this chapter, Sosa and colleagues (2012) identify that women want the midwife or birth supporter to be in the room; in fact they identify 'presence, being with and being available' (p.456) as defining attributes of one-to-one care in labour.

Holly Powell Kennedy has extensively researched the concept of midwifery presence and has developed theory about the way it incorporates philosophy, science and art. She describes combining vigilant attendance in labour with 'the art of doing "nothing" well' (Kennedy, 2000, p.12). In the following text box, we have placed examples of Holly Powell Kennedy's writing about presence, including her reporting on how this contributes to the promotion of normal birth, a subject that we shall return to in subsequent chapters.

Box 1.18   Research Briefing: Exploring the concept of midwifery 'presence'

Kennedy, H.P. (2000). A model of exemplary midwifery practice: results of a Delphi study. *Journal of Midwifery and Women's Health*, 45(*1*), 4–19.

Kennedy, H.P., Shannon, M.T., Chuahorm, U. and Kravetz, M.K. (2004). The landscape of caring for women: a narrative study of midwifery practice. *Journal of Midwifery and Women's Health*, 49(*1*), 14–23.

Kennedy, H.P. and Shannon, M.T. (2004). Keeping birth normal: research findings on midwifery care during labour. *Journal of Obstetric Gynecologic and Neonatal Nursing*, 33(*5*), 554–560.

Cragin, L. and Kennedy, H.P. (2006). Linking obstetric and midwifery practice with optimal outcomes. *JOGNN Clinical Issues*, 35(*6*), 779–785.

Kennedy, H.P., Anderson, T. and Leap, N. (2010). Midwifery Presence: Philosophy, Science and Art. Chapter 7 in D. Walsh and S. Downe (eds), *Essential Midwifery Practice: Intrapartum Care* (pp.105–124). Chichester: Wiley-Blackwell.

Presence: 'being in the birth room'

In many places it seems that women who are allocated one-to-one care in labour do not necessarily get continuous care, which brings us to the issue we shall call 'being in the birth room'. Sosa and colleagues (2012) cite studies showing that the amount of time midwives were in the room providing one-to-one support was minimal, even when they had only one woman allocated to their care:

> It is . . . clear that a one-to-one ratio is not adequate without the motivation of midwives wanting to be present with the woman and raises questions concerning the activities that keep the midwife away from the woman.
>
> (Sosa *et al.*, 2012, p.454)

Record keeping, the giving or receiving of progress reports and the preparation of equipment or drugs are all factors that appear to get in the way of midwives providing continuous support (Sosa *et al.*, 2012). This is reflected in reality TV shows (Morris and McInerney, 2010).

An observational study in Scotland (Ross-Davie *et al.*, 2014) showed that midwives being out of the room was associated with the following factors:

* heightened anxiety for women and their partners, particularly if the midwife did not explain where she was going, why she was leaving or how long she would be away
* women appearing to find the pain of contractions more difficult and having tense interactions with their partner about what was happening
* a reduction in opportunities to build rapport and less supportive care when the midwife *was* in the room
* a reduction in the midwife's ability to monitor the progress of the woman's labour accurately

---

Box 1.19   Reflective Activity: Being in the room with women in labour

In pairs or small groups:
* Watch an episode of a reality TV show about labour and birth and individually make notes about what you see happening when women and their birth companions have left the room.
* Compare notes with your colleagues and discuss what you think it would take to change this culture in maternity units where it has become the norm.

Presence: facilitating safety

Being in the birth room is linked to safety, the argument being that where skilled caregivers are present they are able to observe the course of a woman's labour closely and notice when help may be needed; this can enable referral to a higher level of care in a timely fashion, thus reducing the likelihood of life-threatening emergencies (Centre for Maternal and Child Enquiries, 2011). This is a major consideration in efforts to reduce maternal mortality, particularly in resource-poor countries (WHO *et al.*, 2004).

Box 1.20   Reflective Activity: Continuous support in labour and safety

In pairs or small groups:
- Discuss examples of how continuous care in support in labour might promote safety in the context of your workplace.

In order to discuss these issues in relation to resource-poor countries, we suggest you watch: *Why did Mrs X Die?* This film was made to educate midwives, health workers and decision makers about the key issues associated with safe motherhood. You can access a range of videos and activities related to this film if you search for 'Why did Mrs X Die'.

Supportive care in labour and humanising birth

The Cochrane systematic review of continuous support for women in childbirth (Bohren *et al.*, 2017) identified that, as well as promoting physiological labour, supportive care can enhance women's feelings of control and confidence in their own strength and ability to give birth. The authors suggest that this is an important consideration in addressing concerns about how obstetric interventions and institutional routines can be associated with birth becoming dehumanised.

Respectful care for women in labour

Health facility policies that prohibit birth companions and a lack of any support in labour by care providers still feature in the list of neglectful, abusive and disrespectful treatment of women across the globe (Bohren *et al.*, 2015). In an 'Evidence-to-Action' brief, the World Health Organization (WHO, 2020) states that this can inhibit women from accessing safe care for birth in health facilities, with potentially life-threatening consequences.

Box 1.21   Recommended Resources: Respectful care for women in labour

WHO. (2020). *Companion of choice during labour and childbirth for improved quality of care: Evidence-to-action brief.* Geneva: World Health Organization. https://apps.who.int/iris/bitstream/handle/10665/334151/WHO-SRH-20.13-eng.pdf?ua=1.

Bohren, M.A., Vogel, J.P., Hunter, E.C., Lutsiv, O., Makh, S.K., Souza, J.P., . . . Gülmezoglu, A.M. (2015). The mistreatment of women during childbirth in health facilities globally: a mixed-methods systematic review. *PLoS Med, 12(6)*, e1001847. doi:10.1371/journal. pmed.1001847. https://journals.plos.org/plosmedicine/article?id=10.1371/journal.pmed.1001847.

Freedman, L.P. and Kruk, M.E. (2014). Disrespect and abuse of women in childbirth: challenging the global quality and accountability agendas. *Lancet, 384 (9948)*, e42–e44. doi: https://www.thelancet.com/journals/lancet/article/PIIS0140-6736(14)60859-X/fulltext.

White Ribbon Alliance: Respectful Maternity Care. http://whiteribbonalliance.org/campaigns/respectful-maternity-care.

You can find useful resources, including posters, presentations and short films here.

The International Confederation of Midwives Respect Workshops Toolkit (ICM, 2000) provides a range of resources and ideas for workshops and action to promote Respectful Maternity Care. It includes step-by-step guidance on why and how to run a workshop, and training resources such as a Facilitator Guide and PowerPoint presentation, videos, lesson plans, reference documents and ideas about how these can be adapted for local use. https://www.internationalmidwives.org/our-work/other-resources/respect-toolkit.html.

Box 1.22   Reflective Activity: 'Break the silence' – thinking about respectful maternity care

A short video (four minutes) presents the issues about respectful maternity care in a way that is relevant to all settings:

www.youtube.com/watch?v=K105F9o3HtU.

In pairs or small groups:
- Discuss the issues presented in this video in relation to your own experiences.

Humanising birth

The term 'humanising birth' encompasses the critical need to build systems of care that provide individualised, compassionate and respectful care to all women and their families (Newnham and Page, 2020). Having access to a labour and birth companion of the woman's choice is integral to that principle.

Box 1.23 Recommended Resources: Supportive care and humanising birth

Humanising Birth: A guide for practice e-book. All4Maternity e-book series. Published by Creative World, 2020. https://issuu.com/cwcreativeworld/docs/humanising-birth-ebook-v1.0.

This e-book is a compilation of eight articles published in *The Practising Midwife* in 2019 and 2020. In liaison with other leading maternity experts, lead author Elizabeth Newnham carefully deconstructs dehumanising birth practices. Thereafter, she reconstructs what humanised birth practices are, look like and feel like, and how they can be implemented immediately.

Page, L. (2017). The birth of our humanity. *British Journal of Midwifery*, 25(7), 414–415.
You can watch Lesley Page giving an inspiring talk about 'Humanising Birth' at the Scotland Maternity & Midwifery Festival in 2019: https://www.youtube.com/watch?v=sJI9Z4A3jk4.

Evidence from women: support in labour

We end this chapter by highlighting some women's experiences of support from midwives during their labours. The following quotations are from videoed interviews with women who had midwifery continuity of care throughout pregnancy, labour and the postnatal period (Sandall *et al.*, 2010). The women speak of the potential for this quality of support to have far-reaching consequences in terms of personal growth and confidence in their mothering abilities:

> They expected me to give birth well, they expected me to be a good parent afterwards and I grew to meet that expectation. You know? That's really powerful . . . again, it's the belief in you isn't it. It's like, you're a woman, of course you can give birth, you're designed for it. Why wouldn't you be able to give birth?

> I think for me it's been a big change, because I had two really negative experiences and so I actually didn't think I could deal with the whole process and get to the end, so in terms of growing, sort of emotionally and being able to understand that I can achieve this and have this outcome, this has been huge for me and my partner. And so I think we've both grown in that respect. Yeah, it's very positive.

> The whole time during my labour the midwives kept saying, 'You're fantastic, you're brilliant, you're doing absolutely great', and I just thought, 'Oh well, actually I must be doing fine, I must be doing something right.' So that was really positive, and *they made me come away feeling like, I'll be a fantastic parent, I'll be absolutely fine.*

> *They made me feel everything about me is something I can do* [our emphasis].

Together with Mesepa and Seneuefa's story in the Postcript below, we think those words are a fitting place to end this chapter. If good support helps women to build confidence in their abilities to labour, give birth and nurture their babies, then we can contribute to the ideal set by Barbara Katz Rothman in her oft-cited statement:

> Birth is not only about making babies. Birth is also about making mothers – strong, competent, capable mothers who trust themselves and know their inner strength.
>
> (Katz-Rothman, 1996, pp.253–254)

Postscript

Of Maori and Samoan heritage, Mesepa and Seneufa offer a profound understanding of 'presence' and how to provide support in labour. They reflect on their recent experience of being 'the mothers' supporting Denya ('our Princess') through a long labour at home, with other family members and midwives Jo and Athena in attendance.

Seneuefa: When I first met Jo at the pre-birth visit to Princess, straight away I connected with her in my heart. She was more a heart person in the way she was being with Princess, not so much telling her, but asking the sort of questions to draw responses from Princess. I was very impressed. Just her energy was beautiful. And I felt that Princess was in very good safe hands.

On the actual day of Denya's labour, there were a few things that I was very impressed with about Jo. I think it's more her 'being' rather than 'doing.' She was very present. And I just loved the way she was never *over* Princess. She was sitting in the corner when Princess was in the tub and in my mind I was thinking, 'Oh, should she not come a bit closer, or something?' Until I heard her saying, 'This is your journey Denya. This is your journey and I'm here to support you, but this is your journey. You do it.' And in that moment I feel that when someone says that to me, I receive permission, someone is giving me permission to take hold of my journey. Because really and truly, it's *my* journey. And what I saw when she said that was that Princess went up into the next dimension in herself, as it were, taking her power.

So those words were very empowering. I feel empowering is more powerful than enabling. With 'enabling' it can be as though you think the other person is a victim. But Jo was talking to a very powerful young woman. And she saw that in Denya. And then Denya grabbed that wisdom – because I feel it's wisdom drawn from all Jo's previous experience – she took that wisdom into herself and ran with it. And she went into the zone. I am so impressed with that. If it had been me I would have been screaming around. But she just went inside and worked from there, like she was in her power. And she contained it, like in a vessel, like the alchemy, she contained that wisdom, that energy in herself. The attention was inward now. So when the attention is inward, I am tapping into my power isn't it. But when my attention is outward, the pain takes me outward, so then I'm looking outside and I lose my power.

The way Jo facilitated her birthing was just inspirational. Beautiful. Soft. Gentle. Nothing intruding. Just sit there and be. There were moments when she went and sat in the corridor. She trusted us to be there with Denya so that we become part of the journey. And again, I was following her way of doing things. Not much talk, no talking. Just be there. If she wants our hands somewhere she will ask. There was one moment when I was putting my hands on her back and she said to me in Samoan, 'not that part' [laughter]. So it was like 'Whoa, OK. Where's the point, where's the part where I need to put my hands?' And then I watched Jo putting the hands and I followed her.

I can still feel like a tear of gratitude, you know? For Jo [crying] for the way she guided us and the way she attended to this huge task of bringing a new being into the planet. It was beautiful and such a sacred thing. I see Jo as a 'baby whisperer'. Because no talking. There was hardly any talk.

There was a time when Princess said, 'I feel like there's a change now, I feel like I want to push'. 'Oh, we'd better tell Jo' (because she was in the other room). Princess told her 'I want to push' and Jo said, 'Go for it girl. You push however you want to push.' So again, no more than that. She just gave the power to her.

Mesepa: When I met Jo for the first time, I sort of felt like I'd known her for a long time. There was just an immediate thing that I was at ease. I didn't have to worry. I could see that Denya was in really good hands and I really felt at home.

Athena's presence was so still. She reminded me of a very tall kauri tree. The kauri tree is like the grandmother/grandfather tree of New Zealand. It can span 100 metres wide. Athena's presence was solid – very, very solid. Very still and very quiet. But I was so aware of her presence. Very little said but she was just there.

Like Seneuefa was saying, Jo had this ability to utterly respect and honour Denya at that time. She (Denya) had all that she needed to go in and birth this baby. I saw Jo as the channel that was there to just come in at the time when it was needed to assist with words of encouragement, words of love and words of assurance for Denya. But for the majority of the time, it was really Denya breathing through the whole process, very calmly.

I was really grateful for Jo's calmness because I knew that if she was calm even though it was going on . . . and on . . . and on . . . and on, it was OK. Even if Jo had displayed a little bit of anxiousness, we all would have felt that. It's easy to conjure up in your mind, 'Oh my gosh, is there something wrong?' but there was no display of any anxiousness whatsoever. There was an utter trust in the process and in the journey, a total trust in Denya.

I could actually see the relationship between the two of them that had developed over the duration of Denya's pregnancy. I could actually see how they had really built that. You don't really have to communicate with words, the energy of communication was there and I could see that relationship between the two of them and how that worked. I could feel that. I loved that.

At one point, Jo suggested that we be left alone with Denya. She beautifully said, 'You need to let the Mummas do their thing now'. Seneuefa and I went into the bathroom to be close to Denya, who was just breathing through the process. We were singing our family songs in Samoan and Maori. And I said to Denya, 'When you can hear a sound, or feel a sound, go there and go deep. So we were gently just coaching her to go through to that space. And just as she was quietly beginning to bring that sound out, I did a traditional karanga. It's a traditional call that Maori women do when they're in the sacred spaces. So I started to do the chant, the karanga, Senueufa started singing in Samoan, both cultures were blended in together and then Denya started to breathe differently. That's when she said, 'I feel like I want to go into the other room now, I think I'm ready to push'.

So to witness the silent, grounding presence of Athena and Jo, allowing the family to be in and all around Denya, without actually being close to where Denya was, facilitating from a distance, being present for Denya. And then, when it was the right time, Jo came in when she needed to and that's when we got to witness the most amazing birth of little Sunny Vai.

Even when Denya was holding the baby . . . I myself have sat with all my sisters for their births and I have witnessed and welcomed all my nieces and nephews – I have never experienced a midwife who has allowed the baby to come up, the placenta's still there and she has just sat for almost a good hour, allowing us to just be in awe and present to this beautiful new being. With my own sisters and their children, the midwives have quickly come in, quickly grabbed the clips put them on, told the father, 'Come and cut it off' and then that's it, take the baby off. It was not like that at all.

And the most . . . I'm going to get emotional now [crying.] When I was pregnant with Denya one of the things that my Auntie – who was a midwife – said to my mother was that the most important thing is to grab the placenta, put the placenta on baby's chest, get baby's arms to wrap the placenta, before you cut.

When Jo said during the last antenatal visit, 'Denya is there anything that you would like us to do?' Denya said, 'I would like to do the placenta'. And for Jo to turn round and say to me, 'Would you like to lead that?' I didn't say it at the time, but it was the most . . . I felt like I was heard and that our ancestors and our knowledge was accepted, that she saw that and it was the most honourable thing that she could allow me to do was to do that for Denya and for Sunny Vai.

So Seneuefa and I, as soon as the placenta came through, we lifted the placenta and placed it on Sunny Vai's chest and she started to cry and so we sang a Samoan song, which is really a song of gratitude, 'Fa'afetai Fa'afetai' to say, 'Thank you. Thank you' [crying]. That song it just came to us. We didn't plan it. It's a song about gratitude and acknowledging the one: 'You are the one, you are the one'. Sunny Vai just stopped crying when she heard us singing that song and her hands literally started to massage her placenta.

So the purpose of having the placenta on the baby's chest is so that the baby can embrace its life force and say, 'Thank you to the life that you allowed me to be nurtured; you fed me and you gave me sustenance to grow. So I embrace my life force before I am disconnected from you.'

To see her massaging her own placenta, embracing it – her little hands just went like that to her placenta while we were singing the song over her. To have that as part of the process, it just did something to me. It shifted a whole other part of my being that day. It was very profound. That didn't happen for me when Denya was born. I couldn't do that. So what happened felt like a huge healing for me. A total full circle, a completion, and such an honouring of our culture.

When we finished the song, Jo put the tie on the tube and then it was cut. And we all took a deep breath. And we went, 'Welcome, welcome as you are now an independent individual human being. Welcome to your world.' That was a really powerful thing to experience. That wouldn't have happened if Jo hadn't asked Denya if there was anything else she wanted and if she hadn't acknowledged how important it was.

I can honestly say I am absolutely truly honoured and grateful that it was Jo who was the one who supported Denya in honouring her as a woman and as a mother to be able to give birth to my grandchild.

Aroha Atu, Aroha Mai – Love that is given is love received.

References

Allen, J. (2019). Midwifery continuity of care for specific groups. In C. Homer, N. Leap, P. Brodie and J. Sandall (eds), *Midwifery Continuity of Care*, 2nd edn (pp. 207–230). Australia: Elsevier.

Bohren, M.A., Berger, B.O., Munthe-Kaas, H., Tunçalp, Ö. *et al*. (2019). Perceptions and experiences of labour companionship: a qualitative evidence synthesis. *Cochrane Database of Systematic Reviews*, Issue 3. Art. No.: CD012449. doi:10.1002/14651858.CD012449.pub2.

Bohren, M.A., Hofmeyr, G.J., Sakala, C., Fukuzawa, R.K. and Cuthbert, A. (2017) Continuous support for women during childbirth. *Cochrane Database of Systematic Reviews*, Issue 7. Art. No.: CD003766. doi:10.1002/14651858.CD003766.pub6.

Bohren, M.A., Vogel, J.P., Hunter, E.C., Lutsiv, O., Makh, S.K., Souza, J.P., . . . Gülmezoglu, A.M. (2015). The mistreatment of women during childbirth in health facilities globally: a mixed-methods systematic review. *PLoS Med, 12(6)*, e1001847.

Brodie, P. (1996). Being with women: the experiences of Australian team midwives. Unpublished Masters thesis, University of Technology, Sydney.

Brown, A.E., Middleton, P.F., Fereday, J.A. and Pincombe, J.I. (2016). Cultural safety and midwifery care for Aboriginal women – a phenomenological study. *Women and Birth, 29*, 196–202.

Campbell, D.A., Lake, M.F., Falk, M. and Backstrand, J.R. (2006). A randomized control trial of continuous support in labor by a lay doula. *Journal of Obstetric, Gynecologic and Neonatal Nursing, 35*, 456–464.

Centre for Maternal and Child Enquiries (2011). Saving mothers' lives: reviewing maternal deaths to make motherhood safer: 2006–08. The eighth report on confidential enquiries into maternal deaths in the United Kingdom. *British Journal of Obstetrics and Gynaecology, 118* (Suppl.1), 1–203.

Cooperrider, D.L., Sorensen Jr., P.F., Whitney, D. and Yaeger, T.F. (eds). (2000). *Appreciative Inquiry: Rethinking Human Organization Toward a Positive Theory of Change*. Champaign, IL: Stipes Publishing.

Cragin, L. and Kennedy, H.P. (2006). Linking obstetric and midwifery practice with optimal outcomes. *JOGNN Clinical Issues, 35(6)*, 779–785.

Cross-Sudworth, F. (2007). Racism and discrimination in maternity services. *British Journal of Midwifery, 15(6)*, 327–331.

Darwin, Z., and Greenfield, M. (2019). Mothers and others: the invisibility of LGBTQ people in reproductive and infant psychology. *Journal of Reproductive and Infant Psychology, 37(4)*, 341–343.

Davis Harte, J., Sheehan, A., Stewart S. and Foureur M. (2016). Childbirth supporters' experiences in a built hospital birth environment: exploring inhibiting and facilitating factors in negotiating the supporter role. *Health Environment Research & Design Journal*, 9, 135–161.

Dewar, B., Stulz, V., Buliak, A., Connolly, L., McLaughlin, K., Newport, K., . . . Drayton, N. (2020). Exploring and developing student midwives' experiences (ESME) – an Appreciative Inquiry study. *Midwifery*, 91, 102844.

Durey, A. (2010). Reducing racism in Aboriginal health care in Australia: where does cultural education fit? *Australian and New Zealand Journal of Public Health*, 34, S87–S92.

Eustace, J., Baird, E., Saito, A.S. and Creedy, D.K. (2016). Midwives' experiences of routine enquiry for intimate partner violence in pregnancy. *Women and Birth*, 29(6), 503–510.

Fahy, K., Foureur, M. and Hastie, C. (2008). *Birth Territory and Midwifery Guardianship: Theory for Practice, Education and Research*. Oxford: Elsevier.

Frank, G.D., Fox, D., Njue, C. and Dawson, A. (2021). The maternity experiences of women seeking asylum in high-income countries: a meta-ethnography. *Women and Birth*, 4 January, S1871-5192(20)30390-5. doi:10.1016/j.wombi.2020.12.012. Online ahead of print.

Freedman, L.P. and Kruk, M.E. (2014). Disrespect and abuse of women in childbirth: challenging the global quality and accountability agendas. *Lancet*, 384(9948), e42–e44.

Fortier, J.H. and Godwin, M. (2015). Doula support compared with standard care: meta-analysis of the effects on the rate of medical interventions during labour for low-risk women delivering at term. *Canadian Family Physician*, 61, e284–e292.

Goodwin, L., Hunter, B. and Jones, A. (2018). The midwife–woman relationship in a South Wales community: experiences of midwives and migrant Pakistani women in early pregnancy. *Health Expectations* 21(1): 347–357.

Greenfield, M. (2017). He's not the mother. *AIMS Journal*, 29(2). https://www.aims.org.uk/journal/item/hes-not-the-mother.

Higginbottom, G.M.A., Evans, C., Morgan, M., Bharj, K.K., Eldridge, J. and Hussain, B. (2019). Experience of and access to maternity care in the UK by immigrant women: a narrative synthesis systematic review. *BMJ Open*, 9, e029478-2019-029478.

Homer, C.S.E., Leap, N., Brodie, P. and Sandall, J. (eds). (2019). *Midwifery Continuity of Care*, 2nd edn. Australia: Elsevier.

Homer, C.S.E., Leap, N., Edwards, N. and Sandall, J. (2017). Midwifery continuity of carer in an area of high socio-economic disadvantage in London: a retrospective analysis of Albany Midwifery Practice outcomes using routine data (1997–2009). *Midwifery*, 48, 1–10.

Horn, A. (2020). Racism matters: 'When People Show You Who They Are, Believe Them': why Black women mistrust maternity services. *The Practising Midwife*, 23(8), 15–17.

Hunter, B. (2004). Conflicting ideologies as a source of emotion work in midwifery. *Midwifery*, 20, 261–272.

Johansson, J., Fenwick, J. and Premberg, A. (2015). A meta-synthesis of fathers' experiences of their partner's labour and the birth of their baby. *Midwifery*, 31, 9–18.

Kabakian-Khasholian, T. and Portela, A. (2017). Companion of choice at birth: factors affecting implementation. *BMC Pregnancy and Childbirth*, 17, 265.

Katz-Rothman, B. (1996). Women, providers and control. *Journal of Obstetrics, Gynaecology and Neonatal Nursing*, 25(3), 253–256.

Kennedy, H.P. (2000). A model of exemplary midwifery practice: results of a Delphi study. *Journal of Midwifery and Women's Health*, 45(1), 4–19.

Kennedy, H.P, Anderson, T. and Leap, N. (2010). Midwifery presence: philosophy, science and art. Chapter 7 in D. Walsh and S. Downe (eds), *Essential Midwifery Practice: Intrapartum Care* (pp.105–124). Chichester: Wiley-Blackwell.

Kennedy, H.P and Shannon, M.T. (2004). Keeping birth normal: research findings on midwifery care during labour. *Journal of Obstetric Gynecologic and Neonatal Nursing*, 33(5), 554–560.

Kennedy, H.P., Shannon, M.T., Chuahorm, U. and Kravetz, M.K. (2004). The landscape of caring for women: a narrative study of midwifery practice. *Journal of Midwifery and Women's Health*, 49(1), 14–23.

Klaus, M., Kennell, J. and Klaus, P. (1993). *Mothering the Mother – How a Doula Can Help You Have a Shorter, Easier and Healthier Birth*. New York: Perseus Books.

Klaus, M., Kennell, J., Robertson, S. and Sosa, R. (1986). Effects of social support during parturition on maternal and infant morbidity. *British Medical Journal, 293*, 585–587.

Knight, M., Bunch, K., Tuffnell, D., Shakespeare, J., Kotnis, R., Kenyon, S., . . . (eds). (2020). *Saving Lives, Improving Mothers' Care – Lessons Learned to Inform Maternity Care from the UK and Ireland Confidential Enquiries into Maternal Deaths and Morbidity 2016–18*. Oxford: National Perinatal Epidemiology Unit, University of Oxford.

Kruske, S., Kildea, S. and Barclay, L. (2006). Cultural safety and maternity care for Aboriginal and Torres Strait Islander Australians. *Women and Birth, 19(3)*, 73–77.

Leap, N. (2007, unpublished data). A study to explore how care from Albany midwives may have influenced how women approached and experienced pain in labour. Unpublished data: Florence Nightingale Faculty of Nursing and Midwifery, Kings College London.

Leap, N. (2009). Woman centred care or women centred care: does it matter? *British Journal of Midwifery, 17(1)*, 12–16.

Leap, N. (2010). The less we do the more we give. Chapter 2 in M. Kirkham (ed.), *The Midwife–Mother Relationship*, 2nd edn (pp.17–35). London: Palgrave Macmillan.

Leap, N. (2015, unpublished data). Identifying the experiences of receiving and providing support in labour.

Leap, N. (2020, unpublished data). Interviews to inform the 2nd edition of *Supporting Women for Labour and Birth: A Thoughtful Guide*.

Lokugamage, A. and Meredith, A. (March 2020). Women from ethnic minorities face endemic structural racism when seeking and accessing healthcare. *BMJ Opinion* (online). https://blogs.bmj.com/bmj/2020/03/05/women-from-ethnic-minorities-face-endemic-structural-racism-when-seeking-and-accessing-healthcare/.

Lunda, P., Minnie, C.S. and Benadé, P. (2018). Women's experiences of continuous support during childbirth: a meta-synthesis. *BMC Pregnancy Childbirth, 18*, 167.

Lundgren, I. (2010). Swedish women's experiences of doula support during childbirth. *Midwifery, 26*, 173–180.

Lundgren, I. and Dahlberg, K. (2002). Midwives' experience of the encounter with women and their pain during childbirth. *Midwifery, 18*, 155–164.

Macedo, D.M., Smithers, L.G., Roberts, R.M. and Jamieson, L.M. (2019). Racism, stress, and sense of personal control among Aboriginal Australian pregnant women. *Australian Psychologist, 55*, 336–348.

Mander, R. (2001). *Supportive Care and Midwifery*. London: Blackwell Science.

Migrant and Refugee Women's Health Partnership. (2019a). *Culturally Responsive Clinical Practice: Working with People from Migrant and Refugee Backgrounds*. Canberra: Migrant and Refugee Women's Health Partnership.

Migrant and Refugee Women's Health Partnership. (2019b). *Guide for Clinicians Working with Interpreters in Healthcare settings*. Canberra: Migrant and Women's Health Partnership.

Mohr, B.J. and Magruder Watkins, J. (2002). *The Essentials of Appreciative Inquiry: A Roadmap for Creating Positive Futures*. Waltham, MA: Pegasus Communications.

Morris, T. and McInerney, K. (2010). Media representation and childbirth: an analysis of reality television programs in the United States. *Birth, 37(2)*, 134–140.

Newnham, E. and Page, L. (2020). Humanisation of childbirth 8: where do we go from here? *The Practising Midwife, 23(4)*, 15–17.

NHS. (2019). *The NHS Long Term Plan*. www.longtermplan.nhs.uk.

Page, L. (2017). The birth of our humanity. *British Journal of Midwifery, 25(7)*, 414–415.

Poh, H.L., Koh, S.S. and He, H.G. (2014). An integrative review of fathers' experiences during pregnancy and childbirth. *International Nursing Review, 61(4)*, 543–554.

RCM. (2018) *Midwifery Care in Labour Guidance for All Women in All Settings. RCM Midwifery Blue Top Guidance*. No. 1. London: Royal College of Midwives. https://www.rcm.org.uk/media/2539/professionals-blue-top-guidance.pdf.

Redshaw, M. and Henderson, J. (2013). Fathers' engagement in pregnancy and childbirth: evidence from a national survey. *BMC Pregnancy and Childbirth, 13*, 70.

Robertson, A. (2007). *The Midwife Companion: The Art of Support during Birth*, 2nd edn. Sydney: Birth International.

Rogers, H.J., Hogan, L., Coates, D., Homer, C.S.E. and Henry, A. (2020). Responding to the health needs of women from migrant and refugee backgrounds – models of maternity and postpartum care in high-income countries: a systematic scoping review. *Health and Social Care in the Community, 28,* 1343–1365.

Ross-Davie, M.C. (2012). Measuring the quantity and quality of midwifery support of women during labour and childbirth: the development and testing of the Supportive Midwifery in Labour Instrument (Degree of Doctor of Philosophy), University of Stirling, Scotland. Retrieved from: https://dspace.stir.ac.uk/handle/1893/9796.

Ross-Davie, M.C. and Cheyne, H. (2014). Intrapartum support: what do women want? A literature review to identify how far the nature of labour support shapes women's assessment of their birth experiences. *Evidence Based Midwifery, 12*(2), 52–58.

Ross-Davie, M.C., Cheyne, H. and Niven, C. (2013). Measuring the quality and quantity of professional intrapartum support: testing a computerised systematic observation tool in the clinical setting. *BMC Pregnancy and Childbirth, 13,* 163.

Ross-Davie, M.C., McElligott, M., Little, M. and King, K. (2014). Midwifery support in labour: how important is it to stay in the room? *The Practising Midwife, 17*(6), 19–22(14).

Sandall, J., Leap, N., Grant, J. and Bastos, M.H. (2010). Supporting women to have a normal birth: development and field testing of a learning package for maternity staff. Health and Social Care Research Division, King's College London.

Schmied, V., Burns, E. and Sheehan, A. (2019). Place of sanctuary: an Appreciative Inquiry approach to discovering how communities support breastfeeding and parenting. *International Breastfeeding Journal, 14,* 25.

Sidebotham, M., Fenwick, J., Rath, S. and Gamble, J. (2015). Midwives' perceptions of their role within the context of maternity service reform: an Appreciative Inquiry. *Women and Birth, 28,* 112–120.

Simkin, P. (2002). Supportive care during labor: a guide for busy nurses. *JOGNN, 31*(6), 721–732. doi:10.1177/0884217502239208.

Smith, C.A., Levett, K.M., Collins, C.T. and Crowther, C.A. (2018). Relaxation techniques for pain management in labour. *Cochrane Database of Systematic Reviews,* Issue 3. Art. No.: CD009514. doi:10.1002/14651858.CD009514.pub2.

Sosa, G., Crozier, K. and Robinson, J. (2012). What is meant by one-to-one support in labour: analysing the concept. *Midwifery, 28,* 451–457.

Sosa, R., Kennell, J., Klaus, M., Robertson, S. and Urrutia, J. (1980). The effect of a supportive companion on perinatal problems, length of labour and mother–infant interaction. *New England Journal of Medicine, 303*(11), 597–600.

Stevens, J., Dahlen, H., Peters, K. and Jackson, D. (2011). Midwives' and doulas' perspectives of the role of the doula in Australia: a qualitative study. *Midwifery, 27,* 509–516.

Thorstensson, S., Nissen, E. and Ekstro, A. (2008). An exploration and description of student midwives' experiences in offering continuous labour support to women/couples. *Midwifery, 24,* 451–459.

UNHCR. (2020). Gender based violence. https://www.unhcr.org/gender-based-violence.html.

Vivilaki, V., Soltani, H. and van den Muijsenbergh, M. (eds). (2017). *Practice Guide for Perinatal Health Care of Migrant, Asylum-seeking & Refugee Women (D4.1.).* Co-funded by the Health Programme of the European Union: ORRAMA: Operational Refugee and Migrant Maternal Approach.

Waddell, N. (2019). Trauma histories and childbearing: what maternity care workers need to know. *The Practising Midwife, 22*(10).

WHO. (2018). *WHO Recommendations: Intrapartum Care for a positive Childbirth Experience.* Geneva: WHO.

WHO. (2020). *Companion of Choice during Labour and Childbirth for Improved Quality of Care: Evidence-to-action Brief.* Geneva: WHO.

WHO, ICM and FIGO (2004). Making pregnancy safer: critical role of the skilled attendant – a joint statement by the World Health Organization (WHO), the International Confederation of Midwives (ICM) and the International Federation of Gynecology and Obstetrics (FIGO). Geneva: WHO.

Wren Serbin, J. and Donnelly, E. (2016). The Impact of racism and midwifery's lack of racial diversity: a literature review. *Journal of Midwifery and Women's Health, 61*(6), 694–706.

Xue, W.L., Shorey, S., Wang, W. and He, H.G. (2018). Fathers' involvement during pregnancy and childbirth: an integrative literature review. *Midwifery, 62,* 135–145.

2   Approaches to pain in labour

Introduction

As we discussed in the Prologue to this book, throughout centuries and across the world, women have asked other women to provide them with comfort as they face the uncertainties and challenges associated with labour. The notion of supporting women in labour was to change dramatically after 19 January 1847, when Scottish obstetrician James Young Simpson first administered diethyl ether to facilitate the birth of a baby for a woman with a contracted pelvis. Thus was set in trail the development of obstetric anaesthesia. Popularised initially by the enthusiastic use of chloroform by Queen Victoria for the births of her eighth and ninth babies, access to obstetric anaesthesia became a feminist campaigning issue in the first half of the twentieth century, contributing significantly to the hospitalisation of birth, with the concomitant absence of the woman's chosen supporters from the birthing room.

According to Donald Caton (1999) in his stimulating book, *What a Blessing She Had Chloroform: The Medical and Social Response to the Pain of Childbirth from 1800 to the Present*, ever since Simpson published accounts of his early efforts, debates have continued to rage about the efficacy, safety and ethics associated with pain relief in labour. This controversy continues to be reflected in the attitudes of birth attendants towards how pain in labour should be managed, with a consequential profound effect on how women approach and remember their experiences (Hodnett, 2002; Simkin, 1991, 1992). For this reason, NICE guidelines direct us to consider how our values and beliefs might influence the way in which we support women around 'coping with pain in labour' (NICE, 2020, p.29). This is not as straightforward as it might seem: for birth attendants and women in labour, our attitudes to pain will be influenced by multiple factors, as anthropologist David Morris suggests:

> Pain is never the sole creation of our anatomy and physiology; it emerges only at the intersection of bodies, minds and culture.
>
> (Morris, 1991, p.1)

As you delve into this chapter, we invite you to think about how *your* individual 'body, mind and culture' might affect your values and beliefs, and thus your responses to women around fear and pain in labour. This might include your own experiences of giving birth.

DOI: 10.4324/9781003092520-3

Many of you will be learning about supporting women in labour in maternity units where there is a culture of routinely offering 'pain relief' and promoting epidurals. It can be hard in such circumstances to engage with colleagues – as well as with women and their supporters – in discussions about why we should support women to draw on their inner strength when managing pain. In order to facilitate those conversations and enhance evidence-based practice, we shall explore two distinct but complex and often overlapping approaches to supporting women in labour: 'working with pain' and 'pain relief'. We shall draw on stories from women and midwives to stimulate discussion about these issues.

Pain in labour: research that identifies women's experiences

The starting point for exploring the concepts of 'working with pain' and 'pain relief' is an understanding of what matters to women. In 2002, Ellen Hodnett published a groundbreaking systematic review of pain and women's satisfaction with the experience of childbirth; for the first time, evidence was offered to challenge our thinking and responses to comments such as: 'What really matters is that the mother and baby are healthy . . . satisfaction with the childbirth experience is of secondary importance. . . . If we can control their pain, they will have a positive experience' (Hodnett, 2002, p.S160).

The conclusion of Hodnett's systematic review was that, when women evaluate their experiences of childbirth, four factors appear to be so important that they override all other influences (including the experience of pain, age, socioeconomic status, ethnicity, childbirth preparation, the physical birth environment, immobility, medical interventions and continuity of care):

- personal expectations
- the amount of support from caregivers
- the quality of the caregiver–patient relationship
- involvement in decision making

On the basis of this, Hodnett concluded:

> The influences of pain, pain relief, and intrapartum medical interventions on subsequent satisfaction are neither as obvious, as direct, nor as powerful as the influences of the attitudes and behaviors of the caregivers.
>
> (Hodnett, 2002, p.S160)

Subsequent reviews focusing on women's experiences of ways of managing pain in childbirth have also highlighted how women value supportive relationships with their caregivers to help them overcome the vulnerability and uncertainties that they face during labour (Van der Gucht and Lewis, 2015), including when they have chosen pharmacological pain relief (Thomson *et al.*, 2019).

Box 2.1   Research Briefing: Women's experiences of managing pain during childbirth

Van der Gucht, N. and Lewis, K. (2015). Women's experiences of coping with pain during childbirth: A critical review of qualitative research. *Midwifery, 31*, 349–358.

Two main themes emerged as the most significant influences on a woman's ability to cope with pain in labour:

- the importance of individualised continuous support and an acceptance of pain as part of normal childbirth;
- continuity of care and continuous care in labour, which helped women feel safe and enabled them to avoid feelings of loneliness and fear.

Thomson, G., Feeley, C., Moran, V.H., Downe, S. and Oladapo, O.T. (2019). Women's experiences of pharmacological and non-pharmacological pain relief methods for labour and childbirth: a qualitative systematic review. *Reproductive Health, 16*, 71.

This review provides a comprehensive overview of research related to women's experiences of different pain relief methods. The main conclusions were:

- women report mixed experiences of choosing and using both pharmacological and non-pharmacological pain relief methods;
- pharmacological methods can reduce pain but have negative side effects;
- non-pharmacological methods may not reduce labour pain but can facilitate bonding with professional and birth supporters;
- women need information on risks and benefits of all available pain relief methods.

For over two decades, Nordic researchers have been at the forefront of qualitative research about women's experiences of pain in labour, using the words of women themselves in order to 'bring to life' their experiences. A recurring theme in these studies is that labour is like a journey and that women value the way in which midwives make the journey alongside them, helping them prepare for and manage pain in labour (Halldorsdottir and Karlsdottir, 1996a, 1996b; Karlsdottir *et al.*, 2014; Lundgren and Dahlberg, 1998). We have summarised one of these studies in Box 2.2, which describes the ways in which women reported their attitude to pain changing over the course of the 'journey'.

Box 2.2 Research Briefing: Women's experiences of preparing for and managing pain in labour

Adapted from: Karlsdottir, S. I., Halldorsdottir, S. and Lundgren, I. (2014). The third paradigm in labour pain preparation and management: the childbearing woman's paradigm. *Scandinavian Journal of Caring Sciences*, 28, 315–327.

Summary of findings

Preparing for the journey – getting ready: information from midwives; antenatal classes; creating a special attitude towards pain, 'creative imagination'.

At the journey's commencement – the mental and physical condition is important.

On the journey of no return through pain – the pain was difficult, but manageable with a range of different strategies; the midwife and supportive partner were essential in helping with managing pain.

The demanding and difficult nature of labour pain – described in multiple ways.

The importance of having faith in the body – trusting that the body would know what to do; 'going with the flow of the body'.

Using different strategies in the early stages of labour – 'out to dinner', 'taking a shower', 'a walk with husband', focusing on contractions and the time in between them, relaxing and gathering strength.

Using different strategies during late labour and delivery – moving around; changing positions frequently; music; acupuncture; hot bath; massage; hot and cold pads; counting in the mind; Entonox; support from the midwife when an epidural was the only way to manage.

The essential help of 'a good midwife' in managing the pain – sensitive to needs and chosen strategies; a good partnership to enable feelings of safety, presence, creating a special atmosphere: 'warm, secure and conducive to managing pain'.

The importance of having a supportive partner present to help in managing the pain – for mutual understanding, sharing the experience, understanding needs.

At the journey's end: changed attitudes towards the pain after birth – seeing it as positive, different from other pain experiences; pain had a different meaning in the joy and happiness of having a baby in their arms.

The empowering nature of labour pain – pain changed the women's idea of themselves and strengthened their self-image; since they could manage labour pain, they thought they would be capable of anything in life.

The importance of being at peace with the pain afterwards – enabled by talking about the pain afterwards and thinking that it was worthwhile.

**Box 2.3   Reflective Activity: Stories of women's experiences
of pain in childbirth**

In preparation for this activity, read the papers profiled in Box 2.1 and Box 2.2.

In pairs or small groups:
Discuss the following:
- How do the findings of these studies resonate with the stories of childbirth that you are aware of – in your personal and professional lives?
- In what ways do you think some people might find the findings of these studies challenging or 'counter-intuitive'?
- Make a list of factors that illustrate the suggestion that 'there is a dissonance between what women want in order to enhance their ability to cope with pain and the reality of clinical practice' (Van der Gucht and Lewis, 2015, p.349).
- How might this dissonance be enacted and addressed?

The curious nature of pain in labour

It is not unusual to hear women who have given birth without pharmacological pain relief reflecting, 'It was a different sort of pain', as in this woman's account:

> It's a different sort of pain . . . It's there for a reason, it's productive, every contraction you have is doing something, and I think that's what got me through this time with no pain relief . . . with every pain I was coming closer to having the baby . . . If you really believe in yourself and that it's there for a reason, that something's going to come out of this pain, it's not just pain, then you realise that it's not such a scary pain after all.

> (Mother, Sandall *et al.*, 2010, p.65)

In a similar vein, midwives and childbirth educators often use what we shall call 'The "P" words' to describe the positive purpose of labour pain. The juxtaposition of these 'P' words next to the new definition of pain offered by the International Association for the Study of Pain (IASP, 2020; Raja *et al.*, 2020) offers us food for thought about the paradoxical meanings that individuals may hold in discussions about pain in labour (see Box 2.4).

Box 2.4   Contrasting language used to describe labour pain

The 'P' words of labour pain	The new IASP definition of pain
	An unpleasant sensory and emotional experience associated with, or resembling that associated with, actual or potential tissue damage. International Association for the Study of Pain (IASP, 2020)

- Pain with a Purpose
- Positive Pain
- Pain and Power (empowerment)
- Pain as Physiology

In their review of literature about the nature of labour pain, Laura Whitburn and colleagues (2019) suggest that, where labour pain is conceptualised as negative pain or suffering and therefore managed as pathological, this may influence how women approach labour, their expectations of how labour will be managed, their coping strategies during labour, and the way they describe their experiences. They propose that we consider conceptualising pain in normal labour as different from other types of pain, drawing on alternative paradigms such as 'working with pain' (Leap and Anderson, 2008; Leap *et al.*, 2010), 'functional discomfort' (Sanders, 2015) and 'functional pain' (Dempsey, 2013).

When thinking about these contrasting definitions and reviewing the paper describing the development of the new IASP definition (Raja *et al.*, 2020), you may like to consider how the conditioning of individuals who have worked in nursing and medical environments might influence the culture and practices of hospital maternity care. For nurses and doctors who provide 'person-centred care' for people experiencing chronic or acute pain, ensuring 'adequate pain relief' is seen as essential for good quality care. This ethos then permeates into maternity care, and to some extent may explain the findings of studies where women have described feeling pressured by staff to receive medication or have an epidural (Thomson *et al.*, 2019). Indeed, the culture of providing 'adequate pain relief' may also be one of the factors underpinning the institutional framing of birth as something that needs managing (Newnham *et al.*, 2017).

If we are to explore the nature of labour pain further – and certainly if we are to engage in conversations with colleagues – it may help to contextualise our understanding of labour pain within scientific explanations of the origins and transmission of labour pain stimuli, the hormonal physiology of birth and an appreciation of how physiology is mediated by the complexity of psychosocial, environmental and cultural factors. The papers in Box 2.5 provide a useful resource for considering this complexity of interwoven factors.

Box 2.5   Research Briefing: The nature of pain in labour

Lowe, N.K. (2002). The nature of labor pain. *American Journal of Obstetrics and Gynecology*, *186(5)*, S16–S24.

This important paper is widely studied and quoted because it explains the neurophysiology of labour pain and the complex interaction of a wide variety of multidimensional physiological, psychosocial, spiritual and environmental factors that can influence individual women's responses and experiences. Nancy Lowe provides a fascinating synthesis of literature that explores the different meanings of pain, suffering and comfort in the context of childbirth. She discusses how the profound meanings associated with childbirth encourage us to challenge the popular belief that labour pain is bad and that it should be routinely relieved.

Whitburn, L.Y., Jones, L.E., Davey, M-A. and McDonald, S. (2019). The nature of labour pain: an updated review of the literature. *Women and Birth, 32*, 28–38.

This review provides an update of our understanding of the nature of labour pain, identifying literature published since the review by Nancy Lowe. Drawing on modern pain science, the review explores contemporary issues in relation to cognitive, social and environmental factors that are 'key determinants of this intense, challenging and emotional pain' (p.28).

Mander, R. (2000). The meanings of labour pain or the layers of an onion? A woman-orientated view. *Journal of Reproductive Health and Infant Psychology, 18(2)*, 133–141.

Rosemary Mander explores the multiplicity of meanings that are associated with pain in general as well as pain in labour. She examines the potential influences of religion, philosophy, spirituality, biology, culture and power dynamics that may affect meaning for both pregnant women and their carers. Understanding these individual meanings helps us in our attempts to provide responsive care and facilitate positive experiences of labour for women.

Trout, K.K. (2004). The neuromatrix of pain: implications for selected nonpharmocologic methods of pain relief for labor. *Journal of Midwifery and Women's Health, 49(6)*, 482–488.

Kimberley K. Trout describes the original 'gate theory' of pain developed by Ronald Melzack and explains how this has been expanded to account for multiple influences. She suggests ways in which this relates to midwifery, offering explanations for why non-pharmacological support measures and individualised care can be so effective in supporting women through labour.

Buckley, S.J. (2015) Hormonal Physiology of Childbearing: Evidence and Implications for Women, Babies and Maternity Care. Washington, DC; Childbirth Connection Programs, National Partnership for Women and Babies. Available online: https://www.nationalpartnership.org/our-work/resources/health-care/maternity/hormonal-physiology-of-childbearing.pdf.

This resource offers a comprehensive discussion of how hormonally mediated processes can promote physiological labour, positive experiences and long-term well-being for mothers and babies. Even if we are unable to fully comprehend the complexity of this emerging science, we can respect and marvel at how the swirling interconnectedness of a woman's endogenous hormones, particularly oxytocin and beta-endorphins, helps her to manage pain in labour and how common maternity care practices can undermine this process.

Box 2.6 Reflective Activity: Factors that might influence the way pain in labour is approached and experienced by women

This can be an online or a classroom activity.

In small groups:
- Using original creative art forms and multimedia resources, prepare a presentation or performance to stimulate discussion about factors that might influence the way a woman approaches and experiences pain in labour.
- Provide an annotated bibliography* identifying the resources you drew on in preparing your presentation to circulate to the larger group.

Note: *A few lines describing each resource

Memories of labour pain

Anthropologist David Morris (1991) explores how attempts to describe pain lead to situations where 'language at once runs dry' (Woolf, 1967, p.94). This makes sense when we think about women's recollections of the sensations of labour. We often hear women say that immediately after their baby was born, they could not recall the exact nature of the sensations of labour (though often they describe how that recall switches in as soon as they begin contractions when they are having their next baby). The acclaimed novelist Margaret Atwood describes this experience vividly:

> But who can remember the pain [of childbirth], once it's over? All that remains of it is a shadow, not in the mind even, in the flesh. Pain marks you but too deep to see. Out of sight, out of mind.
>
> (Atwood, 1987, p.135)

Studies that attempt to evaluate women's recall of labour pain are fraught with methodological problems and interacting variables (Niven and Murphy-Black, 2000), not least the problems associated with asking women to focus on pain itself during and after labour. Furthermore, when studies are conducted in institutions where almost all women have epidurals, it is not surprising that researchers conclude that epidurals are not only valuable during labour, but also for modulating memories of labour (Chajut *et al.*, 2014). This leads us to think about the complex topic of how we perceive pain in others.

Being alongside women in labour and reading their experience

Elaine Scarry (1985), a social scientist, takes theory about pain and resistance to language to another level in her exploration of the relationship between the person in pain and the onlooker. Although not talking about labour pain specifically, she states that the person in pain may experience pain as 'the most vibrant example of what it is to have certainty' – pain is 'effortlessly grasped' (that is, even with the most heroic effort it cannot *not* be grasped)' – while, for the onlooker, the other person's pain is so elusive it could be seen as 'the primary model of what it is to have doubt'; here 'what is effortless is not grasping it' (Scarry, 1985, p.4). The inexpressibility of pain can be seen as capable of bringing about an absolute split between one's own sense of reality and the reality of the other person, even when in proximity (as during labour).

This theory about the 'unsharability of pain' (Scarry, 1985, p.4) and the fact that doubting people in pain amplifies their suffering (pp.6–7) is worthy of consideration by all of us who provide support for women in labour. In particular, we can think about this in relation to studies suggesting that there is a mismatch between women's and midwives' assessment of pain, with midwives consistently underestimating women's pain when it is severe (Baker *et al.*, 2001; Chamberlain *et al.*, 1993; Niven, 1994; Rajan, 1993). This may be a coping mechanism for the midwife; however, recognising the severity of pain that a woman is experiencing during labour does not necessarily equate to the need to offer pain relief. In fact, women identify that, when they are in pain, any offer of pain relief is irresistible and potentially undermines their confidence, as expressed by this midwife, reminiscing about what a woman said after her labour:

> I didn't really want an epidural. That wasn't what I was saying. What I wanted was something magic that no one's ever thought of before, that you were going to quickly invent right then to make it all better. But I really didn't want an epidural. It was an expression of my pain.

> (Leap, 1996, p.56)

We can never really know what is going on for a woman in labour; what we can do, though, is respond to cues she gives us in order to offer support and sometimes, suggestions. Primarily, though, the midwife's role is to help the woman identify her own spontaneous strategies for managing pain (Escott *et al.*, 2004), whilst being alert to aspects of care and the environment that potentially disrupt these (Spiby *et al.*, 2003).

Box 2.7   Reflective Activity: Being alongside a woman in labour and reading her experiences

In pairs or small groups:
- Tell a story about a situation you were in where what you thought was going on for a woman in labour was not how she described her experience after giving birth. What did you learn from this?

Responses to pain in labour: universal or culturally determined?

Elaine Scarry (1985) suggests that, when people are in extreme pain, the inexpressibility of pain destroys language, bringing about a reversion to the sounds and cries a person makes before language is learned, transcending the 'narrow margin' (p.5) of variation caused by cultural conditioning. This notion is in opposition to Kitzinger's (1991) description of the language of labour as culturally defined. The examples that Sheila Kitzinger gives, however, refer to the actual words used when women cry out, rather than the overall tones, the noises and the way women breathe and move as they manage pain. When women feel confident and well supported, these noises tend to be rhythmical, low-pitched moaning sounds, different to the sounds when someone is scared, as this midwife explains:

> It's a panic, it's a scream and it's different from the noise they make when they're work-ing with their bodies . . . You don't hear that sound when you know women. You don't hear it at home births.
>
> (Midwife, Leap, 1996, p.42)

Descriptive studies suggest that there is no difference in self-reported childbirth pain intensity ratings across different cultural groups (Lowe, 2002). It is worth remembering, though, that many studies looking at women's experiences of pain in labour do not differentiate between the pain of straightforward labour and the more intense pain associated with contractions that are stimulated with synthetic oxytocin infusion. Furthermore, the harmful effects of cultural stereotyping are often not taken into consideration in discussions about the way care provid-ers interact with women around pain in labour (Henderson *et al.*, 2013).

Cultural stereotyping

Although culturally learned patterns of expected behaviours may affect the way women hav-ing straightforward labours respond to contractions (Callister *et al.*, 2003), this does not always fit with our experience. When women are given free rein to move around and adopt any position they like and when they are told by someone whom they trust that it's OK to make noise if they want, many will behave in spontaneous ways that challenge our cultural stereotyping, as seen in this story about a birth that Nicky attended:

Box 2.8   Han's story

Throughout pregnancy we talked to Han (not her real name) about different positions for giving birth, showed her photographs and explained how upright and all fours posi-tions open the pelvis and help the baby come down. She just laughed and shook her head, saying, 'No, no, women from Vietnam give birth lying on the bed. That's what I did last time and that's what I'll do again.'

As planned, Han's husband calls in the night – 'Come, Han, baby coming.' We arrive at their small council flat to find Han fully clothed, arms stretched upwards, hanging from the doorframe and moaning quietly with contractions. She is obviously in strong labour and acknowledges our presence with a nod. I start getting the bed ready. 'What are you doing?' my midwifery colleague hisses at me, looking perplexed. 'She says women from Vietnam always give birth on the bed', I whisper and continue to prepare the bed.

A rustling noise from the doorway alerts us – Han is still hanging onto the doorframe but her face and noises have changed. Quick as a flash I move to the doorway, where a baby boy emerges into my hands finding his noisy way through Han's garments.

Afterwards, with a mixture of sign language and limited English, Han laughs at me and teases me for thinking that anyone would be so silly as to give birth on a bed!

Box 2.9   Reflective Activity: Women's responses to pain in labour – cultural considerations

Pre-reading: Callister, L.C., Khalaf, I., Semenic, S., Kartchner, R., and Vehvilainen-Julkunen, K. (2003). The pain of childbirth: perceptions of culturally diverse women. *Pain Management in Nursing, 4(4),* 145–154.

In pairs or small groups:
• Drawing on the paper by Callister *et al.* (2003), and your experiences, discuss how you think women's responses to contractions in straightforward labour might vary as a result of cultural socialisation and the nature of the support they receive. What are the implications for practice in considering this?

Racism and discrimination during care in labour

As we discussed in Chapter 1, there is an imperative to examine how our own values and beliefs might contribute to the devastating effects of racism on outcomes and experiences for women from Black, Asian and minority ethnic (BAME) communities in the UK, and Aboriginal women in Australia (Cross-Sudworth, 2007; Knight *et al.*, 2020; Kruske *et al.*, 2006; Lokugamage and Meredith, 2020; Macedo *et al.*, 2019). This is particularly pertinent around pain in labour.

Box 2.10   Research Briefing: Racism and epidural use

Dillaway, H. and Brubaker, S. (2006). Intersectionality and childbirth: how women from different social locations discuss epidural use. *Race, Gender and Class, 13(3–4),* 16–41.

Drawing on two separate qualitative studies, the authors compare differences in how women perceive and decide about epidurals in the hospital setting and argue that feminist critiques of the medicalisation of childbirth should be expanded to address race, class and age as structures of oppression and privilege that shape women's experiences of childbirth.

Morris, T. and Schulman, M. (2014). Race inequality in epidural use and regional anaesthesia failure in labor and birth: an examination of women's experience. *Sexual and Reproductive Healthcare, 5(4),* 188–194.

Compared to 'white women', 'women of colour' were less likely to have their pain and anxiety taken seriously, including when epidurals failed to provide pain relief during labour or caesarean operation. Although 'women of colour' were more likely to want to labour without using epidurals, they experienced more pressure by staff to have one, the inference being that staff were less prepared to offer the degree of support that is required for normal labour.

Approaches to pain in labour: 'pain relief' and 'working with pain'

A small qualitative study aimed at exploring midwifery perspectives on pain in labour (Leap, 1996) offered a new way of exploring approaches to pain in labour. Nicky invited ten midwives from the United Kingdom, Canada, Australia and the Netherlands to address questions that were increasingly being heard in maternity care: 'Why would you not routinely offer all women pain relief in this day and age?' and 'Why on earth would you let women suffer the barbaric pain of childbirth when we have the ultimate form of pain relief in the form of epidurals?' All of the midwives interviewed had experience of attending women giving birth at home and it was presumed that they would have interesting ideas about how to answer these questions.

What the midwives described were two paradigms: the 'pain relief paradigm' and the 'working with pain' paradigm. The word 'paradigm' here refers to typical ways of thinking and being in relation to labour pain. In the interest of using everyday language, we shall talk about approaches rather than paradigms. The features of the two approaches are summarised in the following box.

Box 2.11   Features of 'pain relief' and 'working with pain' approaches

Adapted from *A Midwifery Perspective on Pain in Labour* (Leap, 1996)

The 'pain relief' approach

Ensuring 'adequate pain relief'

Making full use of 'the benefits of modern technology': 'In this day and age, you don't have to suffer . . . you don't have to be heroic'

The culture of informed choice: offering the 'pain relief menu'

The practitioner's own discomfort with pain and noise motivates the offering of pain relief

'Women have unrealistic expectations – primips are ending up feeling guilty and a sense of failure because of the 'natural childbirth lobby'

'It's far more work being with a woman who is agitated and making a noise . . . especially if you're looking after more than one woman in labour'

The 'working with pain' approach

Women *can* cope with contractions in uncomplicated labour with appropriate support

Engaging with uncertainty – associated with empowerment, a positive start to new motherhood

'Normal' and 'abnormal' pain – 'normal' pain is associated with straightforward labour; 'abnormal' pain is associated with malposition/dystocia and is more likely to lead to the need for 'pain relief'

Pain with a purpose, positive pain

Pain as a stimulator of endogenous opioids

Minimising disturbance, creating an environment in which neuro-hormonal physiology can flourish

Pain gives clues to labour progress

The 'pain relief' approach

We shall explore the two approaches outlined in Box 2.11 starting with the 'pain relief' approach. The notion of 'pain relief' thrives in most high-income societies in the risk-averse culture of childbearing (Sanders, 2015; Newnham *et al.*, 2015, 2017). You may be very familiar with a culture that sees and promotes medication as the immediate answer to common ailments like headaches, colds and period pain, even when symptoms are relatively mild.

As we discussed earlier, providing 'adequate pain relief' is the dominant ethos in most Western maternity units and we have all probably seen practitioners who are keen to step in and rescue women from pain in labour:

> My feeling is, from the stories that I hear, that women are sometimes being offered pain relief very directly and quite strongly to help practitioners, not to help the woman herself. A number of women do come back and say, 'I think actually I could have coped a little bit longer but I kept being offered pain relief, and eventually I just said, 'OK I'll take it.'
>
> (Obstetrician, Sandall *et al.*, 2010, unpublished data)

We only have to watch reality television shows about childbirth to get an impression of the prevalent culture of offering 'pain relief' described by this midwife:

> Some midwives give Pethidine because they don't like the fuss and the noise and the agitation and the fact the woman won't settle down. I think that sometimes the midwife isn't coping with the pain either. They think the woman isn't and actually they're not. Because it's a lot more work for a midwife to be interacting with somebody. If someone's agitated and making a lot of noise and being demanding, then you have to be with her all of the time, you can't go and have cups of tea, or whatever.
>
> (Midwife, Leap, 1996, pp.41–42)

In some maternity units the culture of pain relief is so pervasive that it is hard for students to get experience of providing intensive support for women who want to avoid pharmacological 'pain relief':

> I've learnt a lot about the sort of variation of how women cope with pain . . . but I think if you haven't seen that it's very difficult to know what normal might be, and it might be frightening then.
>
> (Midwife, Leap, 1996, p.43)

It is no surprise that, whilst all maternity care providers recognise the value of support in labour, overall, obstetricians tend to have a personal preference for pharmacological pain relief while midwives tend to favour a range of physical support measures (Madden *et al.*, 2013). Generalisations about any one professional group, though, perpetuate stereotyped ideas about colleagues' approaches and warrant caution. For example, you can probably think of midwives who are very keen to offer pharmacological pain relief and anaesthetists who understand the value of supporting women in labour without trying to take away pain, as is the case here:

> Increasingly, when midwives call me to insert an epidural, I get there and it's obvious that, with appropriate support, the woman would soon be pushing her baby out without

needing an epidural. An anaesthetist colleague of mine was reported to the hospital director for refusing to put in an epidural when a woman was nearly fully dilated. The woman was happy but the midwife obviously felt her authority was undermined and said the woman had been denied her choice.

(Anaesthetist, Leap, 2015, unpublished data)

The culture of 'pain relief': global considerations

The culture of 'pain relief' dominates maternity care in most high-income countries and is at its most transparent in research papers reporting on obstetric analgesia in low-income countries. The 'Western' ideal of offering all women epidurals has permeated countries where this form of pain relief is not an option for most women. In such countries, repeated medical research concludes that all women should be offered pain relief, particularly epidurals. The emphasis is often on showing the benefits of pharmacological pain relief for all women (Fyneface-Ogan *et al.*, 2009; Lawani *et al.*, 2014), rather than changing systems to provide better support for women in labour, even when women have identified that this support is what they want (Rachmawati, 2012). There is also not necessarily acknowledgement that the widespread use of synthetic oxytocin to manage labour might contribute to women's pain.

Managing pain: sharing evidence with women

There are many situations in which it is really important to be able to talk through options for pain relief and pain management with a woman and her supporters. This means that we should all have up-to-date knowledge of evidence. A Cochrane systematic review (Jones *et al.*, 2012) provides a useful overview of other systematic reviews regarding non-pharmacological interventions (those that aim to help women cope with pain in labour) and pharmacological interventions (those that aim to relieve the pain of labour).

Box 2.12   Research Briefing: Cochrane systematic review of pain management for women in labour

Jones, L., Othman, M., Dowswell, T., Alfirevic, Z., Gates, S., Newburn, M., Jordan, S., Lavender, T. and Neilson, J. P. (2012). Pain management for women in labour: an overview of systematic reviews. *Cochrane Database of Systematic Reviews*, *2012*(3). Art. No.: CD009234. doi:10.1002/14651858.CD009234.pub2.

Key messages

- Women's experiences of pain during labour vary greatly.
- Factors that influence this include: the ability to adopt different positions in labour and move around, confidence, fear and anxiety.
- During pregnancy, women should be told about the benefits and potential adverse effects on themselves and their babies of the different methods of pain control.

In order to be able to discuss options for managing pain and 'pain relief' with women, drawing on a wider body of evidence than that afforded by the inclusion criteria of studies for Cochrane reviews, we recommend that you engage with the lively discussion provided by Dennis Walsh (2012):

Box 2.13   Recommended Resource: Theory about pain in labour and supportive strategies

Walsh, D. (2012). Pain and labour. Chapter 7 in *Evidence and Skills for Normal Labour and Birth: A Guide for Midwives*, 2nd edn (pp.83–100). London: Routledge.

Midwife Denis Walsh provides an overview of theory about pain in labour and discusses the evidence base for various support strategies under the following headings: psychological methods; physical therapies; sensory methods; complementary therapies; spiritual rituals; and technologies and drugs.

The offering of the 'pain relief menu'

In a culture that privileges the notion of 'informed choice', midwives often see it as part of their role to offer 'the menu' of pain relief options (Leap and Anderson, 2008). As advocated by researchers in the Cochrane review that we have profiled (Jones *et al.*, 2012), this involves a systematic approach to explaining the advantages and disadvantages of each method 'on the menu' with a view to helping a woman to make appropriate choices, usually in advance of labour. This can be tricky because the conscious or subconscious message that women often receive is that some form of pain relief in labour is usually necessary in straightforward labour: 'It is simply a question of choosing the right thing for me'. This assumption that most women will need some form of 'pain relief' also underpins most research in the area and can be seen in the language used in the development of decision-making aids for pain relief in labour (Raynes-Greenow *et al.*, 2007, 2010).

Box 2.14   A typical 'pain relief menu' (not a comprehensive list)

- Methods you control yourself: changing positions, moving around, making noise, baths, showers, breathing techniques, relaxation, mindfulness practice, self-hypnosis, finding a private space;
- Methods with your chosen birth supporter: heat packs, massage, breathing together, counting, chanting, labour coaching, doula support;
- Methods involving complementary therapists: acupuncture, acupressure, reflexology, hypnotism, aromatherapy;
- TENS (transcutaneous electrical nerve stimulation) machine;
- Entonox (inhalation of nitrous oxide);
- Sterile water injections in your back (for back pain);
- Pethidine/morphine, remifentanil (or any equivalent injection of an opiate);
- Epidural anaesthesia.

The concern about the offering of the menu when women are in labour is that, when we start talking about what's on offer, we may inadvertently suggest to the woman that she is not managing pain well and that we think she will need 'something':

> I think midwives feel under pressure to have given women choice to ensure that, if you like, the boxes have been ticked and so they don't want people to think that they're with-holding anything or that they haven't made it clear that they could have this and they could have that. But I'm not sure really what that communicates to women about pain and their ability to cope with it.
>
> (Midwife, Sandall *et al.*, 2010, p.44)

'Realistic expectations'

A systematic review of women's expectations and experiences of pain and pain relief in labour, poignantly called 'More in hope than expectation' (Lally *et al.*, 2008), found that women consistently underestimated the amount of pain they would have. Women who wanted a drug-free labour often found that they needed pharmacological 'pain relief'; similarly, the degree of control and involvement in decision making was less than they had hoped for. The conclusion of this review was that childbirth educators need to address women's 'unrealistic expectations' in order to improve their experience of labour. We think that this avoids the big questions about what these findings mean. The onus is placed on changing the woman's expectations rather than changing systems in order to improve the quality of the relationship with caregivers, as we discussed earlier.

We are left wondering again about the messages women receive when we talk about 'realistic expectations'. A student midwife explored this in relation to women being told that most women will need 'pain relief'. She uses metaphor to encourage discussion about significance and meaning (see Chapter 5):

> When they say we're giving women 'unrealistic expectations' about pain in labour and that most women having first babies will end up with an epidural, it makes me think about this true story. A woman is planning her wedding; she is full of anticipation and excitement about her big day and someone says, 'You know, you do need to have realistic expectations. These days, over half of all marriages end in divorce!'
>
> (Leap, 2012, personal communication: conversation with student midwife after conference presentation)

Box 2.15   Reflective Activity: Discussing evidence about pain management

In pairs or small groups:
- Discuss how you might talk to a pregnant woman about evidence regarding ways of managing pain in labour without adopting a 'menu approach'.
- What do you think are 'realistic expectations' for someone with an uncomplicated pregnancy who is having her first baby?
- How does this vary depending on where the woman decides to give birth and how might you address this?
- Write a script together with fictionalised characters: a short conversation with a woman and her partner in an antenatal clinic about managing pain (maximum five minutes), thinking about every word you use and the potential subliminal messages you are sending (see Chapter 5). Perform your scenario for the larger group and give them a short annotated bibliography – a few lines about each of the resources that informed your script/performance.

The 'working with pain' approach

The 'working with pain' approach that was identified by midwives in Nicky Leap's (1996) study was explored in a chapter she wrote with the late Tricia Anderson (Leap and Anderson, 2008). The phrase is used widely these days to encompasses ways of thinking and being around pain in labour that promote women's confidence in their abilities and strengths. As this midwife describes:

> Rather than going straight to the list of pain relief methods, I say to women, 'If you go into labour spontaneously at term and you have a baby in the right position and you're in a place where you feel safe, you're not going to be sent more pain than you can deal with.' I believe it. I really believe it. . . . by saying it and repeating it, we make it possible for women to do it. What's missing in antenatal care for women in our culture is that completely accurate confidence building reinforcement of their own ability to actually have a baby . . . And the attitudes of midwives will have a profound effect. If you can build up confidence in women that they can definitely get on and do this, then I think they will. I suppose I see it as our responsibility sometimes to believe in women when they don't believe in themselves. It's a protection against all that conditioning.
>
> (Midwife, Leap 1996, p.56.)

The importance of midwives engaging with women in ways that encourage them to trust their bodies and their ability to cope with pain is highlighted in many studies; this often involves conceptualising labour pain as purposeful and productive:

> If a woman can sustain the belief that her pain is purposeful (i.e. her body working to birth her baby), if she interprets her pain as productive (i.e. taking her through a

process to a desired goal) and the birthing environment is safe and supportive, it would be expected that she would experience the pain as a non-threatening, transformative life event.

(Whitburn *et al.*, 2019, p.34)

The concept of 'normal' and 'abnormal' pain

The rationale for encouraging women in their attempts to labour without pharmacological pain relief is underpinned by an understanding of the concept of 'normal and abnormal pain', described here by a midwife in the Netherlands:

> I remember the director of the Dutch midwifery school telling me that for a normal birth there is always normal pain. And it's the art of the midwife to discriminate whether this is normal or abnormal pain. If it's abnormal pain . . . there is something really pathological going on. . . . I was taught in midwifery school that once a woman starts to scream and yell, you the midwife should be happy.
>
> (Midwife, Leap, 1996, pp.43–44)

The concept of 'normal pain' is linked to the idea that women's bodies produce their own, endogenous pain-coping mechanisms (Sanders, 2015). You can study the biological rationale for this in Sarah Buckley's (2015) synthesis of evidence related to the hormonal physiology of childbearing. Experienced midwives say they have 'always known there was something', like this midwife who worked as a community midwife in Battersea, London in the 1930s and 1940s:

> I think myself that the system has a certain amount of sedative in itself that it releases. . . . I'm sure it has, because I've seen people that just looked as if they were half sozzled – and they didn't have anything! Just looked like someone 'gone' – and they hadn't had any dope. I think the body does release something into the system. If it's not interfered with by giving dope, it will work. But I think when you interfere, it won't work then.
>
> (Leap and Hunter, 2013, p.165)

Supporting women who choose to have pharmacological pain relief

Experienced midwives see the offering of 'pain relief' as appropriate when there is 'abnormal pain', as explained here by a Canadian midwife:

> During my experience in West Africa and rural India I learnt the difference between normal and abnormal pain . . . Once I felt that I understood this difference, I began to think it was important, sometimes a critical part of appropriate treatment of abnormal labours, to provide generous chemical pain relief, and that chemical pain relief wasn't necessary for normal labour.
>
> (Midwife, Leap, 1996, p.44)

In subsequent chapters we shall explore the practicalities of how we can support women in labour in ways that maximise the potential for them to have positive experiences of giving birth. This will include support for women who are having pharmacological pain relief in labour (Chapter 8).

Why support for managing pain matters

For women who would like to give birth without interventions, there are far-reaching consequences when they receive support to manage labour without drugs (Sanders, 2015). Culturally diverse women repeatedly relate a sense of achievement and feelings of pride in their ability to cope with the extreme pain of labour, giving rise to positive consequences associated with coping, self-sufficiency, self-esteem and self-efficacy (Callister *et al.*, 2003). As this midwife describes, women can feel a great sense of accomplishment:

> It does a lot for women because it's such a huge thing to go through. Women feel proud of themselves because they've done something very big; there's the satisfaction that they've done something their body's made to do, like running a marathon, a sense of achievement.
>
> (Midwife, Leap, 1996, p.54)

The following quote from a young woman is a typical example of the extreme emotions associated with labour pain and triumph:

> I was requesting for caesarean, I was requesting for everything! . . . As soon as he was born the pain stopped, immediately. I felt strong. I felt like, I've done it! I felt great about myself that I didn't have to go through all that [sic] unnecessary drugs.
>
> (Mother, Sandall *et al.*, 2010, unpublished data)

For all birth attendants, seeing pain in uncomplicated labour as 'normal' helps us deal with our own discomfort and turn to supportive strategies rather than calling for the anaesthetist to come and insert an epidural. Talking to women afterwards helps us build confidence in these skills:

> What gives me confidence is hearing how they feel about it afterwards, because if afterwards they said, 'Listen you b——, I wanted an epidural and you refused to give it to me', and they meant it, then I hope I'd change my approach. . . . Women have told me afterwards that my overview was correct. They were grateful for that and said things like, 'I didn't really mean it. It was an expression of my pain. I'm glad that the relationship we had meant that you could interpret what I was saying'.
>
> (Midwife, Leap, 1996, p.56)

Box 2.16   Reflective Activity: Explaining the rationale for 'working with pain'

In pairs or small groups:
- Discuss how you might you respond if a colleague says to you, 'In this day and age, no woman should have to suffer the barbaric pain of childbirth'?
- Write a paragraph identifying your response and read this out to the larger group in order to promote further discussion.

'I can't believe how strong I am!'

As birth attendants we can build our confidence in supporting women through pain if we understand the profound consequences this can have for each individual woman in terms of how she feels about herself, her body and her capabilities (Thompson, 2004; Lundgren and Karlsdottir, 2009). The strength a woman feels about how she faced the challenges and uncertainties of labour can set her up well for the ongoing challenges and uncertainties of motherhood. To illustrate this, we finish this chapter with a story from a woman whom we shall call Cora, who tells of her two experiences of pain in labour. The first was when she was very young and had no midwifery continuity of care. Subsequently she was booked with midwives she knew and trusted, and was surrounded by a group of people who understood the importance of positive encouragement.

Postscript: Cora's story

Cora's story: 'I know I said I didn't want an epidural, but now I really do'

With my first baby I was a young mum anyway and I think they looked upon that as: 'Young mum, first baby, pop an epidural in'. And that's more or less what happened.

Every time they came in to check on me – 'Would you like an epidural? . . . Is the pain that bad yet?' And I remember thinking, 'No, I'm all right for the moment' and then they said, 'Well as soon as your pain comes press the buzzer and we can come back and sort that out for you'.

And of course I had that set in my mind already, and when that pain came I thought, 'Oh, I remember what the midwife said. Right. OK. Well I'll press the buzzer.' Got the epidural and you know, ended up with the ventouse delivery, which still . . . I still regret now, but that's gone . . .

However, with my second baby I was with the Albany midwives and I actually prepped the midwives, and said, 'Whatever you do, don't give me an epidural'. So I prepped my partner, I prepped my sister, I prepped my mum, I prepped my midwives: 'Do not give me the epidural. I might swear at you. I might shout at you. I might, you know, try and get my dressing gown on and go and get it myself, but don't let me get it.'

So anyway in labour I was approaching second stage – transition actually – and I was going, 'GET ME THAT EFFING EPIDURAL!' really quite loudly, over and over again. And I turned to my sister and I went, 'Don't you ever do this ever again yourself', and I was going to my mum, 'Please, Mum, get me that epidural, you know I really want an epidural'.

And I turned to my midwife and I looked at her and I said, 'I'm not joking now, I really, really want that epidural, please get me that epidural'. Going from shouting at them, then going to being really serious and saying, 'I'm not joking, I'm being really serious, I know we had this discussion . . .'. Trying every tactic.

And everybody was so supportive saying, you know, 'I don't think you need that epidural, you're doing really well, you just need to have your baby, your baby's coming soon'. Everyone was really supportive.

And after I birthed my baby I just lay on the bed and I said to the midwife, 'I'm so glad you didn't give it to me because I can't believe that I did that, I can't believe how strong I am'. Because I've got no pain threshold, and I remember saying in my antenatal visits, 'I've got no pain threshold, I don't know if I'm going to do it, I don't want an epidural, but you know . . .'.

And after I'd done it I was just so proud of myself, really, to this day I think, 'Yay, I did it without an epidural! That's how it's meant to be' (Sandall *et al.*, 2010, unpublished data).

References

Atwood, M. (1987). *The Handmaid's Tale*. London: Virago.

Baker, A., Ferguson, S.A. and Roach, G.D. (2001). Perceptions of labour pain by mothers and their attending midwives. *Journal of Advanced Nursing, 35(2)*, 171–179.

Bewley, S. and Cockburn, J. (2002). Responding to fear of childbirth. Commentary. *The Lancet, 359*, 2128–2129.

Buckley, S.J. (2015) Hormonal Physiology of Childbearing: Evidence and Implications for Women, Babies and Maternity Care. Washington, DC; Childbirth Connection Programs, National Partnership for Women and Babies. Available online: https://www.nationalpartnership.org/our-work/resources/health-care/maternity/hormonal-physiology-of-childbearing.pdf.

Callister, L.C., Khalaf, I., Semenic, S., Kartchner, R. and Vehvilainen-Julkunen, K. (2003). The pain of childbirth: perceptions of culturally diverse women. *Pain Management in Nursing, 4(4)*, 145–154.

Caton, D. (1999). *What a Blessing She Had Chloroform: the medical and social response to the pain of childbirth from 1800 to the present*. New Haven & London: Yale University Press.

Chajut, E., Caspi, A., Chen, R., Hod, M. and Ariely, D. (2014). In pain thou shalt bring forth children: the peak-and-end rule in recall of labor pain. *Psychological Science, 25(12)*, 226–2271.

Chamberlain, G., Wraight, A. and Steer, P. (eds). (1993). *Pain and its Relief in Childbirth: The Results of a National Survey Conducted by the National Birthday Trust*. Edinburgh: Churchill Livingstone.

Cross-Sudworth, F. (2007). Racism and discrimination in maternity services. *British Journal of Midwifery, 15(6)*, 327–331.

Dempsey, R. (2013). *Birth with Confidence. Savvy Choices for Normal Birth*. Fairfield, Australia: Boathouse Press.

Dillaway, H. and Brubaker, S. (2006). Intersectionality and childbirth: how women from different social locations discuss epidural use. *Race, Gender and Class*, 13(3–4), 16–41.

Escott, D., Spiby, H., Slade, P. and Fraser, R.B. (2004). The range of coping strategies women use to manage pain and anxiety prior to and during first experience of labour. *Midwifery, 20(2)*, 144–156.

Fyneface-Ogan, S., Mato, C. and Anya, S. (2009). Epidural anesthesia: views and outcomes of women in labor in a Nigerian hospital. *Annals of African Medicine, 8(4)*, 250–256.

Halldorsdottir, S. and Karlsdottir, S.I. (1996a). Empowerment or discouragement: women's experience of caring and uncaring encounters during childbirth. *Health Care For Women International, 17(4)*, 361–379. doi:10.1080/07399339609516251.

Halldorsdottir, S. and Karlsdottir, S.I. (1996b). Journeying through labour and delivery: perceptions of women who have given birth. *Midwifery, 12(2)*, 48–61.

Henderson, J., Gao, H. and Redshaw, M. (2013). Experiencing maternity care: the care received and perceptions of women from different ethnic groups. *BMC Pregnancy & Childbirth, 13*, 196. http://www.biomedcentral.com/1471-2393/1413/1196.

Hodnett, E.D. (2002). Pain and women's satisfaction with the experience of childbirth: a systematic review. *American Journal of Obstetrics and Gynaecology, 186(5)*, S160–S172.

IASP (2020). The International Association for the Study of Pain Revised Definition of Pain. https://www.iasp-pain.org/PublicationsNews/NewsDetail.aspx?ItemNumber=10475.

Jones, L., Othman, M., Dowswell, T., Alfirevic, Z., Gates S., Newburn, M., Jordan, S., Lavender, T. and Neilson, J.P. (2012). Pain management for women in labour: an overview of systematic reviews. *Cochrane Database of Systematic Reviews, 2012(3)*, Art. No.: CD009234. doi:10.1002/14651858. CD009234.pub2.

Karlsdottir, S.I., Halldorsdottir, S. and Lundgren, I. (2014). The third paradigm in labour pain preparation and management: the childbearing woman's paradigm. *Scandinavian Journal of Caring Sciences, 28*, 315–327.

Kitzinger, S. (1991). Childbirth and society. In I. Chalmers, M. Enkin and M. Keirse (eds), *Effective Care in Pregnancy and Childbirth* (pp.99–109). Oxford: Oxford University Press.

Knight, M., Bunch, K., Tuffnell, D., Shakespeare, J., Kotnis, R., Kenyon, S. *et al.* (eds). (2020). *Saving Lives, Improving Mothers' Care – Lessons Learned to Inform Maternity Care from the UK and*

Ireland Confidential Enquiries into Maternal Deaths and Morbidity 2016–18. Oxford: National Perinatal Epidemiology Unit, University of Oxford.

Kruske, S., Kildea, S. and Barclay, L. (2006). Cultural safety and maternity care for Aboriginal and Torres Strait Islander Australians. *Women and Birth, 19(3)*, 73–77. doi:10.1016/j.wombi.2006.07.001.

Lally, J.E., Murtagh, M.J. and Macphail, S. (2008). More in hope than expectation: women's experience and expectations of pain relief in labour. A review. *BMC Med, 6(7)*. doi:10.1186/1741-7015-1186-1187.

Lawani, L.O., Eze, J.N., Anozie, O.B., Iyoke, C.A. and Ekem, N.N. (2014). Obstetric analgesia for vaginal birth in contemporary obstetrics: a survey of the practice of obstetricians in Nigeria. *BMC Pregnancy and Childbirth, 14*, 140.

Leap, N. (1996). A midwifery perspective on pain in labour. Unpublished MSc dissertation, South Bank University, London. Available on request from nickyleap@me.com.

Leap, N. (2010). The less we do the more we give. Chapter 2 in M. Kirkham (ed.), *The Midwife–Mother Relationship*, 2nd edn (pp.17–35). London: Palgrave Macmillan.

Leap, N. (2012). The power of words re-visited. MIDIRS Focus. *Essentially MIDIRS, 3(1)*, 17–21.

Leap, N. (2015, unpublished data). Identifying the experiences of receiving and providing support in labour.

Leap, N. and Anderson, T. (2008). The role of pain in normal birth and the empowerment of women. Chapter 2 in S. Downe (ed.), *Normal Childbirth: Evidence and Debate*, 2nd edn (pp.29–46). Edinburgh: Churchill Livingstone/Elsevier.

Leap, N., Dodwell, M. and Newburn, M. (2010). Working with pain in labour: an overview of evidence. *NCT New Digest, January(49)*, 22–26.

Leap, N. and Hunter, B. (2013). *The Midwife's Tale: An Oral History from Handywoman to Professional Midwife*, 2nd edn. Barnsley: Pen & Sword.

Leap, N., Sandall, J., Grant, J., Bastos, M.H. and Armstrong, P. (2009). Using video in the development and field-testing of a learning package for maternity staff: supporting women for normal birth. *International Journal of Multiple Research Approaches, 3(3)*, 302–320.

Lokugamage, A. and Meredith, A. (2020). Women from ethnic minorities face endemic structural racism when seeking and accessing healthcare. *BMJ Opinion* (online), 5 March. https://blogs.bmj.com/bmj/2020/2003/2005/women-from-ethnic-minorities-face-endemic-structural-racism-when-seeking-and-accessing-healthcare/.

Lowe, N.K. (2002). The nature of labor pain. *American Journal of Obstetrics and Gynecology, 186(5)*, S16–S24.

Lundgren, I. and Dahlberg, K. (1998). Women's experience of pain during childbirth. *Midwifery, 14(2)*, 105–110.

Lundgren, I. and Karlsdottir, S.I. (2009). Long-term memories and experiences of childbirth in a Nordic context – a secondary analysis. *International Journal of Qualitative Studies on Health and Well-being, 4*, 115–128.

Macedo, D.M., Smithers, L.G., Roberts, R.M. and Jamieson, L.M. (2019). Racism, stress, and sense of personal control among Aboriginal Australian pregnant women. *Australian Psychologist, 55*, 336–348. doi:org/10.1111/ap.12435.

Madden, K.L., Turnbull, D., Cyna, A.M., Adelson, P. and Wilkinson, C. (2013). Pain relief for childbirth: the preferences of pregnant women, midwives and obstetricians. *Women and Birth, 26*, 33–40.

Morris, D. (1991). *The Culture of Pain*. Berkeley, CA: University of California Press.

Morris, T. and Schulman, M. (2014). Race inequality in epidural use and regional anaesthesia failure in labor and birth: an examination of women's experience. *Sexual and Reproductive Healthcare, 5(4)*, 188–194.

Newnham, E., McKellar, L. and Pincombe, J. (2015). Documenting risk: a comparison of policy and information pamphlets for using epidural or water in labour. *Women and Birth, 28*, 221–227.

Newnham, E., McKellar, L. and Pincombe, J. (2017). Paradox of the institution: findings from a hospital labour ward ethnography. *BMC Pregnancy and Childbirth, 17*, 2. doi:10.1186/s12884-016-1193-4.

NICE. (2020). *Intrapartum Care. Care for Healthy Women and Babies. Clinical Guideline (CG190)*. www.nice.org.uk/guidance/cg190.

Nilsson, C. and Lundgren, I. (2009). Women's lived experience of fear of childbirth. *Midwifery, 25*, e1–e9.

Niven, C. (1994). Coping with labour pain: the midwife's role. In S. Robinson and A. Thompson (eds), *Research & Childbirth*. London: Chapman & Hall.

Niven, C. and Murphy-Black, T. (2000). Memory for labor pain: a review of the literature. *Birth, 27(4)*, 244–253.

Rachmawati, I. (2012). Maternal reflection on labour pain management and influencing factors. *British Journal of Midwifery, 20*, 263–270.

Raja, S.N., Carr, D.B., Cohen, M., Finnerup, N.B., Flor, H., Gibson, S., . . . Vader, K. (2020). The revised International Association for the Study of Pain definition of pain: concepts, challenges, and compromises. *Pain, 161*, 1976–1982. © 2020 International Association for the Study of Pain. doi:10.1097/j.pain.0000000000001939.

Rajan, L. (1993). Perceptions of pain and pain relief in labour: the gulf between experience and observation. *Midwifery, 9(3)*, 136–145.

Raynes-Greenow, C.H., Nassar, N., Torvaldsen, S., Trevena, L. and Roberts, C.L. (2010). Assisting informed decision making for labour analgesia: a randomised controlled trial of a decision aid for labour analgesia versus a pamphlet. *BMC Pregnancy and Childbirth, 10(15)*: http://dx.doi.org/10.1186/1471-2393-1110-1115.

Raynes-Greenow, C.H., Roberts, C.L., McCaffery, K. and Clarke, J. (2007). Knowledge and decision-making for labour analgesia of Australian primiparous women. *Midwifery, 23(2)*, 139–145. www.rcog.org.uk/en/news/rcog-statement-on-umbilical-non-severance-or-lotus-birth. London: Royal College of Obsetricians and Gynaecologists.

Sandall, J., Leap, N., Grant, J. and Bastos, M.H. (2010). Supporting women to have a normal birth: development and field testing of a learning package for maternity staff. Health and Social Care Research Division, King's College London.

Sanders, R. (2015). Midwifery facilitation: exploring the functionality of labor discomfort. Commentary. *Birth, 42(3)*, 202–205.

Scarry, E. (1985). *The Body in Pain: The Making and Unmaking of the World*. Oxford: Oxford University Press.

Simkin, P. (1991). Just another day in a woman's life? Women's long term perceptions of their first birth experience. Part 1. *Birth, 18*, 203–210.

Simkin, P. (1992). Just another day in a woman's life? Women's long term perceptions of their first birth experience. Part II: Nature and consistency of women's long term memories of their first birth experience. *Birth, 19*, 64–68.

Spiby, H., Slade, P., Escott, D., Henderson, B. and Fraser, R.B. (2003). Selected coping strategies in labour: an investigation of women's experiences. *Birth, 30(3)*, 189–194.

Thompson, F.E. (2004). *Mothers and Midwives: The Ethical Journey*. Edinburgh: Books for Midwives.

Thomson, G., Feeley, C., Moran, V.H., Downe, S. and Oladapo, O.T. (2019). Women's experiences of pharmacological and non-pharmacological pain relief methods for labour and childbirth: a qualitative systematic review. *Reproductive Health, 16*, 71.

Trout, K.K. (2004). The neuromatrix of pain: implications for selected nonpharmocologic methods of pain relief for labor. *Journal of Midwifery and Women's Health, 49(6)*, 482–488.

Van der Gucht, N. and Lewis, K. (2015). Women's experiences of coping with pain during childbirth: a critical review of qualitative research. *Midwifery, 31*, 349–358.

Walsh, D. (2012). Pain and labour. Chapter 7 in *Evidence and Skills for Normal Labour and Birth: A Guide for Midwives*, 2nd edn (pp.83–100). London: Routledge.

Whitburn, L.Y., Jones, L.E., Davey, M-A. and McDonald, S. (2019). The nature of labour pain: an updated review of the literature. *Women and Birth, 32*, 28–38.

Woolf, V. (1967). On being ill (p.94). *Collected Essays*. New York: Harcourt, Brace and Word.

3 Addressing fear and anxiety about labour and birth

Introduction

The way a woman approaches birth is always laced with the challenge of uncertainty, all the 'what ifs': 'Will my baby be alright?' . . . 'Will either of us be harmed by the process?' . . . 'Will I be able to cope with pain in labour? . . . 'What if I lose control and embarrass myself?' . . . 'Will my partner be able to cope?' Supporting women as they face these and other big issues requires sensitivity and skill on the part of all who provide care and support for them (Gutteridge, 2013, 2020; Haines *et al.*, 2012; Otley, 2011), as this mother vividly describes:

> You're so vulnerable and so suggestible, and so afraid really, even though it's all good and you're feeling strong and womanly, you're afraid. If it's your first baby it's a new experience and you need someone to believe in you, and that's what I felt; I felt that she really believed in me when I didn't believe in myself and that was wonderful, that really stands out for me.
>
> (Mother, Sandall *et al.*, 2010, unpublished data)

In this chapter we explore how we can increase our understanding of women's (and their partners') experiences of anxiety and fear about labour and birth and respond to individual women in supportive ways.

Box 3.1 Recommended Resource: Understanding anxiety, worry and fear in childbearing

Gutteridge, K. (ed.). (2020). *Understanding Anxiety, Worry and Fear in Childbearing: A Resource for Midwives and Clinicians*. Switzerland: Springer.

Consultant midwife and psychotherapist Kathryn Gutteridge has brought together a group of authors who contribute to this definitive textbook and resource for clinicians. Together they explore all aspects of how health professionals and maternity services can engage with fearful pregnant women in supportive ways, drawing on international evidence and experience.

DOI: 10.4324/9781003092520-4

The potential impact of anxiety and fear in pregnancy

It seems that, in high-income countries, women are increasingly anxious about labour and birth (Dennis *et al.*, 2017). Anxiety, stress, depression and a lack of social support contribute to fear of childbirth with potentially serious consequences for women, their babies and families. Studies such as those in Box 3.2 consistently show the following risks associated with women's fear of childbirth:

- Escalating anxiety, depression, insomnia and sleeplessness
- Women requesting caesarean section
- Increased dystocia, instrumental and emergency caesarean births
- Increased admissions to neonatal units
- Increased risk of postnatal depression and post-traumatic stress disorder
- Reduced infant bonding and attachment with potential long-term emotional effects for both mother and baby
- Decisions to have no further pregnancies or a large gap between pregnancies.

Box 3.2   Research Briefing: The potential impact of fear and anxiety in pregnancy

Dencker, A., Nilsson, C., Begley, C., Jangsten, E., Mollberg, M., Patel, H., . . . Sparud-Lundin, C. (2019). Causes and outcomes in studies of fear of childbirth: a systematic review. *Women and Birth, 32(2)*, 99–111.

Dennis, C.L., Falah-Hassani, K. and Shiri, R. (2017). Prevalence of antenatal and postnatal anxiety: systematic review and meta-analysis. *British Journal of Psychiatry: the journal of mental science, 210(5)*, 315–323.

O'Donovan, C. and O'Donovan, J. (2018). Why do women request an elective cesarean delivery for non-medical reasons? A systematic review of the qualitative literature. *Birth, 45(2)*, 109–119.

Simpson, M. and Catling, C. (2016). Understanding psychological traumatic birth experiences: a literature review. *Women and Birth, 29(3)*, 203–207.

Wigert, H., Nilsson, C., Dencker, A., Begley, C., Jangsten, E., Sparud-Lundin, C., . . . Patel, H. (2020). Women's experiences of fear of childbirth: a metasynthesis of qualitative studies. *International Journal of Qualitative Studies on Health and Well-being, 15*, 1.

The impact of an unhappy experience of birth on anxiety and fear in subsequent pregnancies

Women having their first babies are more likely to be scared of labour and birth, but serious fears are more prevalent in women who have already given birth and who have had a childbirth experience that they found traumatic (Dencker *et al.*, 2019). This is often due to having had a complicated labour; however, some women who have had what we might call a straightforward labour have memories of their experience being really traumatic, particularly if they felt that pain relief was inadequate or withheld from them or where there were negative interactions with caregivers (Hollander *et al.*, 2017; Nilsson and Lundgren, 2009). Stories on the websites of the UK and Australian Birth Trauma Associations are a sobering reminder of the devastating ways in which women's experiences of labour are affected by poor support from unsympathetic caregivers who do not listen to them.

Box 3.3   Reflective Activity: Recognising symptoms, risk factors, consequences and treatments of fear of childbirth and PTSD

de Vries, N.E., Stramrood, C.A.I., Sligter, L.M., Sluijs, A.-M. and van Pampus, M.G. (2020). Midwives' practice and knowledge about fear of childbirth and postpartum posttraumatic stress disorder. *Women and Birth, 33* e95–e104.

This study in the Netherlands identified the importance of midwifery education programmes offering the opportunity for students to acquire an in-depth knowledge of fear of childbirth (FoC) and postpartum post-traumatic stress disorder (PTSD). The questions used in Part One of the survey have been adapted here to allow students and maternity care providers to reflect on their knowledge and identify opportunities for learning.

These questions can be used for personal reflection, as a written assignment, or to promote discussion in pairs or small groups:

- Which signs, symptoms and/or signals have you encountered in your daily practice/do you know about indicating women who might have FoC/postpartum PTSD?
- What risk factors have you encountered/do you know about that increase the chances of women developing FoC/postpartum PTSD?
- What negative consequences of FoC/postpartum PTSD have you encountered in your daily practice/do you know about?
- Which effective treatments for postpartum PTSD do you know about?

Women who have had unhappy or traumatic experiences of birth identify that these might have been reduced or prevented with better communication and improved practical and emotional support from caregivers (Hollander *et al.*, 2017). In subsequent pregnancies these women will need additional support to help them regain their trust that maternity caregivers will provide them with good care; also, women who are pregnant for the first time will often need reassurance that the stories they have heard about other women's unhappy experiences with caregivers will not happen to them (Wigert *et al.*, 2020).

Recognising, understanding and addressing women's anxiety and fears

It is understandable that most pregnant women are worried about the unknown challenges that labour might present; indeed, it can be seen as a rational response in the face of uncertainty (Bewley and Cockburn, 2002; O'Connell *et al.*, 2015). The National Childbirth Trust (NCT) (a UK charity providing antenatal support and information for parents), reinforces the idea that being scared of labour is common and suggests some reasons why some women have extreme fear:

* Hormonal changes that make anxiety harder to manage
* Hearing stories from other women close to them who have been through traumatic births
* Fears related to medical care like ineffective pain control, fear of loss of control or death, or lack of confidence in the team providing care
* Psychosocial factors like being a young parent or at a social disadvantage
* Psychological factors like low self-esteem, revival of traumatic memories of childhood or psychiatric disorders like depression or anxiety (NCT, 2018).

Tocophobia – women who have severe fear of childbirth

'Tocophobia', sometimes spelt 'tokophobia' (from the Greek: 'tokos' – childbirth, and 'phobos' – fear), is the term that is used to describe situations where a woman's fears are exaggerated to the point where she has an extreme anxiety disorder and what is seen as an 'irrational' terror of going through labour and giving birth (Hofberg and Brockington, 2000). It is difficult to assess where tocophobia begins on a spectrum of low to high fear, thus there is a move to referring to 'severe fear of childbirth' (O'Connell *et al.*, 2017). Women with extreme fear often describe panic attacks, insomnia and nightmares (O'Connell *et al.*, 2015). Feelings of loneliness, impending danger and being trapped can compound doubts about their abilities to cope with labour and motherhood (Nilsson and Lundgren, 2009).

Tocophobia is classified as 'primary' when the woman is having her first baby and 'secondary' when it is related to a previous experience of giving birth that the woman has found traumatic. Hofberg and Ward (2003) suggest that a third classification is also useful: 'secondary to depressive illness in pregnancy'. Personal characteristics, such as previous psychological trauma, general anxiety, low self-esteem, depression, poor support, social isolation and dissatisfaction with their partner, can all contribute to women suffering extreme fear (Saisto and Halmesmäki, 2003).

Variations in defining and researching childbirth fear make it hard to draw comparisons between countries (Nilsson *et al.*, 2018; O'Connell *et al.*, 2017), but a systematic review suggests that worldwide, the rate of tocophobia is about 14 per cent, with rates varying from 3.7 per cent to 43 per cent in 18 countries (O'Connell *et al.*, 2017).

Box 3.4   Reflective Activity: What are women's worst fears?

Wickham, S. (2017). Thinking outside the box. Untangling tocophobia. *The Practising Midwife*,
   20(7). https://www.all4maternity.com/thinking-outside-box-untangling-tocophobia/.

In this article, Sara Wickham questions whether the term 'tocophobia' takes account
of the complexity of people's fears and suggests that for some, their concerns are more
about fear of the maternity system than fear of birth itself.

A group activity: instructions to participants
1   Before the session: read the article by Sara Wickham and look at a selection of
   videos on YouTube related to fear of birth.
2   Individually, write on a piece of paper *one* statement that you think a pregnant
   woman might make in response to the question, 'What are you most worried
   about?' That is, start your sentence with, 'The thing I'm most worried about is . . .'.
3   Place all the folded pieces of paper in a box to mix them up.
4   In turn, each participant picks a piece of paper out of the box, reads out what it says
   and then facilitates a group discussion about how we might respond if this were a
   conversation during an antenatal visit with a woman who is in early pregnancy.
5   At the end of the session, the group convener facilitates a discussion about what
   people learnt from engaging in this activity.

Understanding, recognising and addressing men's anxiety and fears

Childbirth fear is not uncommon in male partners of pregnant women; for example, a Swedish study found that 13 per cent of men surveyed had an extreme fear of childbirth, and that
this was likely to impact on the woman. In a study carried out in Northern Ireland, the most
common fears for men were that their partner's mental health would suffer as a result of a
traumatic birth; that they would be unable to provide adequate support during labour; and
that their partner or baby would be injured as a result of the birth (Greer *et al.*, 2014). Even
though both men and women expressed a desire to have a normal birth, men saw vaginal
birth as very risky; medical interventions, such as early induction of labour, electronic fetal
monitoring, epidural and planned caesarean section, were seen as resources to address this
risk and help ensure a safe birth.

Fear of birth undoubtedly contributes to expectant fathers wanting their partners to have
an epidural, particularly once they see them in pain in labour (Orbach-Zinger *et al.*, 2008).
Indeed, a study in Italy suggested that epidurals reduce paternal anxiety and stress in labour
and increase paternal involvement and satisfaction with their experiences of childbirth
(Capogna *et al.*, 2007). Bearing that in mind, the following activity challenges us to take a
hard look at the potential effects of partner fear on women in labour.

**Box 3.5   Reflective Activity: Paternal anxiety in labour –
what might be the consequences?**

Pre-reading:

Jomeen, J. (2017). Fathers in the birth room: choice or coercion? Help or hindrance? *Journal of
Reproductive and Infant Psychology*, 35(4), 321–323. doi:10.1080/02646838.2017.1361124.

In this article Julie Jomeen encourages us to discuss how we can facilitate meaningful
engagement with fathers during labour and birth. She suggests it is time to return to
debates about whether fathers being in the birth room is the right option for all couples
and poses the following questions:

- Should 'not being there' become a real option for a father, allowing him to express
  his desire not to be present without censure?
- Should a woman who feels she would better benefit from the support of others in labour
  be able to articulate that wish without feeling judged on the status of her relationship?
- How might such decisions challenge the construct of the 'good mother'/'supportive
  partner'?

In pairs or small groups:
- Discuss what you think about these questions.
- Are there situations where you might discuss these issues with a woman and her partner?
- Do you think the issues are the same where the expectant parents are in a lesbian
  relationship?
- What might you do to encourage partners to express their worries and fears?
- If a woman wants to have a normal birth without intervention, how might you
  engage in a discussion with her partner about the supportive role they can play –
  one that doesn't necessarily go straight to an epidural as a solution?

Antenatal and postnatal anxiety and depression in men

The need for greater engagement of partners in antenatal care and education is widely recognised, but the ways in which anxiety and fear can impede the level of support partners are able
to provide is under-researched. The psychological wellbeing of both partners will impact on the
other. The more dissatisfied the partner is with his life situation, the more anxious the woman
will be; her anxiety will be compounded where there is poor support from her male partner
(Saisto *et al.*, 2001). A systematic review of antenatal and postnatal depression in fathers (Wee
et al., 2011) draws attention to the fact that men were significantly more prone to anxiety and
depression if their partners were anxious or depressed during pregnancy or following birth.
This was compounded where there was low social support. The review identified that a lack of
information about pregnancy and birth was a source of distress for some men and high anxiety
during the antenatal period was the strongest predictor of depression following birth.

Engaging with pregnant women who are fearful of childbirth

Our interactions with pregnant women who are anxious or fearful of labour require sensitivity and good listening skills in order for our perceptions and intuition to help us in the

delicate task of identifying the sort of support that an individual woman might need during pregnancy (O'Connell *et al.*, 2015; Simpson and Catling, 2016). Sometimes it takes many meetings before a woman feels able to disclose or explore the source of her fears; during this time a clue might be that she presents regularly with complaints, such as abdominal pain, that are symptoms of her anxiety (Saisto and Halmesmäki, 2003). Extra time often needs to be set aside to explore the duration and intensity of her anxiety, the meaning that fear has for her, how this impacts on her life and relationships (Melender, 2002), and whether there is a need for more in-depth counselling or referral to other services (Larsson *et al.*, 2019).

Interest from healthcare professionals and an understanding midwife were described as crucial elements of support for women who had an intense fear of childbirth in a Swedish study (Eriksson *et al.*, 2006). We recommend that you read this article, as it helps us understand the difficulties that many pregnant women experience during antenatal consultations with their caregivers:

Box 3.6   Research Briefing: Women's experiences of intense fear of childbirth and interactions with caregivers

Eriksson, C., Jansson, L. and Hamberg, K. (2006). Women's experiences of intense fear related to childbirth investigated in a Swedish qualitative study. *Midwifery*, *22*, 240–248.

Twenty women with intense fear of childbirth described three approaches for dealing with their fear: 'evading', 'processing' and 'seeking help'. These could be used in parallel or were exchangeable, depending on which approach seemed to be most effective at the time. All women talked about how difficult it was to disclose or talk about their fears, and circumstances that hindered this process were identified. The authors of this paper suggest that professionals who provide antenatal care need further training in how to communicate and support women with intense fear of childbirth.

Box 3.7   Reflective Activity: Picking up on the cues when women are fearful

In the article by Eriksson and colleagues (2006), profiled in Box 3.6, women identified the importance of the midwife picking up on cues without them having to express their fear explicitly: 'I don't think I was very clear, I tried a bit cautiously to see if she'd pick up on it' (p.246).

In pairs or in small groups:
- Discuss what sort of cues you think you might pick up on when engaging with a pregnant woman who is not open about her fears.
- How might you respond when you realise that a woman is anxious or fearful of labour?
- Write a 'script' that illustrates this sort of interaction and practise role playing in a similar scenario.

Midwifery continuity of care for women who are fearful

Maternity care providers are, paradoxically, both a major cause of childbirth fear and the most promising mediating factors. Many women are anxious about who will attend them during labour, particularly if they have unhappy memories of the care they received during a previous birth. Changing systems of care so that women can have a known midwife with them during labour, someone with whom they have built a trusting relationship, has been held up as the ideal for decades (Homer *et al.*, 2019) and is a feature of policy documents in the UK (NHS England, 2016; NHS Scotland, 2017; Welsh Government, 2019) and Australia (COAG Health Council, 2019). In the absence of midwifery continuity of care, many women are turning to doulas or other birth workers who will help them work through their fears during pregnancy and guarantee to be with them in labour.

Midwifery continuity of care allows for an in-depth exploration of the woman's individual concerns. Care from a midwife working in a caseload model of care has the potential to alleviate a woman's fears, especially if she also has a known midwife caring for her during labour (Hildingsson *et al.*, 2018, 2019). Particularly in community settings, the midwife can link a woman to services and support networks, whilst keeping an overview of her journey through maternity care and new motherhood (Leap, 2010). This has been shown to be particularly important for women who are most vulnerable and socially disadvantaged, many of whom will be in groups identified as being more prone to being fearful or whose trust has been broken by previous interactions with healthcare professionals (Rayment-Jones *et al.*, 2015, 2019).

Box 3.8   Reflective Activity: Identifying resources in the community for women who fear childbirth

Individually, in pairs or small groups:
Thinking about pregnant women who are anxious or fearful about labour and birth and women who have had unhappy or traumatic experiences of birth: identify services, projects and support groups in the community in your local area that you might tell women about or refer them to. Make a list with notes about each one to share with the larger group.

Interventions to support women who are anxious and fearful about birth

A range of interventions can help fearful pregnant women develop or regain trust in their abilities and increase their knowledge and confidence about giving birth. There are numerous examples of success stories in countries where specialist services offer psychological assessment counselling and planning and support for labour and birth. Services led by midwives are particularly effective in reducing anxiety and fear and improving women's confidence for birth; see, for example, Gamble *et al.* (2005); and Larsson *et al.* (2019). In the following box we have placed one Cochrane protocol, one Cochrane review and a systematic review; these will take you to a wealth of literature related to interventions that address pregnant women's anxiety and fear about birth.

Box 3.9   Research Briefing: Interventions to support women who have antenatal anxiety and fear of childbirth

Dennis, C.L. and Brown, H.K. (2017). Psychosocial, psychological, and pharmacological interventions for treating antenatal anxiety (Protocol). *Cochrane Database of Systematic Reviews,* Issue 11. Art. No.: CD012870. doi:012810.011002/14651858.CD14012870.

O'Connell, M.A., Khashan, A.S., Leahy Warren, P., Stewart, S., O'Neill, S.M. (2021) Interventions for fear of childbirth including tocophobia. Cochrane Database of Systematic Reviews, Issue 7. Art. No.: CD013321.doi:10.1002/14651858.CD013321.pub2.

Stoll, K., Swift, E.M., Fairbrother, N., Nethery, E. and Janssen, P. (2018). A systematic review of nonpharmacological prenatal interventions for pregnancy-specific anxiety and fear of childbirth. *Birth, 45(1),* 7–18.

Recognising, understanding and addressing our own fears

> We cannot hope to begin to deal with women's fear of childbirth unless we are willing to examine our own, and recognise how we can and do contribute to women's fear.
>
> (Dahlen, 2010, p.158)

If we are to support pregnant women to have positive experiences of childbirth and address their fears and anxiety, a good place to start is to look at our own fears about birth:

Box 3.10   Research Briefing: Exploring the roles of trust and fear for practitioners

Dahlen, H. (2010). Undone by fear? Deluded by trust? Commentary. *Midwifery, 26,* 156–162. doi:10.1016/j.midw.2009.11.008.

Hannah Dahlen explores the roles of fear and trust for practitioners and how these relate to safe practice and the facilitation of normal birth. She argues that, whilst both fear and trust are protective for our survival, getting the balance right means reducing manufactured fear and building responsive trust. Identifying our fears and talking about them with trusted colleagues help us shed those fears and not let them get in the way of our ability to trust women's abilities to give birth.

Box 3.11   Reflective Activity: Exploring our own fears

Individual activity:
- After reading the article by Hannah Dahlen (2010) highlighted above, identify your greatest fears and discuss them with a trusted colleague.
- How might these fears affect how you engage with women who are pregnant and giving birth?
- What might help you to address these fears?
- Discuss any situations you have experienced or read about where 'trusting the process' of labour and birth was misplaced.

The social context of fear and anxiety around birth

A study exploring fear of childbirth and its impact on birth choices among women and their partners in Northern Ireland concluded that midwives should be more proactive in offering credible alternatives to medical interventions in order to reduce fears and promote normal birth (Greer *et al.*, 2014). We suggest that it is not that simple: before we can begin to offer such alternatives, we have to consider how cultural norms around fear of birth impact on all of us in our efforts to embrace physiological birth. The following articles provide a rich resource for discussing these issues.

Box 3.12   Research Briefing: The social context of fear and anxiety around birth

Fisher, C., Hauck, Y. and Fenwick, J. (2006). How social context impacts on women's fears of childbirth: a Western Australian example. *Social Science & Medicine*, 63, 64–75.

This research involved in-depth interviews with 22 Australian women, identified as being fearful of birth. The researchers argue that fear of childbirth has social as well as personal dimensions, particularly within the context of the medicalisation of childbirth and prevalence of 'horror stories' and previous birth experiences viewed as 'horrific'. Two main factors mediated against childbirth fear: positive relationships formed with midwives and the support that women received from their informal networks. Working with these factors in mind enables positive interventions to help pregnant women who are fearful.

Reiger, K. and Dempsey, R. (2006). Performing birth in a culture of fear: an embodied crisis of late modernity. *Health Sociology Review*, 15(4), 364–373.

This paper discusses the steady decline in cultural and personal confidence in women's birthing capacity in Western societies. The role of technology, consumerism and the cultural preoccupation with celebrities and choice can be seen to have contributed to a situation where physiological birth is seen as difficult to achieve. The authors examine parallels between the challenges women face in labour with those of the intense creative and physical effort seen in fields such as sport and the arts. They draw on biology, psychology and social theory in proposing a theoretical framework that addresses the crucial role of support for pregnant women, during pregnancy, labour and birth, particularly where they experience a 'crisis of confidence' (p.369).

Childbirth through the lens of reality TV

We cannot consider the social context of birth without looking at the messages about birth portrayed in the media, particularly in reality TV shows (Sanders, 2015). Sensationalist and inaccurate media descriptions of birth are highly influential and potentially contribute to women's fear of giving birth (D'Cruz and Lee, 2014; Vitek and Ward, 2019), as this young woman suggests:

> Television probably plays a big part in shaping the perception of giving birth as you usually see the woman kicking, screaming, swearing and threatening to kill the husband. . . . Hopefully that's not the case in real life.
>
> (Young woman, D'Cruz and Lee, 2014, p.205)

Canadian researchers Kathrin Stoll and Wendy Hall (2013a, 2013b) performed an online survey with over 2,600 university students of mixed ethnicity. With an average age of 22, the students were all women who had not given birth and who identified that they would like to have children at some stage. A summary of the analysis of open-ended questions is presented in Box 3.13. The authors cite the work of Morris and McInerney (2010) in highlighting the negative effect of reality TV shows and conclude that age-appropriate education in primary and secondary schools should be provided as an alternative to mass-mediated information about birth. (We recommend you visit the 'Core of Life' website to view an excellent Australian example of education about birth aimed at 12–17-year-old young people: www. coreoflife.org.au, accessed December 2020.)

Box 3.13   Research Briefing: Young women, childbirth fear and the media

Stoll, K. and Hall, W. (2013a). Vicarious birth experiences and childbirth fear: does it matter how young Canadian women learn about birth? *The Journal of Perinatal Education*, *22(4)*, 226–233.

Stoll, K. and Hall W.A. (2013b). Attitudes and preferences of young women with low and high fear of childbirth. *Qualitative Health Research*, *23(11)*: 1495–1505.

* Students based their attitudes about birth on culturally circulated stories and images as well as their vicarious experiences of being involved in births.
* Overall, 13.6 per cent of the women exhibited high levels of fear.
* Students with high fear of birth described childbirth as a frightening and painful ordeal and viewed obstetric interventions as a means to make labour and birth more manageable.
* Young women whose attitudes towards pregnancy and birth were shaped by the media were 1.5 times more likely to report childbirth fear.
* Three factors that decreased fear of birth were confidence in knowledge of pregnancy and birth, having witnessed a birth and having friends as a source of information.
* Seven per cent had witnessed a birth: on television, in a supportive role with friends or family members or in a professional role. Regardless of the complexity of the birth that they had seen, these women had significantly lower fear scores than women who had not witnessed a birth, especially if the birth had taken place at home.

These findings are congruent with Bandura's (1977) assertion that vicarious experiences can reduce fear.

Analyses of reality TV programmes continue to provide us with food for thought about the messages that women are getting when birth is portrayed as risky and requiring medicalisation to enable safety (Luce *et al.*, 2016; Morris and McInerney, 2010). Conversations with pregnant women about what they've seen recently on television are often useful for opening up discussions about fear and anxiety. We think that it is therefore important that all birth attendants watch these programmes so that they know the messages women are getting and can provide alternative sources of information where appropriate. (Sorry about that folks!)

Box 3.14   Reflective Activity: Conversations about reality TV shows and representations of birth

In pairs:
- Practise conversations about a recently watched reality TV programme with one of you role playing being an anxious pregnant woman.
- Make a list of online resources and films that you might advise women to watch and which have positive messages about birth, with notes about each.
- Circulate this list to other participants and compile a resource to share with others.

When women request planned caesarean section

The reasons for a rise in women asking for elective caesarean sections in the absence of medical indications are complex and context-specific, but negative experiences during previous labours often play a part (O'Donovan and O'Donovan, 2018; Simpson and Catling, 2016). The response of obstetricians to these requests will vary depending on the context. Women in the UK and Nordic countries who request a planned caesarean are likely to be referred to an interdisciplinary team or individual with expertise in counselling (Bewley and Cockburn, 2002; Waldenstrom *et al.*, 2006). In contrast, in Australia, there are reports of obstetricians encouraging women's decisions as a 'safe' and 'responsible' choice, without question (Fenwick *et al.*, 2010).

The NICE Guidelines on Caesarean Birth (2021) set out recommendations for how to respond when a woman requests a caesarean section, including evidence identifying the increased risks of caesarean section compared to vaginal birth when there are no medical indications. The articles profiled in the following boxes provide us with much thought-provoking material in our discussions about planned caesarean section where there is no medical indication.

Box 3.15   Research Briefing: Caesarean upon maternal request

D'Souza, R. and Arulkumaran, S. (2013). To 'C' or not to 'C'? Caesarean delivery upon maternal request: a review of facts, figures and guidelines. *Journal of Perinatal Medicine, 41,* 5–15.

Posing the notion that 'caesarean is the unavoidable consequence of institutionalised birth' (p.5), the authors, both obstetricians, explore sociocultural perspectives and changing attitudes of both women and practitioners to the increasing rise of 'caesarean delivery on maternal request' (CDMR). In exploring whether this trend is justifiable, they present extensive evidence about risk and safety in relation to emergency and elective caesarean and planned vaginal birth, including potential 'reproductive consequences' for each. Medical, ethical and financial dilemmas are discussed.

Box 3.16   Research Briefing: Debates about caesarean section, biology and epigenetics

Dahlen, H.G., Downe, S., Kennedy, H.P. and Foureur, M. (2014). Is society being reshaped on a microbiological and epigenetic level by the way women give birth? *Midwifery*, 1149–1151.

This paper provides a useful background briefing to the documentary film, *Microbirth*: www.oneworldbirth.net/microbirth.

Emerging debates are explored concerning the role of epigenetics in gene expression and the protective role of microbes that colonise a newborn baby's gastrointestinal tract following vaginal birth, skin-to-skin contact and early breastfeeding. The way in which common childbirth interventions – caesarean, induction, augmentation, antibiotics – may inhibit protective processes and pose long-term health risks is highlighted as causing increasing concern.

Box 3.17   Reflective Activity: 'The things that count cannot be counted' – microbiology, epigenetics and birth

There is some debate amongst quotation scholars about whether it was Einstein or someone else who first said this. Leaving the origins of the quotation to one side:

In pairs or small groups:
- Discuss this phrase and what it means to you after reading the articles by D'Souza and Arulkumarum (2013) and Dahlen *et al*. (2014).

This activity will be enhanced if you also watch the documentary film, *Microbirth*, before your discussions: www.oneworldbirth.net/microbirth.

Professional attitudes to planned caesarean section

In the late 1990s, 282 obstetricians working in London NHS maternity units responded to an anonymous postal survey, which included a question asking what sort of birth they would prefer if they or their partners were pregnant for the first time with an uncomplicated, singleton pregnancy (Al-Mufti *et al*., 1997). Overall, 17 per cent chose an elective caesarean (31 per cent of female obstetricians compared with 8 per cent of male obstetricians).

The main reason for choosing caesarean (identified by 88 per cent of the respondents) was fear of perineal damage from vaginal birth with associated perceived long-term sequalae: stress incontinence, anal sphincter damage, impaired sexual function. Fear of damage to the baby was cited by 39 per cent and the desire to choose the time of birth by 27 per cent.

In response to the controversy that was provoked by the reporting of this survey, two obstetricians in the north of England surveyed female midwives and asked them the same question (Dickson and Willett, 1999). Almost all (129 of 135 midwives) said they would prefer to have a vaginal birth in the absence of complications.

This survey was undertaken in an era where planned caesarean in the absence of medical indication was not part of maternity service culture in NHS Britain. In response to a similar survey in the USA, where elective caesarean section was already much more common, 56.5 per cent of male obstetricians and 32.6 per cent of female obstetricians said they would prefer to have a caesarean section (Gabbe and Holzman, 2001).

Box 3.18   Reflective Activity: Professional attitudes to planned caesarean or vaginal birth

In the years since the surveys were carried out identifying obstetricians' and midwives' preferences for vaginal or caesarean birth, caesarean rates have increased considerably in high-income countries, including those for planned caesarean in the absence of medical indications. Recent studies also show that women are increasingly fearful of birth.

In pairs or small groups:
- Do you think that maternity care providers are more fearful than they were in the 1990s?
- Conduct a straw poll with colleagues from different disciplines asking them what sort of birth they would prefer if they or their partners were pregnant for the first time with an uncomplicated, singleton pregnancy.
- Discuss the implications of what you learn.

Talking about contractions – 'The Midwifery Wave'

In this chapter we have looked at why women may feel anxious and fearful about labour and birth, how they may show this and how we can help them. It is important to remember that there are some very simple things that we can do in our interactions to support them, build trust and reduce fear. We finish this chapter by highlighting the most common way that midwives and birth workers are able to help anxious women who have not had a labour to feel more confident. It's as simple as explaining the rhythmic patterns of contractions. Nicky calls this 'The Midwifery Wave' because all over the world, in whatever language midwives are using, they do the same things with their hands – forming a wave pattern with an emphatic gesture denoting the rests in between, as they say:

- It starts slowly.
- It builds to a peak.
- It starts to fade.
- It lasts about a minute.
- And then there's a REST.

Box 3.19   Reflective Activity: Practising 'The Midwifery Wave'

Practising 'The Midwifery Wave' with students and colleagues opens up useful discussions about the potential messages that it gives and how it might be received.

In pairs or groups:
- With colleagues, practise doing The Midwifery Wave, speaking it out loud with the hand movements showing the wave and rest patterns. Discuss what you think women hear and see when you do this. Why do you think it might be useful in changing women's perceptions of how they will manage labour?

The following box contains examples of phrases that midwives and obstetricians identified that they would use when talking to a woman who would like to have a normal birth without interventions, but is scared about how she will cope with labour (Sandall *et al.*, 2010). It may be useful to practise saying them out loud, particularly if you are doing the activity that we have placed in the postscript to this chapter.

Box 3.20   Reflective Activity: Encouraging words when talking to a pregnant woman about labour

In pairs:
In turn, practise saying each of these phrases out loud. Discuss how you think each one might be received by a pregnant woman or her birth supporters and the ensuing conversations you might have.

- 'Contractions build to a peak and then tail off, lasting about a minute, and there are rests in between – it's not a constant pain.'
- 'Every contraction's really important and doing good work – each one brings you a little closer to having your baby.'
- 'You can focus on one contraction at a time, staying in the present.'
- 'There are lots of things you can do to bring your baby to you: moving around, getting into good positions, kneeling, sitting on the toilet, squatting, rocking.'
- 'You'll have strong contractions for less than a day in your whole life – your body is going to keep you going through that.'
- 'Your body's got all these hormones designed to help you in labour and it's going to keep you going right until the end, no matter how tired you feel, how exhausted you feel, you'll just keep going, because you're designed to do that – and then you're going to have your baby.'
- 'Labour pain is a really different kind of pain because it's a special pain, it's not like a pain where you break your arm or you break your leg, it's a pain that's bringing your baby, it's a really wonderful thing that you're doing and every pain that you have brings you just a little bit closer to having your baby.'
- 'Your body works on a build-up effect, so it starts off fairly mild, kind of spaced out, and then gradually it will get closer together and stronger, so that your body's got time to get used to it, to cope with it, and your body's got time to release its own endorphins, its natural painkillers, to help you through the process; your body's working with you to help you have your baby, not against you. And it's that thing about trusting your body to do that.'
- 'Your contractions are going to get stronger and more powerful, but you're going to get much better at dealing with them, you're going to find it much easier, and you'll go with it and it will be something that you'll be able to do.'
- 'I'm going to tell you all these things today and it's really important that you go home and relay all that to your partner, so that they understand what's happening as well.'
- 'Good support is better than any epidural. Good support, and then that feeling afterwards of achievement.'

In the next chapter, we shall be looking at some structured approaches to what is commonly described as 'childbirth education'. We will explore ways of engaging with women during pregnancy that may help them develop a sense of control and agency in how they approach birth and put in place appropriate support structures.

Postscript: scenario-based workstation (OSCE*) – addressing a pregnant woman's anxiety

This scenario-based OSCE was developed as a six-week follow-up activity to an interdisciplinary workshop for NHS maternity staff in the UK: 'Supporting women to have a normal birth: development and field testing of a learning package for maternity staff' (Leap *et al.*, 2009; Sandall *et al.*, 2010). It can be adapted for a range of scenarios involving interaction between pregnant women and their caregivers. *We suggest that you invite the actors to substitute names of their choice for the pregnant woman, her partner and sister and that these names are changed in the following instructions for the activity.*

Note: * OSCE: Objective Structured Clinical Examination

The instructions for the activity are in three parts:

1   Participant instructions
2   Instructions for the actor playing an anxious pregnant woman
3   Workstation scoring sheet

---

1   Participant instructions (midwife or doctor)

You have just finished a routine antenatal check with a pregnant woman called 'Tracy' who is having her first baby. She is reassured that all is well with her baby and her pregnancy.

As she is about to leave, she says, 'Can I ask you about something? Everything's fine and I'm really hoping I'll have a normal birth without using any drugs or the epidural – but I'm very worried about how I'll cope with pain in labour. Do you have any tips?'

In the informal discussion that follows you may want to draw on your experience (stories), and include the following:

•   the nature of contractions;
•   endogenous hormones that can help;
•   the 'transition' phase of labour;
•   your confidence in her abilities and self-help strategies that women and their birth supporters can employ.

This role play will be followed by a constructive five-minute discussion where you, the observer and the actor will give your impressions of how the role play went. You will be encouraged to reflect on how you addressed the woman's fears, including the information you gave her, the language you used and your communication skills. After you have left, the observer and actor will together complete the scoring sheet (see below), which will be given to you later so that you can reflect further on how you engaged in the OSCE.

---

2   Instructions for the actor playing an anxious pregnant woman

The observer will introduce the participant and check that they have read the instructions and understand the process before starting the role play.

You are 'Tracy Walker', a 38-year-old woman having your first baby, and you are 36 weeks' pregnant. Everything has gone well in this pregnancy and you have recently taken maternity leave from your job as a hotel receptionist. You have been receiving care at the antenatal clinic at this maternity unit.

You and your husband, 'Ron', have not been to any antenatal classes. You are thinking you might ask your sister, 'Karen', who had a normal birth, to come and support you and 'Ron' during labour.

You would really like to have a normal birth without using any drugs but you don't think you'll be able to cope because you have a low pain threshold. Also, you have heard some very frightening stories from your sister and friends.

You are attending an antenatal appointment and decide to ask the midwife/doctor about something that's bothering you. After the check-up – which shows that all is well with your baby and your pregnancy – you say, 'Can I ask you about something? Everything's fine and I'm really hoping I'll have a normal birth without using any drugs or the epidural – but I'm very worried about how I'll cope with pain in labour. Do you have any tips?'

During a (maximum) eight-minute, informal conversation with the medical student/ midwife/doctor participant you can include the following questions:

- I've heard that labour pain's really terrible. What will the contractions feel like?
- I'm a bit of a wimp – I've got a really low pain threshold. Do you think this means I won't be able to cope?
- If you (or your partner) were having a baby, would you have an epidural?

This role play will be followed by a constructive five-minute discussion with the midwife/doctor participant, observer and actor giving their impressions of how the role play went. After this the participant leaves.

Following this, the actor and the observer will discuss the participant's performance and fill in the scoring sheet, a copy of which will be given to the participant (maximum seven minutes).

TOTAL TIME ALLOCATED: 20 minutes

3   Scenario-based workstation scoring sheet

PARTICIPANT NAME:

OBSERVER: ACTOR:

Instructions for actors: You have just finished a routine antenatal check with a pregnant woman called 'Tracy' who is having her first baby. She is reassured that all is well with her baby and her pregnancy. As she is about to leave, she says, 'Can I ask you about something? Everything's fine and I'm really hoping I'll have a normal birth without using any drugs or the epidural – but I'm very worried about how I'll cope with pain in labour. Do you have any tips?'

You have an informal discussion during which you draw on your experience (stories) and talk about: the nature of contractions; endogenous hormones that can help; the 'transition' phase of labour; your confidence in her abilities and self-help strategies that women and their birth supporters can employ.

Scoring: 2 = Good, 1 = Adequate, 0 = Not done/inadequate	*Actor*	*Observer*
Listens to 'Tracy', does not interrupt		
Acknowledges her fears		
Eye contact, open body language		
Explains the nature of contractions: lasting a minute, building to a peak, breaks between contractions		
Describes endogenous hormones that can help		
Reassures re: 'low pain threshold'		
Describes practical strategies for pain		
Draws on experience/stories		
Articulates confidence in 'Tracy'		
Asks about her birth supporters		
Scoring: 5 = Very good, 4 = Good, 3 = Pass, 2 = Borderline, 1 = Fail		
OBSERVER GLOBAL RATING Overall competence of candidate	5 4 3 2 1	
ROLE PLAYER GLOBAL RATING Overall competence of candidate	5 4 3 2 1	

References

Al-Mufti R., McCarthy, A. and Fisk, M.N. (1997). Survey of obstetricians' personal preference and discretionary practice. *European Journal of Obstetrics and Gynecology and Reproductive Biology, 73*, 1.

Bandura, A. (1977). Self efficacy: toward a unifying theory of behavioural change. *Psychology Review, 84*, 191–215.

Bewley, S. and Cockburn, J. (2002). Responding to fear of childbirth. Commentary. *The Lancet, 359*, 2128–2129.

Capogna, G., Camorcia, M. and Stirparo, S. (2007). Expectant fathers' experience during labor with or without epidural analgesia. *International Journal of Obstetric Anaesthesia, 16(2)*, 110–115.

COAG Health Council. (2019). *Woman-centred Care: Strategic Directions for Australian Materntiy Services*. Canberra: Australian Government Department of Health.

Dahlen, H.G. (2010). Undone by fear? Deluded by trust? Commentary. *Midwifery, 26*, 156–162.

Dahlen, H.G., Downe, S., Kennedy, H.P. and Foureur, M. (2014). Is society being reshaped on a micro-biological and epigenetic level by the way women give birth? *Midwifery*, 1149–1151.

D'Cruz, L. and Lee, C. (2014). Childbirth expectations: an Australian study of young childless women. *Journal of Reproductive and Infant Psychology, 32(2)*, 196–208.

Dencker, A., Nilsson, C., Begley, C., Jangsten, E., Mollberg, M., Patel, H., . . . Sparud-Lundin, C. (2019). Causes and outcomes in studies of fear of childbirth: a systematic review. *Women and Birth, 32(2)*, 99–111.

Dennis, C.L. and Brown, H.K. (2017). Psychosocial, psychological, and pharmacological interventions for treating antenatal anxiety. *Cochrane Database of Systematic Reviews*, Issue 11. Art. No.: CD012870. doi:10.1002/14651858.CD012870.

Dennis, C.L., Falah-Hassani, K. and Shiri, R. (2017). Prevalence of antenatal and postnatal anxiety: systematic review and meta-analysis. *British Journal of Psychiatry: The Journal of Mental Science, 210(5)*, 315–323.

de Vries, N.E., Stramrood, C.A.I., Sligter, L.M., Sluijs, A.-M. and van Pampus, M.G. (2020). Midwives' practice and knowledge about fear of childbirth and postpartum posttraumatic stress disorder. *Women and Birth, 33*, e95–e104.

Dickson, M.J. and Willett, M. (1999). Midwives would prefer a vaginal delivery. *British Medical Journal, 319(7215)*, 1008.

D'Souza, R. and Arulkumaran, S. (2013). To 'C' or not to 'C'? Caesarean delivery upon maternity request: a review of facts, figures and guidelines. *Journal of Perinatal Medicine, 41*, 5–15.

Eriksson, C., Jansson, L. and Hamberg, K. (2006). Women's experiences of intense fear related to childbirth investigated in a Swedish qualitative study. *Midwifery, 22*, 240–248.

Fenwick, J., Staff, L., Gamble, J., Creedy, D.K. and Bayes, S. (2010). Why do women request caesarean section in a normal, healthy first pregnancy? *Midwifery, 26*, 394–400.

Fisher, C., Hauck, Y. and Fenwick, J. (2006). How social context impacts on women's fears of childbirth: a Western Australian example. *Social Science & Medicine, 63*, 64–75.

Gabbe, S.G. and Holzman, G.B. (2001). Obstetricians' choice of delivery. *The Lancet, 357*, 722.

Gamble, J., Creedy, D.K, Moyle, W., Webster, J., McAllister, M. and Dickson, P. (2005). Effectiveness of a counseling intervention after a traumatic childbirth: a randomized controlled trial. *Birth, 32(1)*, 11–19.

Greer, J., Lazenbatt, A. and Dunne, L. (2014). 'Fear of childbirth' and ways of coping for pregnant women and their partners during the birthing process: a salutogenic analysis. *Evidence Based Midwifery, 12(3)*, 95–100.

Gutteridge, K. (2013). Who's afraid of the big bad birth? *MIDIRS Midwifery Digest, 23(4)*, 441–446.

Gutteridge, K. (ed.). (2020). *Understanding Anxiety, Worry and Fear in Childbearing: A Resource for Midwives and Clinicians*. Switzerland: Springer.

Haines, H.M., Rubertsson, C., Pallant, J.F. and Hildingsson, I. (2012). The influence of women's fear, attitudes and beliefs of childbirth on mode and experience of birth. *BMC Pregnancy and Childbirth, 12*, 55.

Hildingsson, I., Rubertsson, C., Karlström, A. and Haines, H. (2018). Caseload midwifery for women with fear of birth is a feasible option. *Sexual & Reproductive Healthcare, 16*, 50–55.

Hildingsson, I., Rubertsson, C., Karlström, A. and Haines, H. (2019). A known midwife can make a difference for women with fear of childbirth-birth outcome and women's experiences of intrapartum care. *Sexual & Reproductive Healthcare*, *21*, 33–38.

Hofberg, K. and Brockington, I. (2000). Tokophobia: an unreasoning dread of childbirth. A series of 26 cases. *The British Journal of Psychiatry*, *176*, 83–85.

Hofberg, K. and Ward, M.R. (2003). Fear of pregnancy and childbirth. *Postgraduate Medical Journal*, *79*, 505–510.

Hollander, M.H., van Hastenberg, E., van Dillen, J., van Pampus, M.G., de Miranda, E. and Stramrood, C.A.I. (2017). Preventing traumatic childbirth experiences: 2192 women's perceptions and views. *Archives of Women's Mental Health*, *20(4)*, 515–523.

Homer, C.S.E., Leap, N., Brodie, P. and Sandall, J. (ed.). (2019). *Midwifery Continuity of Care*, 2nd edn. Chatswood, NSW: Elsevier Australia.

Jomeen, J. (2017). Fathers in the birth room: choice or coercion? Help or hindrance? *Journal of Reproductive and Infant Psychology*, *35(4)*, 321–323.

Larsson, B., Hildingsson, I., Ternström, E., Rubertsson, C. and Karlström, A. (2019). Women's experience of midwife-led counselling and its influence on childbirth fear: a qualitative study. *Women and Birth*, *32(1)*, e88–e94.

Leap, N. (2010). The less we do the more we give. Chapter 2 in M. Kirkham (ed.), *The Midwife–Mother Relationship*, 2nd edn (pp.17–35). London: Palgrave Macmillan.

Leap, N, Sandall J, Grant, J, Bastos, M.H. and Armstrong, P. (2009). Using video in the development and field-testing of a learning package for maternity staff: supporting women for normal birth. *International Journal of Multiple Research Approaches*, *3(3)*, 302–320.

Luce, A., Cash, M., Hundley, V., Cheyne, H., van Teijlingen, E. and Angell, C. (2016). 'Is it realistic?' The portrayal of pregnancy and childbirth in the media. *BMC Pregnancy and Childbirth*, *16*, 40.

Melender, H.-L. (2002). Fears and coping strategies associated with pregnancy and childbirth in Finland. *Journal of Midwifery & Women's Health*, *47(4)*, 256–263.

Morris, T. and McInerney, K. (2010). Media representation and childbirth: an analysis of reality television programs in the United States. *Birth*, *37(134–140)*.

NCT. (2018). Tokophobia: how to get over extreme fear of giving birth. https://www.nct.org.uk/pregnancy/how-you-might-be-feeling/tokophobia-how-get-over-extreme-fear-giving-birth.

NHS England. (2016). *Better Births: Improving Outcomes of Maternity Services in England. A Five Year Forward View for Maternity Care. National Maternity Review*. https://www.england.nhs.uk/wp-content/uploads/2016/02/national-maternity-review-report.pdf.

NHS Scotland. (2017). *The Best Start: a Five Year Forward Plan for Maternity and Neonatal Care in Scotland*. Edinburgh: NHS Scotland. https://www.gov.scot/publications/best-start-five-year-forward-plan-maternity-neonatal-care-scotland/.

NICE (2021). Caesarean birth. *National Institute for Health and Clinical Excellence*. www.nice.org.uk/guidance/ng192.

Nilsson, C., Hessman, E., Sjöblom, H., Dencker, A., Jangsten, E., Mollberg, M., . . . Begley, C. (2018). Definitions, measurements and prevalence of fear of childbirth: a systematic review. *BMC Pregnancy & Childbirth*, *18(1)*, 28.

Nilsson, C. and Lundgren, I. (2009). Women's lived experience of fear of childbirth. *Midwifery*, *25*, e1–e9.

O'Connell, M.A., Leahy-Warren, P., Khashan, A.S. and Kenny, L.C. (2015). Tocophobia – the new hysteria? *Obstetrics, Gynaecology and Reproductive Medicine*.

O'Connell, M.A., Leahy-Warren, P., Khashan, A.S., Kenny, L.C., and O'Neill, S.M. (2017). Worldwide prevalence of tocophobia in pregnant women: systematic review and meta-analysis. *Acta Obstetricia et Gynecologica Scandinavica*, *98(8)*, 907–920.

O'Connell, M.A., Khashan, A.S., Leahy Warren, P., Stewart, S., O'Neill, S.M. (2021) Interventions for fear of childbirth including tocophobia. Cochrane Database of Systematic Reviews, Issue 7. Art. No.: CD013321.doi:10.1002/14651858.CD013321.pub2.

O'Donovan, C. and O'Donovan, J. (2018). Why do women request an elective cesarean delivery for non-medical reasons? A systematic review of the qualitative literature. *Birth*, *45(2)*, 109–119.

Orbach-Zinger, S., Bardin, R., Berestizhevsky, Y., Sulkes, J., David, Y., Elchayuk, S., Peleg, D. and Eidelman, L.A. (2008). A survey of attitudes of expectant first-time fathers and mothers toward epidural analgesia for labor. *International Journal of Obstetric Anaesthesia, 17*, 243–246.

Otley, H. (2011). Fear of childbirth: understanding the causes, impact and treatment. *British Journal of Midwifery, 19(4)*, 215–220.

Rayment-Jones, H., Harris, J., Harden, A., Khan, Z. and Sandall, J. (2019). How do women with social risk factors experience United Kingdom maternity care? A realist synthesis. *Birth, 46(3)*, 461–463.

Rayment-Jones, H., Murrells, T. and Sandall, J. (2015). An investigation of the relationship between the caseload model of midwifery for socially disadvantaged women and childbirth outcomes using routine data – a retrospective, observational study. *Midwifery, 31(4)*, 409–417.

Reiger, K. and Dempsey, R. (2006). Performing birth in a culture of fear: an embodied crisis of late modernity. *Health Sociology Review, 15(4)*, 364–373.

Saisto, T. and Halmesmäki, E. (2003). Fear of childbirth: a neglected dilemma. *Acta Obstetrica et Gynecologica Scandinavia, 82*, 201–208.

Saisto, T, Salmela-Aro, K., Nurmi, J.E. and Halmesmäki, E. (2001). Psychosocial characteristics of women and their partners fearing vaginal childbirth. *British Journal of Obstetrics and Gynaecology, 108*, 492–498.

Sandall, J., Leap, N., Grant, J. and Bastos, M.H. (2010). Supporting women to have a normal birth: development and field testing of a learning package for maternity staff. Health and Social Care Research Division, King's College London.

Sanders, R. (2015). Midwifery facilitation: exploring the functionality of labor discomfort. Commentary. *Birth, 42(3)*, 202–205.

Simpson, M. and Catling, C. (2016). Understanding psychological traumatic birth experiences: a literature review. *Women and Birth, 29(3)*, 203–207.

Stoll, K. and Hall, W. (2013a). Vicarious birth experiences and childbirth fear: does it matter how young Canadian women learn about birth? *The Journal of Perinatal Education, 22(4)*, 226–233.

Stoll, K. and Hall, W. (2013b). Attitudes and preferences of young women with low and high fear of childbirth. *Qualitative Health Research, 23(11)*, 1495–1505.

Stoll, K., Swift, E.M., Fairbrother, N., Nethery, E. and Janssen, P. (2018). A systematic review of non-pharmacological prenatal interventions for pregnancy-specific anxiety and fear of childbirth. *Birth, 45(1)*, 7–18.

Vitek, K. and Ward, L.M. (2019). Risky, dramatic, and unrealistic: reality television portrayals of pregnancy and childbirth and their effects on women's fear and self-efficacy. *Health Communication, 34(11)*, 1289–1295.

Waldenstrom, U., Hildingsson, I. and Ryding, E.L. (2006). Antenatal fear of childbirth and its association with subsequent cesarean section and experience of childbirth. *British Journal of Obstetrics and Gynaecology, 113*, 638–646.

Wee, K.Y., Weea, K.Y., Skouteris, H., Pier, C., Richardson, B. and Milgrom, J. (2011). Correlates of ante- and postnatal depression in fathers: a systematic review. *Journal of Affective Disorders, 130*, 358–377.

Welsh Government (2019) Maternity Care in Wales: a Five Year Vision for the Future (2019–2024). https://gov.wales/sites/default/files/publications/2019-06/maternity-care-in-wales-a-five-year-vision-for-the-future-2019-2024.pdf.

Wickham, S. (2017). Thinking outside the box. Untangling tocophobia. *The Practising Midwife, 20(7)*. Accessed via Sara Wickham's blog 9 January 2021: https://www.sarawickham.com/articles-2/untangling-tocophobia/.

Wigert, H., Nilsson, C., Dencker, A., Begley, C., Jangsten, E., Sparud-Lundin, C., . . . Patel, H. (2020). Women's experiences of fear of childbirth: a metasynthesis of qualitative studies. *International Journal of Qualitative Studies on Health and Well-being, 15(1)*, 1704484.

4 Supporting women preparing for labour and birth

Introduction

Kerreen Reiger and Rhea Dempsey (2006) have likened the support that women need in preparation for birth to the sort of support that is required when producing a creative theatrical performance or striving to achieve optimal performance in a sporting activity. They suggest that the type of psychological and physiological processes encountered in preparing for such events are highly individual, but always involve others:

> As the self is social, the role of support becomes critical to sustaining self-direction and to maintaining confidence in the capacity to accomplish the task.
>
> (p.369)

In this chapter, we shall explore various approaches to helping pregnant women and their birth companions prepare for labour and birth, including thinking through what sort of support they might need. We begin with a brief description of the evolving nature of 'childbirth education' (referred to by a variety of names, including, for example, 'antenatal education' or 'preparation for parenthood').

Preparation for childbirth: changing attitudes and practices

The genesis of 'childbirth education'

Prior to organised 'childbirth education', in most cultures, women learnt about birth and baby care from female relatives (Nolan, 1997). This persisted during the early decades of the twentieth century in Western countries at a time when healthcare systems were evolving and professional 'experts' (physiotherapists, health visitors and midwives) began to see it as their role to 'educate' pregnant women through didactic, strict instructions about diet, exercise, infant feeding and baby care.

In 1933, Grantly Dick-Read (1890–1959) published *Childbirth Without Fear: The Principles and Practice of Natural Childbirth* and launched the concept of eliminating the cycle of 'fear, tension and pain' through counteractive education and training. Gentle, coached breathing and relaxation, with the emphasis on collaboration with the coach, were to play a vital role in keeping the woman on course through labour (Dick-Read, 1933). (This classic text was reissued in 2013 by Pinter & Martin with a new Foreword by Ina May Gaskin. The publicity for the book claims that: 'In an age where birth has often been overtaken by obstetrics, Dr Dick-Read's philosophy is still as fresh and relevant as it was when he originally wrote this book.')

DOI: 10.4324/9781003092520-5

The development of childbirth education 'classes'

From the 1950s, *Childbirth Without Fear* provided a foundation for community-organised programmes or 'classes' focused on preparing women to give birth 'naturally'. In her autobiography, Sheila Kitzinger (2015) describes how women in the UK who wanted to promote Grantly Dick-Read's teaching formed the Natural Childbirth Association in 1956 (later to become the National Childbirth Trust). Across the Western world, the sharing of information on a mother-to-mother basis soon incorporated a package of breathing and relaxation techniques known as 'psychoprophylaxis', developed by French obstetrician Fernand Lamaze after visiting Russia in the early 1950s (Michaels, 2014; Shilling and Bingham, 2010).

The Active Birth movement

In the late 1980s, in high-income countries, childbirth education gradually adopted less structured approaches to preparation for labour and birth than simply psychoprophylaxis. The concept of 'Active Birth' (Balaskas, 1983) embraced the benefits of women being supported to follow their instincts, move around, adopt different positions and use water for comfort in labour; this happened many years before these activities were validated by research evidence.

'Active Birth' became the mainstay of childbirth education across the Western world, developing further with emerging understandings of the complex influences of psychology, sexuality and the environment on the neuro-hormonal physiology of labour (Buckley, 2009, 2010, 2015; Buckley and Uvnäs Moberg, 2019; Foureur, 2008; Odent and Odent, 2015; Uvnäs Moberg, 2019; Walsh, 2006). For many of us, this has meant an imperative to share with women and their birth companions the important evidence of creating an environment of non-disturbance and privacy in labour.

Box 4.1   Reflective Activity: Enabling 'Active Birth' and 'non-disturbance' in labour

In pairs or small groups:
- Make a list of the points you would make when talking to women and their birth companions about 'Active Birth' and 'non-disturbance' in labour. Provide an annotated bibliography of key texts and resources related to these concepts. These could be compiled into a resource to share with colleagues.

'Classes' offered by maternity services and the notion of 'choice'

Over recent decades, the emphasis of childbirth education classes provided by maternity services has shifted towards offering information to equip women to make 'informed choices'. This has often meant a strong focus on information about pharmacological pain relief – the 'menu' that we discussed in Chapter 2 – and explaining common medical interventions, rather than a focus on advising women about how they can optimise their chances of having a straightforward labour and birth (Bergström *et al.*, 2009; Lothian, 2008; Morton and Hsu, 2007).

Anecdotal evidence provides examples of situations where midwives have come under pressure from their employers to maintain the status quo and avoid any challenges to the policies and practices of the maternity service (Walker *et al.*, 2009). Out of respect for women and the notion of 'informed choice', there is sometimes a reluctance to advocate for the value of normal birth, particularly where this involves challenging the choices they make (Morton and Hsu, 2007).

Box 4.2   Recommended Resource: Midwives as childbirth educators

Wickham, S. and Davies, L. (2005). Are midwives empowered enough to offer empowering education? Chapter 5 in M. Nolan and J. Foster (eds), *Birth and Parenting Skills* (pp. 69–83). Edinburgh: Churchill Livingstone.

In asking this thorny question, the authors offer some useful ideas about what an empowering model of childbirth education might look like, whilst recognising the pressures and challenges that many employed midwives face when facilitating classes and groups.

Birth plans: negotiations and choice for women?

The idea of women making a 'birth plan' was pioneered by Sheila Kitzinger in the 1960s and 1970s as a way of stimulating discussion and negotiations between women and their caregivers and enabling women to have more control over their birth experiences (Kitzinger, 1962, 2015).

Box 4.3   Research Briefing: Birth plans

Lothian, J. (2006). Birth plans: the good, the bad, and the future. *Journal of Obstetric, Gynecologic and Neonatal Nursing, 35*(2), 295–303. doi:10.1111/J.1552-6909.2006.00042.x.

Judith Lothian explores the history, purpose and potential of birth plans. She suggests that the tensions between health professionals and childbearing women caused by birth plans reflect the larger problems within contemporary maternity care, including conflicting ideologies about birth.

As the notion of 'choice' became increasingly prevalent in documents related to childbirth, in many places, the concept of a 'birth plan' became visible in maternity care notes. Today, this is often one section within the notes with prescribed tick-boxes or check lists identifying specific choices that the woman can make about her care. This is in contrast to the original concept of an individualised birth plan made by the woman and her partner to stimulate discussion with staff about their wishes.

Box 4.4   Reflective Activity: Thinking about birth plans and choice

The NHS Choices website offers an interactive resource for women wishing to make a birth plan. In order to prepare for this, links are provided to information and short videos on a large range of topics:

www.nhs.uk/conditions/pregnancy-and-baby/pages/birth-plan.aspx#close.

- As you explore the resources and watch the video clips, imagine that you are a pregnant woman who wants to make a birth plan and is anxious about how she and her partner will cope with labour.

In pairs or small groups:
- Discuss how you felt as you explored the website, particularly in relation to pain in labour and support.
- What did you learn from this activity in terms of how you discuss making a birth plan with pregnant women?
- Discuss how this resource sits with the critique of birth plans provided by Judith Lothian (Box 4.3 and her suggestion that the three questions that birth plans should address are:

  - What will I do to stay confident and feel safe?
  - What will I do to find comfort in response to my contractions?
  - Who will support me through labour, and what will I need from them?

(Lothian, 2006, p.300)

Preparing for childbirth via the Internet

Undoubtedly the main source of information for pregnant women and their partners today is the Internet (Ahmadian *et al.*, 2020; Johansson *et al.*, 2010; Larsson, 2009; Romano, 2007; Sayakhot and Carolan-Olah, 2016). It is therefore important that antenatal educators are familiar with the main websites that prospective parents visit and have a short list of web resources to recommend (Romano, 2007). We would add that this applies to all birth workers who engage with pregnant women and that we should also be familiar with the reality TV shows that are informing women's understanding of labour and birth.

A systematic review of studies identifying the ways in which pregnant women use the Internet suggests that women tend not to discuss the information they are accessing during antenatal consultations unless a discussion is initiated by the maternity care provider. Unless we ask, we remain oblivious to potentially inaccurate information or mistaken beliefs about pregnancy that women are accessing (Sayakhot and Carolan-Olah, 2016). There is an imperative to guide pregnant women to high-quality, evidence-informed, web-based resources and to take the opportunity to discuss this information with them during antenatal visits

(Larsson, 2009). The following activity challenges us to explore the sort of conversations this might involve.

Box 4.5   Reflective Activity: Discussing Internet information sources with a pregnant woman

Pre-reading:

Sayakhot, P. and Carolan-Olah, M. (2016). Internet use by pregnant women seeking pregnancy-related information: a systematic review. *BMC Pregnancy and Childbirth, 16(65).* doi:10.1186/s12884-016-0856-5.

Cutajar, L., Miu, M., Fleet, J-A., Cyna A.M. and Steen, M. (2020). Antenatal education for childbirth: labour and birth. *European Journal of Midwifery, 4,* 11. doi:10.18332/ejm/120002.

This activity could be a student assignment* or an activity for individuals, pairs or small groups.

- Choose a topic that you think a pregnant woman who is worried about labour might access via the Internet. Identify at least six websites that she is likely to find, and for each write a short paragraph, critiquing the information provided and the language and images that are used in terms of positive and negative suggestions.
- Drawing on your research, write a short script of a conversation you might have with a woman during an antenatal consultation that has the following features. In response to her mentioning her concerns, you ask her what she has seen on the Internet about the topic she just mentioned; she tells you about a website that you know contains misinformation and negative messages. Discuss the information that the woman has seen, being aware of how best to counter any misinformation, and include a recommendation of other Internet resources she might find useful.
- See Chapter 5 for ideas about language that may promote women's confidence in their abilities.
- Share the resources you have identified in this activity with others in your learning group.

* Note to educators: This activity can be configured as an assignment similar to that described in Chapter 5: 'Communication and thoughtful encouragement'.

Childbirth education in the face of increasing obstetric intervention

The psychological and physiological benefits of normal birth for women and families are widely acknowledged and education initiatives to promote normal birth have been identified as an urgent global imperative (Amis, 2016). As obstetric intervention increasingly pervades maternity care, childbirth educators who are not employed by maternity services tend to continue to prepare women and their partners for birth in ways that seek to potentiate their efforts to have a normal birth. There is little evidence to suggest that this approach alone is successful in terms of decreasing caesarean operations and epidural rates; such changes would require systematic change in the culture and practices of obstetric care (Bergström *et al.*, 2009;

Chen *et al.*, 2018). In light of this, educators feel obliged to share information about routine hospital practices that might constrain a woman's wish to have an active, physiological labour and birth.

Navigating the system

In *Birth with Confidence: Savvy Choices for Normal Birth*, Rhea Dempsey describes navigating the 'technocratic' system of maternity care (Davis-Floyd, 2001) as 'birthing against the odds in the labour-bypass era' (2013, p.35). She suggests that it is not enough to want a normal birth; a 'savvy' woman will plan for appropriate birth companions to support her through any 'crises of confidence' that she might face during labour and attempt to ensure that her wishes are not undermined by the technocratic birth system.

Drawing on her experience of over 30 years of being a childbirth educator and labour companion, Rhea Dempsey explores how a woman's life experiences and personal attitudes to pain will affect how she approaches and prepares for birth. She suggests that, if we are to support women, there is value in understanding a spectrum of approaches to pain in labour. At one end, there are women who make an unwavering choice to avoid all pain in labour and some who have a passive acceptance of 'pain relief' as the status quo proposed by 'experts'. At the other end of the spectrum, 'willing women' embrace pain as part of promoting normal birth and may or may not have thought about the particular sort of support they might need to achieve this. In the middle of the spectrum are women who adopt a 'wait and see' approach, unaware that their pain tolerance can be affected by the sort of support they receive:

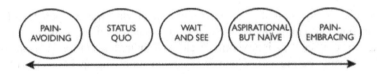

Figure 4.1 'Pain attitudes'

Source: Dempsey, 2013, p.110. Reproduced with kind permission of the author.

Box 4.6   Reflective Activity: Identifying women's individual needs for support in labour

In pairs or small groups:

- Devise five short 'scripts' for conversations (each lasting less than five minutes) that you could have with women who have uncomplicated pregnancies and whose attitudes to pain in labour concur with each of the five approaches outlined in Figure 4.1. Start each script with the question: 'Have you thought about having your baby in the local (free-standing) midwifery-led birth centre or at home?' and see where that takes you in terms of conversations about approaches to managing pain in labour. Include in your script discussions about the sort of labour support that the woman thinks she will need.
- You could share these scripts with others in a classroom or workshop activity through performance and discussion.

Supporting parents to challenge and avoid unnecessary interventions

Most women want to have a physiological labour and birth, but if interventions are necessary, they want to maintain a sense of personal achievement and control through active decision making (Downe *et al.,* 2018). In the USA, the importance of 'shared decision making' is highlighted in initiatives to reduce caesarean birth rates and unnecessary interventions in labour (Wharton *et al.,* 2017; Caughey *et al.,* 2014, 2016). However, leading antenatal educator Penny Simkin has challenged the notion of 'shared decision making', suggesting that this cannot happen when most women do not have a clear understanding of what interventions are and whether they are likely to be beneficial or harmful. She cites the large nationwide survey in the USA, *Listening to Mothers III* (Declercq *et al.,* 2013), which showed that: 'Most women trust their caregivers to give good care; yet caregivers often give inaccurate, incomplete advice; women usually follow their caregiver's recommendation, but feel they made their own decisions; and generally women are poorly informed' (Simkin, 2017, p.293).

Box 4.7   Recommended Resource: Childbirth education for 'shared decision making'

Simkin, P. (2017). Should ACOG support childbirth education as another means to improve obstetric outcomes? Response to ACOG Committee Opinion # 687: approaches to limit intervention during labor and birth. *Birth, 44,* 293–297. doi:10.1111/birt.12306.

In this article, Penny Simkin provides a table identifying the components of childbirth education that equip parents to engage in 'shared decision making' and avoid the following unnecessary interventions: elective induction before 41 or 42 weeks; hospital admission before active labour; induction following spontaneous rupture of membranes when there are no indications; admission to hospital for exhaustion, anxiety or pain in latent labour; and early and coached pushing in second stage.

Supporting pregnant women who have had a previous caesarean birth

Hesitation or reluctance to promote normal birth is, perhaps, most evident in discussions with women who have had a previous caesarean birth. In spite of evidence that vaginal birth after caesarean (VBAC) is a safe and satisfying option for most women, low and declining rates of VBAC are evident in most maternity units in high-income countries (Keedle *et al.,* 2019, 2020). The potential danger of not encouraging women to consider VBAC is that, over time, the repertoire of reassurance about caesarean birth becomes the pervasive ideology.

There are many lessons to be learnt from countries with high VBAC rates (Sweden, Finland and the Netherlands), not least the need for clinicians and services to reflect on their approach to VBAC in order to develop a 'pro-VBAC culture'; this involves a united voice in strengthening women's trust in VBAC (Lundgren *et al.,* 2015, 2020). Women want personalised discussions about their options (Chen and Hancock, 2012) and, for many of them, this includes discussing information that they have accessed via the Internet (Dahlen and Homer, 2013; David *et al.,* 2010):

Box 4.8   Reflective Activity: Learning from women through VBAC blogs

Dahlen, H. and Homer, C. (2013). 'Motherbirth or childbirth'? A prospective analysis of vaginal birth after caesarean blogs. *Midwifery*, *29*, 167–173.

In pairs or small groups:

- After reading this paper, access blogs with women's stories about VBAC and discuss how these reflect the themes of either 'motherbirth' or 'childbirth'.
- Make a list of websites or blogs that you would recommend to women who have had a previous caesarean birth. For each of these, add a few lines identifying why you have chosen to recommend this resource. Consider pooling your annotated lists to form an online resource to share with others.
- Discuss the implications of using the following terms: 'caesarean section'; 'caesarean birth'; or 'caesarean operation' when talking to pregnant women.

Whether it is decision making about VBAC or other choices that they are faced with in pregnancy, the reality is that most women have limited choice and little autonomy as they engage with contemporary maternity services. We could also argue that the way in which information is given heavily influences the choices that women make (Edwards, 2005; Gregg, 1993; Leap and Edwards, 2006; Nolan, 2005, 2010).

'Talking up' positive birth

In an effort to avoid making women feel guilty about birth by caesarean, both women and birth workers often report feeling tentative about 'talking up' the advantages of normal birth:

> At my NCT class, I wanted to talk about the positive sides of birth and how you can manage it without focusing on needing drugs etc. And the teacher actually took me to one side and said, 'I think it's lovely that you feel like that but you have to remember these people are not going to have the experience you're going to have; they haven't got any continuity of care, and you're in a sense giving them false expectations.' And rightly so, I think, in that, out of six of us, the other five all had interventions at some level. So at the class reunion, again I felt silenced; I felt I couldn't talk about my beautiful, life-changing birth at home.
>
> (Mother, Leap, 2007, unpublished data)

Through her website 'Tell me a good birth story', doula and Active Birth teacher Natalie Meddings challenges this code of silence and connects pregnant women with mothers who have positive stories to share about a range of birth experiences (including those that involved obstetric intervention):

> Given so many women today have difficult or even traumatic births, it's not surprising that women with good memories feel the need to keep quiet, or to imply they got lucky. But this is a missed opportunity. Given there's such little knowledge around birth, and

even less confidence, NOT talking to a mother with a good birth story is to waste a really valuable resource . . . Listening to a good birth story is powerful. It's a simple message – 'I did it, so can you.'

In recent years there has been a shift towards talking about 'positive birth' in order to acknowledge that positive experiences of birth are not limited to stories of normal birth. The Positive Birth Movement is a global network connecting pregnant women through groups and social media to share stories, expertise and positivity around birth.

Box 4.9   Recommended Resources: Promoting Positive Birth

We think the websites and books associated with 'Tell me a good birth story' and 'The Positive Birth Movement' are inspiring resources for pregnant women, their families and all birth workers who engage in conversations about how to prepare and support women for labour and birth.

How to have a baby: mother gathered guidance on birth and new babies
Meddings, N. (2017). Founder of 'Tell me a good birth story':
http://www.tellmeagoodbirthstory.com/resources.

The Positive Birth Handbook: A New Approach to Pregnancy, Birth and the Early Weeks.
Give Birth Like a Feminist: Your Body, Your Baby, Your Choices
Hill, M. (2017, 2019). Founder of 'The Positive Birth Movement':
https://www.positivebirthmovement.org.

Childbirth education: moving from classes to groups

Evaluations of childbirth education are fraught with methodological difficulties due to confounding variables and differences in the aims, content and processes in the delivery of programmes (Ferguson *et al.*, 2013; Gagnon and Sandall, 2007; Gilmer *et al.*, 2016). There is little consensus about what should be taught and learnt, other than that multiple approaches are required to suit local parents' needs and that programmes should be interactive and address adult learning principles (Entsieh and Hallström, 2016; Gilmer *et al.*, 2016; Nolan, 2021).

Increasingly, studies show that parents want equal emphasis placed on preparation for giving birth and parenting (Ahldén *et al.*, 2012; Barimani *et al.*, 2018; Entsieh and Hallström, 2016). This evidence has contributed to discussions about the need for a radical rethink in the way that childbirth education classes are offered (Lothian, 2008; Morton and Hsu, 2007; Nolan, 2021, Walker *et al.*, 2009). Emerging from such debates are strong arguments for midwives and other birth workers to set up small, interactive groups in which pregnant women and their partners can come together, share ideas and information and build friendship networks (Koushede *et al.*, 2017; Leap, 2010; Nolan, 2009, 2010; Rising *et al.*, 2004; Schrader McMillan *et al.*, 2009). This approach is summarised by renowned childbirth educator Mary Nolan:

> Education for birth and early parenting is, and needs to be seen as, a primary preven-
> tion measure, with the potential to reduce physical and psychological trauma related to
> labour and to increase sensitive parenting of infants . . . The educator can help parents

anticipate and prepare for the transformative experience of labour and for the challenges that come with a new baby; promote healthy parent–child relationships and secure attachment in babies; increase parents' confidence in their own problem solving, and build a support network amongst the individuals taking the antenatal programme which will reduce their isolation following the birth of their babies.

(Nolan, 2021, p.235)

Box 4.10   Research Briefing: Approaches to childbirth education that are valued by women and their partners

Nolan, M. (2009). Information giving and education in pregnancy: a review of qualitative studies. *The Journal of Perinatal Education, 18(4),* 21–30.

This review confirms women's preference for a small-group learning environment, in which they can talk to each other and the facilitator and relate information to their individual circumstances. Women value a facilitator who is skilled in sharing information in a way that promotes discussion, allows time to practise skills and encourages women to get to know and support each other.

The Deptford Group model – 'groups not classes'

The antenatal group model pioneered by midwives in Deptford (the South East London Midwifery Group Practice) is an example of a service developed through community participation. Later embedded in the NHS service provided by the Albany Midwives (Homer *et al.*, 2017; Nolan and Foster, 2005; Reed and Walton, 2009), the model has been adapted in a variety of settings across the world (Homer *et al.*, 2019; Leap, 2010).

Unlike 'drop in' groups where women can call in to a group session at a time that suits them, these free antenatal groups start and finish at an arranged time. The group is there every week and women can attend at any stage of their pregnancy, as often as they want. There is no fixed agenda for these groups: the content of the discussion and information sharing evolves during the course of each session and is usually triggered by a woman returning to the group with her new baby and telling her story of pregnancy, birth and new motherhood. Women are motivated to continue to enjoy the close friendships that are formed in the antenatal group; therefore they transition to postnatal groups and continue to meet and support each other (Leap, 1991, 2010):

> I think they're probably friends that you'll have for life, even though we're all so different. I would have been very isolated otherwise . . . we formed a network of women who met up outside of the group and carried on meeting for years.
>
> (Mother, Leap, 1991, VHS Video)

Individualised '36-week birth talks'

Another feature of preparation for birth pioneered by midwives in the South-East London Midwifery Group Practice was the 'birth talk' (Reed and Walton, 2009). This is a one-off individualised session in the woman's home when she is 36 weeks' pregnant, which brings together anyone in her family and friendship group who may be involved in supporting her during labour and in the early postnatal period.

The '36-week birth talk' provides an opportunity for midwives to explore choices that the woman might like to make, for example: revisiting the option of birth at home or in a birth centre if her pregnancy is uncomplicated; whether she wants photographs of her labour and birth; what she wants to do with her placenta; or any particular wishes related to her culture or religion. If other children are likely to be involved during the labour, appropriate arrangements can be made for their support.

During a 36-week birth talk, midwives can explain that they will be there during labour as a 'safety net'; they can explain the purpose and nature of pain in labour and their reasons for not offering pain relief routinely. Particular attention can be given to talking through the concept of early labour and building the support group's confidence in their ability to support the woman until labour is well established (phoning the midwives if they have any concerns). Situations that warrant calling the midwife can be discussed as well as giving a simple list of instructions, detailing what to do if the baby is arriving in a hurry before the midwife arrives.

Practical support in the early weeks following birth can be discussed, including the concept of 'bring food, not flowers' and making sure that the new parents have as much rest as possible and private time with their new baby. Rotas (rosters) can be suggested for visiting friends to take responsibility for one prearranged evening each where they will come in and cook, clean, shop or take away washing.

In a study of the role of the 36-week birth talk in the Albany Midwifery Practice, Joy Kemp and Jane Sandall (2010) concluded that the effectiveness of 36-week birth talks cannot be separated from the philosophy and relational continuity offered by the midwives. Their study reinforces the value of embedding 36-week birth talks in caseload practice models of care.

Box 4.11   Research Briefing: 36-week birth talks

Kemp, J. and Sandall, J. (2010). Normal birth, magical birth: the role of the 36-week birth talk in caseload midwifery practice. *Midwifery*, *26*, 211–221. doi:10.1016/j.midw.2008.07.002.

The authors observed midwives communicating an underpinning philosophy that birth is both normal and transformational and that it is an important social and cultural event. Three main themes were identified: a new philosophy for birth ('don't forget the magic'); the construction of authoritative midwifery knowledge ('they make you believe that you can have what you want'); and achieving a sense of coherence ('making sense of the birth').

Incorporating preparation for birth and social support in group antenatal care

Group antenatal care: CenteringPregnancy®

The CenteringPregnancy® model was developed by midwife Sharon Schindler Rising (1998), who piloted it in a Connecticut clinic in 1993–1994. Health assessment (antenatal care), education and support are combined in a structured group programme that replaces the usual schedule of one-to-one antenatal visits. Eight to 12 women – plus or minus partners – who are all at the same stage of pregnancy receive their antenatal care within a group setting where they are also able to engage in facilitated information-sharing sessions and build friendship networks. The same two midwives (or doctors/other maternity care staff) facilitate all the sessions, which usually last about two hours. Women with complicated pregnancies can also attend extra visits with an obstetrician or other specialist (Rising and Quimby, 2017).

Summaries of research articles demonstrating the potential for CenteringPregnancy to improve outcomes and experiences for women and babies can be found on the Centering Healthcare website. The model has been adapted in both high- and low-income countries, with mainstream implementation in the Netherlands (Rijnders *et al.*, 2019). Group antenatal care is recommended by the World Health Organization (WHO, 2018) as an alternative to standard antenatal care where appropriate resources are available, and women's choices are taken into consideration. There is a plethora of videos on YouTube identifying examples of 'group prenatal care' in the USA.

'Preparation for Birth and Beyond' resource

In identifying the need for active learning and social support to take place through participative antenatal groups, researchers at the University of Warwick in the UK have suggested that groups should have a strong focus on relationship building and exploring the complex individual transitions to parenthood experienced by both women and men (Schrader McMillan *et al.*, 2009). Drawing on this research, the Department of Health in the UK (2011) commissioned an interactive, online learning resource:

Box 4.12   Recommended Resource: 'Preparation for Birth and Beyond'

Department of Health, NCT, One Plus One and The Fatherhood Institute (2011). Preparation for Birth and Beyond: a resource pack for leaders of community groups and activities.

https://assets.publishing.service.gov.uk/government/uploads/system/uploads/attachment_data/ file/215386/dh_134728.pdf.

This resource provides a summary of the evidence supplied by Schrader McMillan, Barlow and Redshaw (2009) and aims to support health professionals in developing ideas for running successful groups with the participation of local communities. The overarching goal is to promote initiatives that have the potential to reduce inequalities and support parents to give their children the best start in life.

The framework for facilitating groups using the 'Preparation for Birth and Beyond' approach is outlined, including an overview of associated concepts and theories.

Section 3 of the resource covers the planning of groups: addressing local contexts and actively engaging parents and community support; planning an appropriate programme; and theory about skilful group facilitation.

Six themes form the content of the 'Preparation for Birth and Beyond' programme: 'Our Developing Baby'; 'Changes for Me and Us'; 'Giving Birth and Meeting Our Baby'; 'Caring for Our Baby'; 'Our Health and Wellbeing'; and 'People Who Are There for Us'.

Box 4.13   Reflective Activity: Identifying values in childbirth education

Before engaging in this activity, all participants should access the 'Preparation for Birth and Beyond' resource via the Internet and be familiar with its content.

Agree/disagree activity: large group classroom or workshop activity

Instructions for facilitators:
- Place two large signs, 'Agree' and 'Disagree', at either end of the room and prepare a list of value statements.
- Give the following instructions and keep time:

    1   After I've read out a statement go and stand at either end of the room, depending on whether you agree or disagree with the statement, or stand somewhere in between (in the middle) if you tend to agree/tend not to agree or are not sure.
    2   Talk to someone close to you for *ONE minute* about why you've stood where you are.
    3   Go and stand next to someone in an opposite or different position for *ONE minute* and see if you can persuade them to come and stand with you.

Keep the activity moving on fast, with lots of different value statements, and then finish with a whole group discussion about what they learnt from the activity.
    Some suggestions for value statements (you can make up others):

- Labour and birth are only one day in a woman's life. So the main focus of childbirth education programmes should be on relationships and parenting, not preparing for labour.
- Doulas provide a better quality of support than most male partners.
- Women who want a normal birth should be encouraged to hire a doula.
- The word 'pain' should not be used in childbirth education. Contractions should be referred to as 'surges' or 'rushes'.

Preparing for labour and birth: teaching and learning theories

Having thought about changing attitudes and practices in childbirth education, we will now explore some of the underpinning theories and concepts that inform our efforts to enable situations in which women and their partners can feel empowered as they approach birth and new parenthood.

To help us with this, the 'Preparation for Birth and Beyond' resource, profiled in Box 4.12, provides useful overviews and references about the following topics:

- foetal and early infant development: development of the human brain;
- attachment theory;
- self-efficacy and behaviour change;
- social support and social capital;
- adult learning principles;
- skilful group facilitation.

Skilful group facilitation

Although we may have studied the principles of adult learning (Henderson, 2005; Knowles *et al.*, 2014), many of us have had few opportunities to learn about group facilitation. If this applies to you, we encourage you to attend courses or workshops that will help you develop these skills.

The following activity provides an opportunity to think about how group facilitation skills differ from didactic teaching styles.

Box 4.14   Reflective Activity: Group facilitation – honouring women's expertise

The whole ethos of the antenatal group was about sharing and women having kind of equal expertise. It wasn't about 'experts/novices, women/us'. It was about women who were going through the experience of childbirth and we were all seen as having a valuable contribution to make; we were seen as having our own expertise really to share amongst each other. Somehow that meant that we took more risks, we shared more and therefore, I think, developed deeper friendships.

(Mother, Leap, 1991, VHS Video)

Classroom or workshop activity; in small groups:

• Make a list of responses that you might use when facilitating an antenatal group in order to adopt a facilitative style, one that encourages the contributions of women in the group, as described by the woman in the above quote. (For example: 'That's an interesting idea. What do the rest of you think?')
• List as many potential initial responses as you can to address each of the following situations (you may think of others):

1   Someone asks you what the best position is for giving birth.
2   A woman says she's heard that breastfeeding means the father is less involved with the baby.
3   During a discussion about the latest TV episode of 'One Born Every Minute', someone asks you what you think about women who choose to have an elective caesarean section.
4   A partner says he thinks women are made to feel guilty if they end up having a caesarean.
5   Someone says they've heard that having sex can help get you into labour if you're overdue.
6   A woman says that she doesn't like the idea of doing the perineal massage that someone just spoke about.
7   Someone asks you if it's true that men are more likely to be violent towards their partners if they're pregnant.
8   Someone in the group is taking up a lot of space and obviously needs to talk to you after the group about her particular relationship issues and concerns.

Take it in turns to practise being the facilitator in these situations and any others that you have discussed (initial responses only). Compare and discuss your responses in a facilitated discussion with the whole group.

Self-efficacy and preparation for labour and birth

Self-efficacy refers to an individual's confidence in their ability to exert control over their motivation, behaviour and social environment in order to manage prospective situations. The theory of 'self-efficacy' was developed by psychologist Albert Bandura (1977, 1986, 1997, 2012) and has been applied in a large body of research related to how women approach the challenges of labour and parenting.

Perceived self-efficacy is an important determinant of behaviour; it influences the choices people make and how they feel and behave when facing challenges. The higher someone's self-efficacy, the more likely they are to exert effort around intentions and try previously feared actions (Ajzen and Madden, 1986; Gollwitzer, 1993).

Research related to childbirth education and self-efficacy

Nancy K. Lowe first identified maternal confidence in coping with labour as a self-efficacy concept in 1991; she subsequently pioneered the development of the 'Childbirth Self-Efficacy Inventory' (CBSEI), a self-reporting instrument that measures women's perceived self-efficacy for coping with an approaching birth (Lowe, 1991, 1993, 2000). The CBSEI has been used in many studies in both high and low-income countries. This overall consistency in how childbirth self-efficacy is defined and measured facilitates international comparison and synthesis (Tilden *et al.*, 2016). Childbirth education activities appear to make a significant positive difference in maternal perinatal self-efficacy, for both nulliparous and multiparous women. This results in a wide variety of improved perinatal outcomes, including: a reduction in fear and anxiety in pregnancy and labour; decreased use of pharmacological pain relief in labour; a reduction in depression and anxiety in the postnatal period; and enhanced adaptation to motherhood (Tilden *et al.*, 2016; Timmermans *et al.*, 2019).

Bandura's self-efficacy model

A person's self-efficacy can change as a result of learning and experience; hence the relevance to preparation for labour and birth. According to Albert Bandura (1977, 1997), apart from initiatives that reduce stress and anxiety, there are three main factors that can increase a person's self-efficacy expectancies:

- *performance accomplishments* – successful coping experiences in the past and/or building confidence through simulation or practising tasks;
- *vicarious experience* – opportunities to learn from others, including observation of their successful coping experiences;
- *social or verbal persuasion* – encouragement from someone who is influential and respected.

Box 4.15   Recommended Resource: Researching women's self-efficacy for labour and birth

Campbell, V. and Nolan, M. (2019). 'It definitely made a difference': a grounded theory study of yoga for pregnancy and women's self-efficacy for labour. *Midwifery*, *68*, 74–83.

This paper is an interesting example of how qualitative research findings about an initiative for pregnant women can be mapped against Nancy K. Lowe's and Albert Bandura's (1997) self-efficacy models. Summarised by the paper's authors in Table 1 and Figure 4 , this mapping brings to life the theory of self-efficacy as it relates to 'real-life' women's voices and experiences. We think this paper is particularly useful for sharing with students who are learning about self-efficacy as well as those who have an interest in yoga for pregnancy research.

Childbirth education: core components of programmes

As we discuss some of the core components of most childbirth education programmes, we will offer some examples of how these may be addressed in practice.

De-mystifying the physiology of childbirth

Prospective parents appreciate having explanations about the physiological processes associated with labour. A childbirth educator and birth supporter explains how these explanations enhance understanding:

> It's about talking to the woman about labour and about her body and explaining what's going to happen, so that she understands why she's doing it, what the contractions actually mean. So, showing her diagrams of what's happening inside her body . . . this is what the contractions are doing at this stage of labour, this is what's happening.
> (Childbirth educator/birth supporter, Sandall *et al.*, 2010, p.47)

This process of de-mystification can be particularly useful in building women's confidence in their abilities if explanations are woven into discussions throughout pregnancy in groups or consultations with a midwife (Finlayson *et al.*, 2015).

Physical skills for labour

In hospital environments instinctive behaviours that enhance oxytocin levels are often compromised; it is therefore important to teach and practise physical skills for labour that women can resort to, such as position changes that enhance gravity, massage and working with the rhythm of their breathing (Nolan, 2021). This involves helping partners practise skills that they may need to support the woman in achieving an 'Active Birth'.

Breathing, relaxation and adopting different positions

Traditionally, childbirth education classes have included practising slow breathing, relaxation and adopting different positions.

Box 4.16   Research Briefing: Breathing, relaxation and postures

Slade, P., Escott, D., Spiby, H., Henderson, B. and Fraser, R.B. (2000). Antenatal predictors and use of coping strategies in labour. *Psychology and Health*, *15*(*4*), 555–569. doi:10.1080/08870440008402013.

Researchers at the University of Sheffield in the UK aimed to see if the coping strategies for labour taught in a class were actually used by women subsequently in labour. Women were likely to use the slow breathing strategy, but the use of relaxation and different postures was limited. The discussion section of this paper offers some useful suggestions for why this might have been the case.

Encouraging women to find their own coping strategies

The group of researchers profiled in Box 4.16 have published subsequent research suggesting that pregnant women should be encouraged to explore a wider range of strategies than breathing, relaxation and adopting different postures. They suggest cognitive-based strategies, enabling women to find their own coping strategies, drawing on what instinctively feels right at the time, and their unique knowledge of how they have coped with pain and anxiety in previous situations (Spiby *et al.*, 2003; Escott *et al.*, 2004; Escott *et al.*, 2009).

Speaking from our experience, it is usually not helpful to suggest to women that they should relax during strong contractions and breathe in a certain way:

> We were given the impression that if we could relax and breathe slowly throughout each contraction we would be able to manage. That was OK in early labour but when the contractions got strong I couldn't relax and felt like I wasn't coping.
>
> (Mother, Leap, 2015, unpublished data)

Both of us have attended labours where women have met the intensity of contractions with equally intense physical actions, before sinking into relaxation and slow breathing *between* contractions. For example, we have been with women who have run up and down on the spot throughout contractions; women who have shouted rhythmically or beat their fists on a pillow; a singer who soared from low to high in a crescendo that threatened to shatter windows – to name just a few intense behaviours that some women have discovered as their coping mechanisms.

We suggest that the key message for pregnant women should be that their bodies will tell them which positions will be most helpful and that, with appropriate support and a conducive environment, they will find ways of managing contractions.

Perhaps the most useful phrases to embed in women's minds when practising any strategies for labour are these: 'You've got a contraction coming now, relax, breathe, *go with it*. . . . The contraction has gone, take a deep breath to blow it away, relax and enjoy the rest'. Anecdotally, women who practise this say they remembered the words as each contraction started and that 'going with it' encompassed either finding, or being supported to try, a range of rhythm activities, such as, for example, rocking, swaying, moving, tapping, moaning or roaring (Escott *et al.*, 2009; Escott *et al.*, 2004). We shall discuss this more in subsequent chapters when we talk about support during labour.

Box 4.17 Recommended Resource: Heli, S. (2021) *Give Birth*
Without Fear: Practical Tools for a Confident Birth.
London: Clink Street Publishing.

Originally published as *Confident Birth*, this book by physiotherapist and doula
Susanna Heli offers some simple techniques linking emotions and birth physiology:
breathing, relaxation, the voice and the mind. These techniques can be explored with
pregnant women and their birth partners to help them practise physical skills for labour
and build confidence as they approach birth.

The 'Robertson Flexible Pelvis Activity'

Ina May Gaskin (2003, p.193) describes Andrea Robertson's demonstration of how the pelvis opens when we are on hands and knees as 'a wonderfully empowering exercise for creating awareness of this ability'. Many people (including obstetricians) in Andrea's workshops
have found it surprising how much their hands move as they feel an increase in the distance
between their pubic bone and tailbone after leaning forward. This helps them understand
and remember the importance of upright and all fours positions when supporting women for
labour and birth. As Andrea explained to Nicky:

> My goal is for this activity to become widespread so that pregnant women know how
> well their bodies are designed for giving birth and for men to appreciate this as well so
> they can be supportive when the time comes.
>
> (Leap, 2015, personal communication with Andrea Robertson)

Figure 4.2 'Learning about the pelvis'

Source: Robertson, 2006a, p.146. Reproduced with permission of the author.

If you have a model of a pelvis handy you can use it to demonstrate how the reverse of this opening up movement applies when a woman is lying semi-prone or sitting:

Figure 4.3 'Learning about the pelvis'

Source: Robertson, 2006a, p.146. Reproduced with permission of the author.

Box 4.18   Recommended Resource: 'Skills for Childbirth Educators' DVD

This DVD is in two sections: 'Learning About the Pelvis' and 'Using Models Effectively.' Andrea Robertson (2006b) demonstrates how information can be presented and how to use teaching resources like a doll and pelvis and knitted uterus effectively with individuals or in a group setting.

Available from: Birth International. https://birthinternational.com/product/skills-for-childbirth-educators-dvd-ntsc/.

Box 4.19   Reflective Activity: Demystifying physiology

In pairs or small groups:

- Take it in turns to practise doing the 'Robertson Flexible Pelvis Activity' as if you were showing a pregnant woman and her partner how to do it.
- Develop a 'script' that incorporates the activity in a discussion about 'helpful' positions for labour and birth.
- Whilst engaging in this activity, consider the language you use, with reference to the New Zealand study, 'Women's perspectives of the stages and phases of labour' (Dixon *et al.*, 2013), which suggests that talking to pregnant women about labour using the language of 'stages of labour' and 'cervical dilatation' is not helpful, particularly for fostering women's innate understanding of how their labour progresses.
- Make a list of the points you could cover in a session describing the physiology of labour and birth, including labour progress and the hormonal physiology of childbirth. What teaching aids might you use to help you and where might you access these?

(You might want to knit a uterus if you do not already have one – see pattern for this resource at the end of this chapter.)

In filmed interviews (Sandall *et al.*, 2010), women identified that learning about physiology was particularly useful when it was incorporated into activities such as: storytelling; the sharing of birth photos; and the 'acting out' of potential labour behaviours and sounds by the midwife. We shall explore each of these activities in turn.

Storytelling in antenatal groups

In reflecting on their experiences of antenatal groups, women have described the impact of hearing a woman talk about her labour 'with her baby in her arms'. This appeared to affect the way they processed descriptions of pain and the challenges of labour and enabled links to be made between 'abstract information' and real-life experience:

> As a woman was telling her story about how her baby had got stuck, the midwife picked up a doll and pelvis and showed what had been going on. It stayed in my head because it was attached to real people. It wasn't abstract information you were getting. It was associated with women in the group so it got absorbed differently.
>
> (Leap, 1991, VHS Video)

Women remembered these stories during labour and saw them as a useful frame of reference and source of encouragement, even when they were about complicated labours:

> But even the sort of negative birth stories in the antenatal group were positive, that's the weird thing. . . . Even though they ought to have been traumatised by the experience. They sort of weren't, they were still incredibly positive and joyful about it . . . which made me feel very confident as well.
>
> (Mother, Sandall *et al.*, 2010, p.40)

Talking about birth using photos

In antenatal groups, at 36-week birth talks, or during discussions that arise informally in an antenatal visit, women appreciate looking at photos depicting women's experiences of labour and birth (Leap *et al.*, 2010; Sandall *et al.*, 2010, p.43). A combination of stories and photos can provide a sense of 'reality' that counteracts some of the sanitised or calamitous views of birth in the media. Women have talked about remembering the photographs when trying different positions and using water during labour. Photos were also useful for their partners in helping them prepare to offer labour support:

> He's a bit squeamish to be honest, [laughs] . . . but the midwives made him feel that it wasn't just, 'Look at these birth photos', you know, they were talking through them and explaining everything, and I think that really helped him to realise that it was all quite normal, and it wasn't going to be scary at all . . . they really did make us both feel at ease.
> All the pain and agony in the pictures before and then afterwards it was all gone, just these beautiful, clear faces. That was one thing that stood out.
>
> (Mother, Sandall *et al.*, 2010, p.43)

There are some excellent images of labour and birth available for purchase from organisations that sell childbirth teaching aids. It is worth considering, however, that these tend to set up a dynamic where the facilitator is 'teaching' about what is going on using a teaching aid. The sharing of small photos and a related story – whether by the woman herself or the facilitator (with permission from the woman) – is quite different from the use of large, professional photographs. As one woman put it: 'It was like someone sharing their holiday snaps and we were able to have a good look and ask questions about what happened'. In our experience, the focus on people in the photos can feel a safer way to promote discussion than relying on participants to raise personal queries about abstract information.

Box 4.20   Reflective Activity: Using birth photos in groups

If you do not have labour and birth photos, you can access some from websites that offer free downloads of childbirth images.

In small groups:
- Practise sharing these photos with the group and use them to tell a story (this can be imaginary).
- Discuss how the images triggered discussion and information sharing about labour, birth and new parenthood.

Simulating labour behaviours and sounds

It is not unusual to see midwives and childbirth educators simulating the noises, movements and behaviours that women might make when managing contractions. This can promote the adoption of appropriate positions for labour and giving birth and stimulate discussion on a range of issues, including comfort measures:

> I think that people find that a good way of learning, it's not frightening and threatening in the way that sometimes watching a woman giving labour might be on a DVD or TV . . . they don't mind me pretending to be a labouring woman, and it makes them laugh some-times, and it might make them a bit uncomfortable too, but they take on board how women might be in labour.
>
> (Childbirth educator/birth supporter, Sandall *et al.*, 2010, unpublished data)

Box 4.21   Reflective Activity: Simulating labour behaviour and sounds

In pairs:
- Make a list of the salient points you might include in both the acting out and infor-mation sharing around each of the following phases of labour:
  - early labour
  - established labour
  - transition
  - expulsive contractions
  - crowning
  - the moment of birth
  - physiological third stage

In turn, practise 'acting out' each of these and then discuss:
- how comfortable you feel 'acting out' each of these experiences;
- the responses you might encounter from the woman and her birth companions and how these might stimulate discussion.

Emerging models of childbirth education

Increasingly in high-income countries, pregnant women are turning to programmes that have an integrated 'mind-body' focus, using mindfulness meditation, yoga and self-hypnosis techniques (Simkin, 2002). We suggest that you access information about such programmes via the Internet, including any that are in your local area, as this is often how women both learn about and describe their experiences of these programmes.

Mindfulness-based childbirth and parenting

Increasingly, studies are identifying the potential for mindfulness-based childbirth education programmes to increase women's feelings of self-efficacy, reduce fear of labour, and improve maternal mental health, with positive effects on the health of children (Braeken *et al.*, 2017; Byrne *et al.*, 2014; Duncan *et al.*, 2017). Several small studies have shown that pregnant women who receive mindfulness training find it beneficial for helping them cope with stress and anxiety (Duncan and Bardacke, 2010; Guardino *et al.*, 2014; Vieten and Astin, 2007). In all of these studies, women particularly valued reductions in their anxiety when coping with the challenges of new motherhood.

Box 4.22   Research Briefing: Mindfulness and preparation for childbirth

Hughes, A., Williams, M., Bardacke, N., Duncan, L.G., Dimidjian, S. and Goodman, S.H. (2009). Mindfulness approaches to childbirth and parenting. *British Journal of Midwifery, 17(10)*, 630–635. Available via Open Access PMC: www.ncbi.nlm.nih.gov/pmc/articles/PMC3846392.

This article presents a useful overview of how mindfulness meditation has been used in healthcare and the potential of mindfulness approaches for parents preparing for childbirth. Three areas are highlighted: managing pain during pregnancy and labour; reducing the risk of perinatal depression; and increasing the 'availability' of attention for the infant. Case studies help to illuminate each of these areas. The authors conclude that there is sufficient evidence to suggest that mindfulness has an important contribution to make, both for reducing vulnerability in high risk groups and as a universal intervention.

In 1998, Nancy Bardacke, an American certified nurse-midwife, developed the ten-session Mindfulness-Based Childbirth and Parenting (MBCP) programme, incorporating childbirth education and the teaching of mindfulness skills. A detailed description of the MBCP programme is provided in the reporting of a pilot study exploring the potential effects on labour, birth and parenting (Walker *et al.*, 2009).

In *Mindful Birthing: Training the Mind, Body and Heart for Childbirth and Beyond*, and on her website (www.mindfulbirthing.org), Nancy Bardacke (2012) explains how MBCP aims to enhance joy and well-being and promote women's self-coping mechanisms so that they can address anxiety, stress, fear and the physical symptoms that may be challenging during pregnancy, labour and early parenting.

Box 4.23   Recommended Resource: 'Mindful birthing'

Bardacke, N. (2012). *Mindful Birthing: Training the Mind, Body and Heart for Childbirth and Beyond*. New York: Harper One.

In this book, Nancy Bardacke speaks in the first person to a pregnant woman. With an immediacy and warmth, she shares experiences, information, evidence and stories about the potential of mindfulness to enhance pregnancy, labour and birth, and early parenting. This is an informative and useful resource for students, midwives, childbirth educators and all others who are engaged in supporting women through childbirth and new motherhood.

Mindfulness practice in preparation for labour: 'being in the moment'

Women who are able to be in the moment without being judgemental about their thoughts and sensations may be less fearful of birth (Byrne *et al.*, 2014; Dunn *et al.*, 2012) and more willing to experience the intensity of contractions. They may also be able to engage positive thoughts when labour does not go according to their expectations, for example if they decide to use pain relief after all or require interventions (Byrne *et al.*, 2014; Duncan and Bardacke, 2010).

It is possible that, instead of being overwhelmed by fear and loss of control in labour, women who have engaged in mindfulness practice are able to accept each contraction as it comes, working with the pain, rather than resisting it or focusing on pain relief (Hughes *et al.*, 2009). According to an Australian study, there is value in encouraging all women to adopt this 'being in the moment' approach (Hughes *et al.*, 2009). The researchers concluded that a mindfulness state of mind may be ideal to help women avoid catastrophising when facing the individual challenges posed by labour. This point has significant implications for supporting women in labour, since the majority will not have had mindfulness training. The approach is in keeping with the traditional words of encouragement used by midwives and birth companions: 'Welcome the contraction . . . go with it, concentrate on each one as it comes.'

Box 4.24   Reflective Activity: Explaining 'mindfulness' approaches in labour

In pairs or small groups:
- Discuss how you might describe 'mindfulness' approaches in labour to a pregnant woman and her birth companions.
- How might this be different (or not) if you were talking to a sceptical midwifery or medical colleague?

Yoga for pregnancy

The value of yoga for enabling women to feel calm and use pain management strategies effectively in labour is gaining attention (Jones *et al.,* 2012). If you search for studies of yoga for pregnancy, you will find a plethora of articles. You may want to return to Box 4.15 where we profiled a grounded theory study identifying how the benefits of yoga in pregnancy relate to building women's self-efficacy (Campbell and Nolan, 2019). Commenting on an earlier part of this study, Virginia Campbell and Mary Nolan (2016) suggest that it was not just the traditional elements of yoga that played a part in building women's self-efficacy: the beneficial effects of safe, women-only groups, where women can share anxieties, experiences and stories, and where pain-coping strategies for labour can learn be learned and practised, should not be underestimated.

'Hypnobirthing' and 'calm birth'

Many pregnant women who want to have a normal birth are attending programmes with a focus on 'self-hypnosis', which is generally referred to as 'hypnobirthing' (Whitburn *et al.,* 2014). Also based on subconscious mind therapies are courses called 'calm birthing'. There are websites that address the confusion about the difference between 'hypnobirthing' and 'calm birthing' courses. The common aim is to provide programmes where prospective parents can engage in a method that helps them release the fear and negativity of social conditioning around childbirth and replace it with calm confidence; thus they are able to engage with the experience of pregnancy and birth in a joyful and positive way, including when birth brings unexpected challenges (Walker *et al.,* 2009).

Hypnobirthing and calm birth programmes enable women and their birth companions to practise using relaxation, visualisation and focused attention techniques. This prepares women to enter a hypnotic or 'trance'-like state in labour that increases their receptivity to positive verbal and non-verbal communications, referred to as 'suggestions' (Graves, 2012). As we shall explore in the next chapter, pregnant women have an increased ability to respond to subconscious messages; this means an enhanced opportunity to engage in self-hypnosis techniques in preparation for childbirth (Cyna *et al.,* 2004).

The Internet is a rich source of information about hypnobirthing and calm birthing, especially YouTube postings, where parents from different countries describe their experiences. In order to begin to appraise research around this subject we suggest you access the following articles:

Box 4.25   Research Briefing: Self-hypnosis for labour and birth

Madden, K., Middleton, P., Cyna, A.M., Matthewson, M. and Jones, L. (2016). Hypnosis for pain management during labour and childbirth. *Cochrane Database of Systematic Reviews 2016*, Issue 5. Art. No.: CD009356. doi:10.1002/14651858.CD009356.pub3.

Phillips-Moore, J. (2012). Birthing outcomes from an Australian HypnoBirthing programme. *British Journal of Midwifery, 20(8)*, 558–564.

Finlayson, K., Downe, S. and Hinder, S. (2015). Unexpected consequences: women's experiences of a self-hypnosis intervention to help with pain in labour. *BMC Pregnancy and Childbirth, 15(229)*.

Box 4.26   Reflective Activity: Discussing hypnobirthing and calm birthing with women and their birth companions

In pairs or small groups:
- Read the papers in the research briefings above.
- Access women's accounts of using self-hypnosis and calm birthing for labour via personal experience and/or on the Internet, including YouTube.
- Discuss how the research findings compare with women's accounts.
- Using evidence from all of these sources, write a short 'script' together, describing the words you might use when a woman in early pregnancy asks you, 'What do you think about hypnobirthing/calm birthing? We've been reading about it on the Internet and were wondering whether we should do it.'

We shall return to self-hypnosis in Chapter 6, where we explore how we can support women in labour who have prepared using hypnobirthing methods.

Complementary therapies in preparation for labour and birth

As we discussed earlier there is no conclusive evidence that antenatal education counteracts rising epidural and caesarean rates. In Box 4.27 we highlight a notable exception that is attracting attention.

Box 4.27   Research Briefing: A complementary therapies course to reduce interventions

Levett, K.M, Smith, C.A, Bensoussan, A. and Dahlen, H.G. (2016). Complementary therapies for labour and birth study: a randomised controlled trial of antenatal integrative medicine for pain management in labour. *BMJ Open Access, 6.* doi:10.1136/ bmjopen-2015-010691.

In this randomised controlled trial, women who attended a two-day course involving acupressure, visualisation and relaxation, breathing, massage, yoga techniques and facilitated partner support were significantly less likely to use epidurals, with reduced rates of augmentation, caesarean section, length of second stage, any perineal trauma and resuscitation of the newborn.

Levett, K.M. (2016). The complementary therapies for labour and birth study making sense of labour and birth – experiences of women, partners and midwives of a complementary medicine antenatal education course. *Midwifery, 40,* 124–131.

In the qualitative arm of the study, women and their partners described how the knowledge they had gained about normal birth physiology helped them make sense of labour and to use the techniques they had learned to support normal birth and reduce interventions in labour.

Conversations about birth: opening and closing doors

Mary Nolan highlights a key challenge confronting anyone engaged in childbirth education in its broadest sense:

> The resources needed for normal birth are those which women already possess. Their internal resource is their instinctive understanding of how to give birth to their babies, and their external resource is the support provided by the people who are with them during labour. Both of these resources operate more powerfully when birth takes place in a social or family context, such as a home-like birth centre or the woman's own home, where she is looked after by professionals who understand and trust the normal process of birth . . . Convincing parents-to-be of these truths is the challenge confronting antenatal education.
>
> (Nolan, 2021, p.237)

Whether or not we provide structured 'childbirth education', we all engage in conversations about labour and birth with pregnant women and their families during our professional and everyday lives. The way we provide information can have a profound effect on the way women and their partners approach birth and grapple with all the uncertainties around decision-making (Leap and Edwards, 2006).

'Keeping an open mind' about possibilities

We have probably all seen colleagues talk about 'keeping an open mind' in a way that encourages confidence about the choices women can make, for example around giving birth at home, where this is an option:

> You meet lots of women who say, 'Really? Am I allowed to have a home birth? I've got that choice?' So, it's kind of planting that seed in their mind early on. . . . So you talk about it throughout the antenatal period but also they can decide in labour, because that's the time when they know how they're going to feel, especially with first babies.
>
> (Midwife, Sandall *et al.*, 2010, p.35)

We may also have heard 'keeping an open mind' used in a way that sends a message that we think women may have 'unrealistic expectations' (Lally *et al.*, 2008), as identified by a woman describing her initial conversation with a midwife in an antenatal clinic, after she expressed interest in giving birth in the local free-standing, midwifery-led unit:

> She said, 'Well it's your first baby and a lot can happen in pregnancy that might mean you're no longer suitable, so let's keep an open mind about that. If there are no problems in your pregnancy, you could think about going there later, but you do have to consider that about 40% of women having first babies who go to birth centres have to transfer to the hospital during labour – and that's not much fun.'
>
> (Mother, Leap, 2015, unpublished data)

In order to practise some ways in which we open doors to possibilities, we will stay with the theme of interacting with women around their choice of birth in a carousel activity.*

Promoting choices about where to give birth

In preparation for this carousel activity, participants should access the NICE guideline: Intrapartum care: care of healthy women and their babies during childbirth (NICE, 2014) and be familiar with the evidence and recommendations regarding information that should be shared with pregnant women to inform their choices about where to give birth (Section 1.1 'Place of Birth', pp.10–22).

Box 4.28   Reflective Activity: Talking to women about choice of birthplace

Classroom or workshop activity: carousel; facilitator instructions:
- Explain that the purpose of the activity is to practise initial reactions, not to get anything 'right' – they will only have one minute to begin a conversation:

  - Half the group form an inner circle with their chairs facing outwards.
  - The other half form an outer circle facing the people in the inner circle.
  - The inner circle will be midwives, doulas or childbirth educators.
  - The outer circle will be women having their first babies, with healthy pregnancies, who start a conversation with the midwives, doulas or childbirth educators by saying, 'I've heard the transfer rates are really high if you choose to have your baby at home or in the new birth centre. So maybe it's not such a great idea?'
  - Call time after one minute and all participants in the outer circle move on one place in a clockwise direction and start a similar conversation with the next person they are sitting opposite.
  - Repeat this for some time and then get participants to swap seats and roles. Repeat the activity.

Eventually, bring everyone back into a large circle and discuss what it felt like to be the woman/birth worker.

- Without naming names, what were the phrases that were helpful when you were pretending to be the woman?
- What was the learning from this activity?

Note: * This activity can be adapted to explore and practise our initial interactions with pregnant women around many other questions that they might ask, including those that we might find challenging.

Encouraging conversations with pregnant women and their partners:
some examples to practise

We finish this chapter with some examples of the sort of things midwives say to encourage women in their abilities as they contemplate the uncertainties of labour and birth, drawing on filmed interviews with midwives (Sandall *et al.*, 2010, unpublished data).

If you are not familiar with these kinds of phrases, it may be helpful to read them out loud, perhaps as a classroom activity, in order to remember them and think about how you might adapt them to your own style of communication.

The rests in between contractions

It's not going to be a constant thing, you know . . . you get a contraction, it's there for a minute and then you get a rest in between, and every contraction brings you a little bit closer to you having your baby so every one's really important and it's doing really good work.

Working with your body

Your body helps you. Labour starts off fairly mild and gradually contractions will get closer together and stronger, so that your body's got time to get used to it, to cope with it. And your body's got time to release its own endorphins, its natural painkillers, to help you through the process. Your body's working with you to help you have your baby, not against you. So trust your body.

Movement and rhythm

When you're in labour it's really important that you're able to move around, get into good positions, be able to kneel, to sit on the toilet, to squat, to rock, to do slow dancing, you know, all things like that are going to help your labour to progress and to bring your baby more quickly. And actually, you know, if you have an epidural you're not going to be able to do those things.

One contraction at a time

All you've got to worry about is that one contraction that you're in and not kind of project ahead as to how many more hours am I going to be going through this? It's that one, and by breathing through it and getting really focused on that one contraction you'll come to the end of it and it will be like, that's one less, that's one behind me . . . don't worry about the length of the process, stay very present, and it will become a lot easier.

Transition – look at the midwife

Women say all kinds of things that they don't really mean; it can be a really tricky time in their labour that they find really hard. . . . So it's good to remind your partner to know that it's a really normal part of labour. . . . We always say to partners: 'Look at the midwife'. The midwife will be saying, 'It's OK, it's all right, it's all normal'. So look at the midwife and she will give you lots of encouragement. She'll tell you if there's anything to be worried about.

Good support and feelings of achievement

Good support is better than any epidural. . . . Good support and then that wonderful feeling afterwards of achievement.

These phrases from midwives lead us into the next chapter, where we explore the complex dimensions of how we communicate with pregnant women and their families through 'thoughtful encouragement'.

Postscript

We leave this chapter with a few of our favourite free resources for sharing information with prospective parents and colleagues.

Simkin, Penny. Comfort in Labour: How You Can Help Yourself to a Normal Satisfying Childbirth

This 14-page leaflet, written by renowned childbirth educator and birth supporter Penny Simkin, provides a succinct, practical guide to labour support for parents and birth attendants, illustrated with beautiful line drawings. It was published originally by Childbirth Connection, a non-profit organisation in the USA that works to improve the quality of maternity care through research, education, advocacy and policy. Childbirth Connect is now a programme of the National Partnership for Women and Families. You can download Penny Simkin's leaflet from their website:

https://www.nationalpartnership.org/our-work/resources/health-care/maternity/comfort-in-labor-simkin.pdf.

Buckley, Sarah (2015). Hormonal Physiology of Childbearing: Evidence and Implications for Women, Babies, and Maternity Care

Sarah Buckley is a well-known author, birth activist and GP, who has had a profound influence on how we understand the hormonal physiology of childbirth. This groundbreaking report is a valuable resource for prospective parents, birth workers and childbirth educators. Sarah explains the scientific evidence and rationale for enabling situations in which hormonal physiology can thrive, including the negative impact that common maternity care interventions can have on disturbing these processes. We agree with the experts who wrote the Foreword: 'This report . . . will be retrospectively evaluated as one of the most revolutionary and influential publications on maternity and newborn care ever issued'. Commissioned by Childbirth Connect and now published by National Partnership for Women and Families, the report is free to download at:

https://www.nationalpartnership.org/our-work/resources/health-care/maternity/hormonal-physiology-of-childbearing.pdf.

The issues in the report are presented in a simplified format in a brochure for parents: Pathway to a Healthy Birth: How to Help Your Hormones Do Their Wonderful Work:

https://www.nationalpartnership.org/our-work/resources/health-care/maternity/pathway-to-a-healthy-birth-booklet.pdf.

All4Birth: https://www.all4birth.com

All4Birth is an online, free resource for sharing of information and resources related to childbirth and maternity care. The resource is for pregnant women, mothers, partners, families, maternity care workers, childbirth activists, childbirth educators and anyone interested in normal, physiological childbirth. Created by a global community of birth practitioners, women and families, the objectives of All4Birth are to gather resources into one, accessible space, to increase awareness of and knowledge relating to normal physiological childbirth, to transfer and share knowledge between locations, individuals and countries, and to maximise the potential for optimal outcomes for mothers and babies. Resources include real-life stories and evidence-informed fact sheets, articles and free-flow blog articles, providing links to publications, research reports, websites, media and films, guidelines, toolkits and consensus papers.

Knitted uterus pattern

Finding a pattern on the Internet for a knitted uterus that is suitable for teaching purposes is becoming increasingly difficult, so we provided one here which we have used:

Box 4.29   Knitted uterus for teaching purposes

Materials:

Yarn: 8 ply, 'double knitting' or 4 ply doubled: 2 ounces
1 set double-pointed needles, 4mm (Size 8 UK, Size 6 USA)

Directions:

Cast on 48 stitches. Divide evenly on three needles. Join yarn, knit in the round
Knit 2, Pearl 2 until cuff measures 2 inches.
First round: increase 1 stitch in every 6th stitch – 56 stitches.
Knit evenly for 6 rounds.
8th round: increase 1 stitch in every 7th stitch – 61 stitches
Knit evenly for 6 rounds
15th round: increase 1 stitch in every 8th stitch – 72 stitches
Knit evenly for 6 rounds
22nd round: increase 1 stitch in every 9th stitch – 80 stitches
Knit evenly for 6 rounds
29th round: increase 1 stitch in every 10th stitch – 88 stitches
Knit evenly for 6 rounds
36th round: increase 1 stitch in every 11th stitch – 96 stitches
Knit evenly for 6 rounds
43rd round: increase 1 stitch in every 12th stitch – 104 stitches
Knit evenly for 6 rounds
Continue knitting 104 stitches evenly for 5 inches.
Decrease:
First needle *Knit 11 stitches, slip knit, pass slip stitch over, repeat from * for entire round
Next round, *Knit 10 stitches, slip, knit, pass slip stitch over, repeat from * for entire round
Next round, *Knit 8 stitches, skip, knit, pass slip stitch over, repeat from * for entire round
Next round, *Knit 7 stitches, slip, knit, pass slip stitch over, repeat from * for entire round
Next round, *Knit 5 stitches, slip, knit, pass slip stitch over, repeat from * for entire round
Next round, *Knit 4 stitches, slip, knit, pass slip stitch over, repeat from * for entire round
Next round, *Knit 3 stitches, slip, knit, pass slip stitch over, repeat from * for entire round
Next round, *Knit 2 stitches, slip, knit, pass slip stitch over, repeat from * for entire round
Next round, *Knit 1 stitch, slip, knit, pass slip stitch over, repeat from * for entire round
Next round, * slip, knit, pass slip stitch over, repeat from * for entire round

Finishing: Draw yarn through remaining 8 stitches and fasten.

References

Ahldén, I., Ahlehagen, S., Dahlgren, L.O., Josefsson, A. (2012). Parents' expectations about participating in antenatal parenthood education classes. *The Journal of Perinatal Education, 21(1)*, 11–17.

Ahmadian, L., Khajouei, R., Kamali, S., Mirzaee, M. (2020). Use of the Internet by pregnant women to seek information about pregnancy and childbirth. *Informatics for Health and Social Care, 45(4)*, 385–395.

Ajzen, I. and Madden, T.J. (1986). Prediction of goal-directed behaviour: attitudes, intentions and perceived behavioural control. *Journal of Experimental Social Psychology, 22*, 453–474.

Amis, D. (2016). The role of the childbirth educator in supporting vaginal birth and reducing primary cesareans: highlights from the California maternal quality care collaborative toolkit. *Journal of Perinatal Education, 25*, 208–214.

Balaskas, J. (1983). *Active Birth*. London: Unwin Paperbacks.

Bandura, A. (1977). Self efficacy: toward a unifying theory of behavioural change. *Psychology Review, 84*, 191–215.

Bandura, A. (1986). *Social Foundations of Thought and Action: A Social Cognitive Theory*. Englewood Cliffs, NJ: Prentice-Hall.

Bandura, A. (1997). *Self-efficacy: The Exercise of Control*. New York: Freeman.

Bandura, A. (2012). On the functional properties of perceived self-efficacy revisited. *Journal of Management, 38(1)*, 9–44.

Bardacke, N. (2012). *Mindful Birthing: Training the Mind, Body and Heart for Childbirth and Beyond*. New York: Harper One.

Barimani, M., Forslund Frykedal, K., Rosander, M. and Berlin, A. (2018). Childbirth and parenting preparation in antenatal classes. *Midwifery, 57*, 1–7.

Bergström, M., Kieler, H. and Waldenstrom, U. (2009). Effects of natural childbirth preparation versus standard antenatal education on epidural rates, experience of childbirth and parental stress in mothers and fathers: a randomised controlled multicentre trial. *British Journal of Obstetrics and Gynaecology, 116*, 1167–1176.

Braeken, M.A.K.A., Jones, A., Ottte, R.A., Nyklíček, I. and Van den Bergh, B.R.H. (2017). Potential benefits of mindfulness during pregnancy on maternal autonomic nervous system function and infant development. *Psychophysiology, 54*, 279–288.

Buckley, S.J. (2009). *Gentle Birth, Gentle Mothering: A Doctor's Guide to Natural Childbirth and Early Parenting Choices*. Berkeley, CA: Celestial Arts Press.

Buckley, S.J. (2010). Sexuality in labour and birth: an intimate perspective. Chapter 12 in D. Walsh and S. Downe (eds), *Essential Midwifery Practice: Intrapartum Care* (pp.213–234). Chichester: Wiley-Blackwell.

Buckley, S.J. (2015). *Hormonal Physiology of Childbearing: Evidence and Implications for Women, Babies, and Maternity Care*. Washington, DC: Childbirth Connection Programs, National Partnership for Women and Families.

Buckley, S.J. and Uvnäs Moberg, K. (2019). Nature and consequences of oxytocin and other neurohormones during childbirth. Chapter 2 in S. Downe and S. Byrom (eds), *Squaring the Circle. Normal Birth Research, Theory and Practice in a Technological Age* (pp. 19–32). London: Pinter & Martin.

Byrne, J., Hauck, Y., Fisher, C., Bayes, S. and Schutze, R. (2014). Effectiveness of a mindfulness-based childbirth education pilot study on maternal self-efficacy and fear of childbirth. *Journal of Midwifery and Women's Health, 59*, 192–197.

Campbell, V.R. and Nolan, M. (2016). A qualitative study exploring how the aims, language and actions of yoga for pregnancy teachers may impact upon women's self-efficacy for labour and birth. *Women and Birth, 29*, 3–11.

Campbell, V.R. and Nolan, M. (2019). 'It definitely made a difference': a grounded theory study of yoga for pregnancy and women's self-efficacy for labour. *Midwifery, 68*, 74–83.

Caughey, A.B., Cahill, A.G., Guise J.M. and Rouse D.J. (2014, reaffirmed 2016). Safe prevention of the primary cesarean delivery. Obstetric Care Consensus No. 1. American College of Obstetricians and Gynecologists & Society for Maternal-Fetal Medicine. *American Journal of Obstetrics & Gynecology, 10*, 179–193.

Chen, I., Opiyo, N., Tavender, E., Mortazhejri, S., Rader, T., Petkovic, J., . . . Betran, A.P. (2018). Non-clinical interventions for reducing unnecessary caesarean section. *Cochrane Database of Systematic Reviews*, Issue 9. Art. No.: CD005528.

Chen, M.M. and Hancock, H. (2012). Women's knowledge of options for birth after caesarean section. *Women and Birth*, *25*, e19–e26.

Cutajar, L., Miu, M., Fleet, J-A., Cyna, A.M. and Steen, M. (2020). Antenatal education for childbirth: Labour and birth. *European Journal of Midwiery*, *4*, 11.

Cyna, A.M., McAuliffe, G.L. and Andrew, M.I. (2004). Hypnosis for pain relief in labour and childbirth: a systematic review. *British Journal of Anaesthesia*, *93(4)*, 505–511.

Dahlen, H.G and Homer, C.S.E. (2013). 'Motherbirth or childbirth'? A prospective analysis of vaginal birth after caesarean blogs. *Midwifery*, *29*, 167–173.

David, S., Fenwick, J., Bayes, S. and Martin, T. (2010). A qualitative analysis of the content of telephone calls made by women to a dedicated 'Next Birth After Caesarean' antenatal clinic. *Women and Birth*, *23*, 166–171.

Davis-Floyd, R. (2001). The technocratic, humanistic and holistic paradigms of childbirth. *International Journal of Gynaecology & Obstetrics*, *75*, S5–S23.

Declercq, E., Sakala, C., Corry, M.P., Applebaum, S. and Herrlich, A. (2013). *Listening to Mothers III: Pregnancy and Birth. Report of the Third National U.S. Survey of Women's Childbearing Experiences*. New York: Childbirth Connection.

Dempsey, R. (2013). *Birth with Confidence. Savvy Choices for Normal Birth*. Fairfield, Australia: Boathouse Press.

Department of Health (Producer). (2011). Preparation for Birth and Beyond: a resource pack for leaders of community groups and activities. www.gov.uk/government/uploads/system/uploads/attachment_data/file/215386/dh_134728.pdf.

Dick-Read, G. (1933). *Childbirth Without Fear: The Principles and Practice of Natural Childbirth*. London: Heineman. Republished by Pinter & Martin, 2004.

Dixon, L., Skinner, J. and Foureur, M. (2013). Women's perspectives of the stages and phases of labour. *Midwifery*, *29*, 10–17.

Downe, S., Finlayson, K., Oladapo, O.T., Bonet, M. and Gülmezoglu, A.M. (2018). What matters to women during childbirth: a systematic qualitative review. *PLoS ONE*, *13(4)*, e0194906.

Duncan, L.G. and Bardacke, N. (2010). Mindfulness-based childbirth and parenting education: promoting family mindfulness during the perinatal period. *J. Child Fam. Stud.*, *19(2)*, 190–202. doi:10.1007/s10826-009-9313-7.

Duncan, L.G., Cohn, M.A., Chao, M.T., Joseph G., Cook, J.G., Riccobono, J. and Bardacke, N. (2017). Benefits of preparing for childbirth with mindfulness training: a randomized controlled trial with active comparison. *BMC Pregnancy and Childbirth*, *17*, 140.

Dunn, C., Hanieh, E., Roberts, R. and Powrie, R. (2012). Mindful pregnancy and childbirth: effects of a mindfulness based intervention on women's psychological distress and wellbeing in the perinatal period. *Archives of Women's Mental Health*, *15(2)*, 139–143.

Edwards, N.P. (2005). *Birthing Autonomy: Women's Experiences of Planning Home Birth*. London: Routledge.

Entsieh, A.A. and Hallström, I.K. (2016). First-time parents' prenatal needs for early parenthood preparation – a systematic review and meta-synthesis of qualitative literature. *Midwifery*, *39*, 1–11.

Escott, D., Slade, P. and Spiby, H. (2009). Preparation for pain management during childbirth: the psychological aspects of coping strategy development in antenatal education. *Clinical Pschology Review*, *29*, 617–622.

Escott, D., Spiby, H., Slade, P. and Fraser, R.B. (2004). The range of coping strategies women use to manage pain and anxiety prior to and during first experience of labour. *Midwifery*, *20(2)*, 144–156.

Ferguson, S., Davis, D. and Browne, J. (2013). Does antenatal education affect labour and birth? A structured review of the literature. *Women and Birth*, *26*, e5–e8.

Finlayson, K., Downe, S. and Hinder, S. (2015). Unexpected consequences: women's experiences of a self-hypnosis intervention to help with pain in labour. *BMC Pregnancy and Childbirth*, *15(229)*.

Foureur, M. (2008). Creating birth space to enable undisturbed birth. Chapter 5 in K. Fahy, M. Foureur and C. Hastie (eds), *Birth Territory and Midwifery Guardianship: Theory for Practice, Education and Research*. Edinburgh: Heinemann/Elsevier.

Gagnon, A. and Sandall, J. (2007). Individual or group antenatal education for childbirth or parenthood, or both. *Cochrane Database of Systematic Reviews*, Issue 3. Art. No.: CD002869. doi:10.1002/14651858.CD002869.pub2.

Gaskin, I.M. (2003). *Ina May's Guide to Childbirth*. New York: Bantam Books.

Gilmer, C., Buchan, J., Letourneau, N., Bennett, C., Shanker, S., Fenwick, A. and Smith-Chant, B. (2016). Parent education interventions designed to support the transition to parenthood: a realist review. *International Journal of Nursing Studies*, *59*, 118–133.

Gollwitzer, P.M. (1993). Goal achievement: the role of intentions. *European Review of Social Psychology*, *4*, 141–185.

Graves, K. (2012). *The Hypnobirthing Book: An Inspirational Guide for a Calm, Confident, Natural Birth*. Marlborough: Katherine Publishing.

Gregg, R. (1993). 'Choice' as a double-edged sword. *Women & Health, 20*(*3*), 53–73.

Guardino, C.M., Dunkel Schetter, C., Bower, J.E., Lu, M.C. and Smalley, S.L. (2014). Randomised controlled pilot trial of mindfulness training for stress reduction during pregnancy. *Psychology and Health, 29*(*3*), 334–349.

Heli, S. (2021) *Give Birth Without Fear: Practical Tools for a Confident Birth*. London: Clink Street Publishing.

Henderson, W. (2005). Context and purpose: learning styles and priniciples of adult education. Chapter 2 in *Birth and Parenting Skills: New Directions in Antenatal Education* (pp.17–31). Edinburgh: Churchill Livingstone.

Hill, M. (2017). *The Positive Birth Handbook: A New Approach to Pregnancy, Birth and the Early Weeks*. London: Pinter & Martin.

Hill, M. (2019). *Give Birth Like a Feminist: Your Body, Your Baby, Your Choices*. London: HarperCollins.

Homer, C.S.E., Cheah, S.L., Rossiter, C., Dahlen, H., Ellwood, D., Foureur, M., . . . Scarff, V.L. (2019). Maternal and perinatal outcomes by planned place of birth in Australia 2000–2012: a linked population data study. *BMJ Open Access, 9*, e029192. doi:10.1136/bmjopen-2019-029192.

Homer, C.S.E., Leap, N., Edwards, N. and Sandall, J. (2017). Midwifery continuity of carer in an area of high socio-economic disadvantage in London: a retrospective analysis of Albany Midwifery Practice outcomes using routine data (1997–2009). *Midwifery, 48*, 1–10.

Hughes, A., Williams, M., Bardacke, N., Duncan, L.G., Dimidjian, S. and Goodman, S.H. (2009). Mindfulness approaches to childbirth and parenting. *British Journal of Midwifery, 17*(*10*), 630–635.

Johansson, M., Rubertsson, C. and Rådestad I. (2010). The Internet: one important source for pregnancy and childbirth information among prospective fathers. *Journal of Men's Health, 7*(*3*).

Jones, L., Othman, M., Dowswell, T., Alfirevic, Z., Gates S., Newburn, M., Jordan, S., Lavender, T. and Neilson, J.P. (2012). Pain management for women in labour: an overview of systematic reviews. *Cochrane Database of Systematic Reviews 2012*, Issue 3. Art. No.: CD009234. doi:10.1002/14651858.CD009234.pub2.

Keedle, H., Peters, L., Schmied, V., Burns, E., Keedle, W. and Dahlen, H.G. (2020). Women's experiences of planning a vaginal birth after caesarean in different models of maternity care in Australia. *BMC Pregnancy & Childbirth, 381*. doi:org/10.1186/s12884-020-03075-8.

Keedle, H., Schmied, V., Burns, E. and Dahlen, H.G. (2019). A narrative analysis of women's experiences of planning a vaginal birth after caesarean (VBAC) in Australia using critical feminist theory. *BMC Pregnancy Childbirth, 19*, 142. doi:org/10.1186/s12884-019-2297-4.

Kemp, J. and Sandall, J. (2010). Normal birth, magical birth: the role of the 36-week birth talk in caseload midwifery practice. *Midwifery, 26*, 211–221. doi:10.1016/j.midw.2008.07.002.

Kitzinger, S. (1962). *The Experience of Childbirth*. London: Victor Gollancz.

Kitzinger, S. (2015). *A Passion for Birth. My Life: Anthropology, Family and Feminism*. London: Pinter & Martin.

Knowles, M.S., Holton, E.F. and Swanson, R. (2014). *The Adult Learner: The Definitive Classic in Adult Education and Human Resource Development*, 8th edn. London: Routledge.

Koushede, V., Brixval, C.S., Thygesen, L.C., Axelsen, S.F., Winkel, P., Lindschou, J., . . . Due, P. (2017). Antenatal small-class education versus auditorium-based lectures to promote positive transitioning to parenthood – a randomised trial. *PLoS ONE*, *12*(*5*), e0176819.

Lally, J.E, Murtagh, M.J. and Macphail, S. (2008). More in hope than expectation: women's experience and expectations of pain relief in labour. A review. *BMC Med*, *6*(*7*).

Larsson, M. (2009). A descriptive study of the use of the Internet by women seeking pregnancy-related information. *Midwifery*, *25*(*1*), 14–20.

Leap, N. (1991, VHS Video). Helping you to make your own decisions – antenatal and postnatal groups in Deptford SE London. Available in mp4 format from: nickyleap@me.com.

Leap, N. (2007, unpublished data). A study to explore how care from Albany midwives may have influenced how women approached and experienced pain in labour. Unpublished data: Florence Nightingale Faculty of Nursing and Midwifery, Kings College London.

Leap, N. (2010). The less we do the more we give. Chapter 2 in M. Kirkham (ed.), *The Midwife–Mother Relationship*, 2nd edn (pp.17–35). London: Palgrave Macmillan.

Leap, N. (2015, unpublished data). Identifying the experiences of receiving and providing support in labour.

Leap, N. and Edwards, N. (2006). The politics of involving women in decision making. Chapter 5 in L.A. Page and R. Campbell (eds), *The New Midwifery: Science and Sensitivity in Practice*, 2nd edn. London: Churchill Livingstone/Elsevier.

Leap, N., Sandall, J., Buckland, S. and Huber, U. (2010). Journey to confidence: women's experiences of pain in labour and relational continuity of care. *Journal of Midwifery and Women's Health*, *55*(*3*), 235–242.

Levett, K.M. (2016). The complementary therapies for labour and birth study making sense of labour and birth – experiences of women, partners and midwives of a complementary medicine antenatal education course. *Midwifery*, *40*, 124–131.

Levett, K.M., Smith, C.A., Dahlen, H.G. and Bensoussan, A. (2014). Acupuncture and acupressure for pain management in labour and birth: a critical narrative review of current systematic review evidence. *Complementary Therapies in Medicine*, *22*, 523–540.

Lothian, J.A. (2006). Birth plans: the good, the bad, and the future. *Journal of Obstetric, Gynecologic and Neonatal Nursing*, *35*(*2*), 295–303.

Lothian, J.A. (2008). Childbirth education at the crossroads. *Journal of Perinatal Education*, *17*(*2*), 45–49.

Lowe, N.K. (1991). Maternal confidence in coping with labor: a self-efficacy concept. *Journal of Obstetric Gynecologic and Neonatal Nursing*, *20*, 457–463.

Lowe, N.K. (1993). Maternal confidence for labor: development of the childbirth self-efficacy inventory. *Research in Nursing and Health*, *16*, 141–149.

Lowe, N.K. (2000). Self-efficacy for labor and childbirth fears in nulliparous pregnant women. *Journal of Psychosomatic Obstetrics & Gynecology*, *21*(*4*), 219–224.

Lundgren, I., Morano, S., Nilsson, C., Sinclair, M. and Begley, C. (2020). Cultural perspectives on vaginal birth after previous caesarean section in countries with high and low rates – a hermeneutic study. *Women and Birth*, *33*, e339–e347.

Lundgren, I., van Limbeek, E., Vehvilainen-Julkunen, K. and Nilsson, C. (2015). Clinicians' views of factors of importance for improving the rate of VBAC (vaginal birth after caesarean section): a qualitative study from countries with high VBAC rates. *BMC Pregnancy & Childbirth*, *15*(*196*).

Madden, K., Middleton, P., Cyna, A.M., Matthewson, M. and Jones, L. (2016). Hypnosis for pain management during labour and childbirth. *Cochrane Database of Systematic Reviews 2016*, Issue 5. Art. No.: CD009356. doi:10.1002/14651858.CD009356.pub3.

Meddings, N. (2017). *How to Have a Baby: Mother Gathered Guidance on Birth and New Babies.* Chipping Norton: Eynham Press.

Michaels, P. (2014). *Lamaze: An International History.* Oxford: Oxford University Press.

Morton, C.H. and Hsu, C. (2007). Contemporary dilemmas in American childbirth education: findings from a comparative ethnographic study. *Journal of Perinatal Education*, *16*(*4*), 25–27.

NICE (2014). Intrapartum care: care of healthy women and their babies during childbirth. Clinical guideline 190. National Collaborating Centre for Women's and Children's Health UK. Commissioned by the National Institute for Health and Care Excellence (NICE): www.nice.org.uk/guidance/cg190.

Nolan, M. (1997). Antenatal education – where next? *Journal of Advanced Nursing, 25,* 1198–1204.

Nolan, M. (2005). Childbirth and parenting education: what the research says and why we may ignore it. In M. Nolan and J. Foster (eds), *Birth and Parenting Skills: New Directions in Antenatal Education.* London: Churchill Livingstone.

Nolan, M. (2009). Information giving and education in pregnancy: a review of qualitative studies. *The Journal of Perinatal Education, 18(4),* 21–30.

Nolan, M. (2010). Childbirth education: politics, equality and relevance. Chapter 3 in D. Walsh and S. Downe (eds), *Essential Midwifery Practice: Intrapartum Care* (pp.31–44). Chichester: Wiley-Blackwell.

Nolan, M. (2021). Antenatal education: sustaining healthy families. In L. Davies, R. Daellenabach and M. Kensington (eds), *Sustainability, Midwifery and Birth,* 2nd edn (pp.235–247). Abingdon: Routledge.

Nolan, M. and Foster, D.A. (2005). The Albany practice, South-East London: antenatal and postnatal groups. Chapter 7 in M. Nolan and D.A. Foster (eds), *Birth and Parenting Skills: New Directions in Antenatal Education* (pp.110–112). Edinburgh: Churchill Livingstone.

Odent, M. and Odent, P. (2015). Essay: from homo superpredator to homo ecologicus. https://www.wombecology.com/home/from-homo-superpredator-to-homo-ecologicus.

Phillips-Moore, J. (2012). Birthing outcomes from an Australian HypnoBirthing programme. *British Journal of Midwifery, 20(8),* 558–564.

Reed, B. and Walton, C. (2009). The Albany midwifery practice. In R. Davis-Floyd, L. Barclay, J. Tritten and B.A. Daviss (eds), *Birth Models that Work.* London: University of California Press.

Reiger, K. and Dempsey, R. (2006). Performing birth in a culture of fear: an embodied crisis of late modernity. *Health Sociology Review, 15(4),* 364–373.

Rijnders, M., Jans, S., Aalhuizen, I., Detmar, S. and Crone, M. (2019). Women centered care: Implementation of CenteringPregnancy® in The Netherlands. *Birth, 46,* 450–460.

Rising, S. (1998). CenteringPregnancy: an interdisciplinary model of empowerment. *Journal of Nurse-Midwifery, 43(1),* 46–54.

Rising, S., Kennedy, H. and Klima, C. (2004). Redesigning prenatal care through CenteringPregnancy. *Journal of Midwifery & Women's Health, 49(5),* 398–404.

Rising, S.S. and Quimby, C.H. (eds). (2017). *The CenteringPregnancy Model: The Power of Group Health Care.* New York: Springer Publishing Company.

Robertson, A. (2006a). *Empowering Women: Teaching Active Birth.* Sydney: Birth International.

Robertson, A. (2006b). Skills for childbirth educators, DVD. Sydney: Birth International.

Romano, A.M. (2007). A changing landscape: implications of pregnant women's Internet use for childbirth educators. *Journal of Perinatal Education, 16(4),* 18–24.

Sandall, J., Leap, N., Grant, J. and Bastos, M.H. (2010). Supporting women to have a normal birth: development and field testing of a learning package for maternity staff. Health and Social Care Research Division, King's College London.

Sayakhot, P. and Carolan-Olah, M. (2016). Internet use by pregnant women seeking pregnancy-related information: a systematic review. *BMC Pregnancy and Childbirth, 16,* 65.

Schrader McMillan, A., Barlow, J. and Redshaw, M. (2009). *Birth and Beyond: A Review of the Evidence about Antenatal Education.* Warwick: University of Warwick.

Shilling, T. and Bingham, S. (2010). Revisiting the classics in childbirth education. *The Journal of Perinatal Education, 19(3),* 73–78. doi:10.1624/105812410X514477.

Simkin, P. (2002). Supportive care during labor: a guide for busy nurses. *JOGNN, 31(6),* 721–732. doi:10.1177/0884217502239208.

Simkin, P. (2017). Should ACOG support childbirth education as another means to improve obstetric outcomes? Response to ACOG Committee Opinion # 687: approaches to limit intervention during labor and birth. *Birth, 44,* 293–297.

Slade, P., Escott, D., Spiby, H., Henderson, B. and Fraser, R.B. (2000). Antenatal predictors and use of coping strategies in labour. *Psychology and Health, 15(4),* 555–569.

Spiby, H., Slade, P., Escott, D., Henderson, B. and Fraser, R.B. (2003). Selected coping strategies in labour: an investigation of women's experiences. *Birth, 30(3)*, 189–194.

Tilden, E.L., Caughey, A.B., Lee, C.S. and Emeis, C. (2016). The effect of childbirth self-efficacy on perinatal outcomes. *Journal of Obstetric, Gynecologic and Neonatal Nursing, 45*, 465–480.

Timmermans, E., Timmermans, O., Mestdagh, E. and Bogaerts, A. (2019). The effect of prenatal interventions on self-efficacy in women during childbirth – a systematic review *Journal of Gynecology and Women's Health, 16(5)*, ID.555946.

Uvnäs Moberg, K. (2019). *Why Oxytocin Matters*. London: Pinter & Martin.

Vieten, C. and Astin, J. (2007). Effects of a mindfulness-based intervention during pregnancy on prenatal stress and mood: results of a pilot study. *Archives of Women's Mental Health, 11*, 67–74.

Walker, D.S., Visger, J.M. and Rossie, D. (2009). Contemporary childbirth education models. *Journal of Midwifery & Women's Health, 54(6)*, 469–476.

Walsh, D. (2006). 'Nesting' and 'matrescence' as distinctive features of a free-standing birth centre in the UK. *Midwifery, 22(3)*, 289–239.

Wharton, K.R., Ecker, J.L. and Wax, J.R. (2017). Approaches to limit intervention during labor and birth. Committee Opinion No 687. American College of Obstetriciand and Gynecologists. *Obsterics and Gynecology, 129*, e20–e28.

Whitburn, L.Y., Jones, L.E., Davy, M-A. and Small, R. (2014). Women's experiences of labour pain and the role of the mind: an exploratory study. *Midwifery*, 1029–1035.

WHO. (2018). *WHO Recommendation on Group Antenatal Care*. The WHO Reproductive Health Library: Geneva: WHO.

Wickham, S. and Davies, L. (2005). Are midwives empowered enough to offer empowering education? Chapter 5 in M. Nolan and J. Foster (eds), *Birth and Parenting Skills* (pp.69–83). Edinburgh: Churchill Livingstone.

5 Communication and thoughtful encouragement

Introduction

In this chapter, we explore ways of communicating that encourage pregnant women to believe in their abilities in the face of uncertainty – literally: 'the promotion of courage'. This encouragement is important for all pregnant women: those who sail though childbirth on the wings of prosperity and good health as well as those who face challenges and need the help of medical interventions.

The opportunities for building trusting relationships and reducing fear and anxiety are optimal when we are providing midwifery continuity of care, doula support or meeting women regularly in antenatal groups or preparation for birth sessions (Dahlen *et al.*, 2020; Homer *et al.*, 2019; Leap, 2010; Leap and Edwards, 2006; Leap *et al.*, 2010). Significantly, the value of sharing positive stories about birth in our everyday interactions with people can be far-reaching. People remember stories, and stories have the potential to open up new ways of understanding (Kirkham, 1997; Callister, 2004). It has been suggested, though, that stories can limit women's exploration of choices when the dominant narrative suggests that having a healthy baby depends on care in a hospital setting with full technological support (Kay *et al.*, 2017). In our experience, even in fleeting interactions (for example, with cab drivers or hairdressers), most people have their own stories to share (or they want to discuss something they've seen in the latest reality TV show about birth). These interactions can lead to penetrating discussions about birth, including whether it is (or should be) valued as a social or medical event.

All of us receive messages from multiple sources at both a conscious and subconscious level that can have either 'placebo' (positive) or 'nocebo' (negative) effects on how we approach labour and birth. We touched on this in the previous chapter when exploring research by Lisa Cutajar and colleagues who have studied the potential effects of phraseology used in antenatal education (Cutajar and Cyna, 2018; Cutajar, Steen *et al.*, 2020; Cutajar, Miu *et al.*, 2020). In this chapter, we take time to think about how our verbal and communication might be received, drawing on an emerging body of research from the disciplines of neuroscience and social psychology. Communication is highly complex and multidimensional, as Prineas *et al.* (2011, p.4) observe:

> The many human dimensions of communication – the practical, the social, the linguistic, the lyrical, the subliminal, its ability to soothe and to injure, to inform, to entertain, to terrify – are what make this topic so challenging.

Theory about the psychophysiology of emotion, cognition, perception, semantics and metaphor can play an important part in increasing our awareness of how we can support women in a way that promotes positive experiences of birth. We shall touch on some of this theory

DOI: 10.4324/9781003092520-6

in this chapter and also direct you to other resources that you can turn to in order to study this area more closely.

Starting with first impressions

Within less than a second of meeting someone for the first time we make enduring value judgements about their personality (Naumann *et al.*, 2009), whether we are prepared to trust them (Yu *et al.*, 2014) and whether we find them attractive, likeable, trustworthy, competent or aggressive (Willis and Todorov, 2006). A range of value judgements are formed swiftly through the subliminal processing of a complex range of clues arising from our senses, stored memories and social conditioning (Gilron and Gutchess, 2009). This affects how we all communicate with each other, every day, all of the time.

It can be confronting for a woman when there is an element of surprise in the appearance of the midwife, particularly if that challenges her idea of what a midwife is. This might be about the midwife's features, body shape, expression, body language, speech, accent, ethnicity, skin colour and clothing (Deprez-Sims and Morris, 2010; Hu *et al.*, 2018; Naumann *et al.*, 2009;); it might also be about the fact that the midwife is a man or appears rather young.

In her study of midwives who do not have children, Chris Bewley (2000, 2010) explored situations where, on first meeting, women ask midwives to confirm their assumptions that they do or do not have children. Anxiety about the midwife's experience often underpins the question, 'Do you have children?', particularly if the midwife is young. For midwives who have not had children this can feel challenging, especially where they have experienced pregnancy loss or the loss of potential motherhood.

As we make value judgements about women, based on how they present to us, so they make value judgements about us, particularly in relation to the clothes we wear if we are not wearing uniforms. We would probably all draw the line about what is acceptable in terms of how much individuality we should be able to express in the way we present ourselves in different places. How short is too short a skirt? What about those tattoos? Are piercings acceptable if they are in ears, but what about nose, tongue, eyebrow and lip piercing? What is acceptable wear on a continuum of subdued to flamboyant? How much leeway do we need in order to feel able to express our individuality? And should we all just stick to navy blue trousers and a white patterned shirt – or simply, uniforms – in the interest of a 'professional look'?

Along the same line, debates still continue about wearing 'scrubs' (operating theatre clothing) in birthing areas. We may be very attached to the comfort of those loose-fitting garments, but no one can deny that they give a strong message that we're about to go to theatre. Some people think that wearing scrubs is acceptable in spite of that, especially as it eliminates laundry problems for the midwife. Many suggest that scrubs inspire confidence in the skill and capabilities of the midwife, especially when decorated by the accessory of a stethoscope around the neck. Others argue that, if the scrubs are a deep colour, rather than the pale blue of television soap operas, they can accommodate individuality and are acceptable. Certainly the subconscious messages induced by colour are a consideration when attending a birth. Many of us who attend home births think about the colours and mood messages of the clothes we wear when going to someone's home as well as the practicalities of comfort.

In the debates about how we present to the women (and their 'families') for whom we provide care, consensus is unlikely as the very nature of the discourse revolves around our individuality and some strongly held opinions about what constitutes professionalism. We suggest that, nevertheless, there is value in exploring these issues with colleagues, particularly in terms of how first impressions may impact on how we support women in labour.

Box 5.1   Reflective Activity: First impressions and communication with pregnant women and their families

Group activity; instruction to facilitator/s:
- Prepare a set of photographs aimed at stimulating discussion about first impressions. Alternatively, you could ask each participant to bring a photograph to share in a discussion about: 'First impressions that might affect communication with pregnant women and their families'.
- Place the images in a pile face down and ask each person in turn to take one and lead a discussion in relation to the issues we have discussed above.

The LAURS of communication: a framework for thoughtful encouragement

A resource that we have found particularly useful in thinking about communication is a textbook written for anaesthetists.

Box 5.2   Recommended Resource: A communication handbook

Cyna A.M., Andrew, M.I., Tan, S.G.M. and Smith, A.F. (eds). (2011). *Handbook of Communication in Anaesthesia and Critical Care. A Practical Guide to Exploring the Art.* Oxford: Oxford University Press.

This edited textbook has much to offer all who support women through childbirth, in particular its lively sections on the principles and structures of communication; how words can hurt; language and the subconscious; narrative and metaphor; communication in the context of maternity care; critical incidents; and communication with colleagues.

With permission from the authors, we have adapted information about a framework to guide effective communication from Chapter 2 of *Handbook of Communication in Anaesthesia and Critical Care* (Cyna *et al.*, 2011, pp.17–29). This framework – the **LAURS** of communication (Cyna, 2019) – can be especially useful if we are feeling confused about how to approach an interaction, since it can easily be remembered:

- **Listening reflectively**
- **Acceptance**
- **Utilisation**
- **Reframing**
- **Suggestion**

Each of the components of LAURS can be used individually or as part of a whole, but the first skill embedded in LAURS – 'Listening reflectively' – is paramount:

The three steps to improving communication skills are:

Step 1	Listen.
Step 2	Listen.
Step 3	Listen.

LAURS: Listening reflectively

The steps for effective listening are:

1 Observe yourself and recognise your role as a listener.
2 Note whether you are thinking about your response to the person who is talking, rather than listening to what is being said.
3 Resist the temptation to interrupt or second-guess what the other person is thinking.
4 Recognise that silences or pauses can be useful.
5 'Check in' to seek clarification regarding your understanding of what the person means and their understanding of what you mean.

Listening reflectively involves listening while observing: the other person's body language, the words they use and the tone, pace, volume and pitch of their voice. There are four questions to bear in mind when listening reflectively:

- Did you hear what was said?
- Did you understand what was meant?
- Does the other person know that she/he has been heard?
- Does the other person know that she/he has been understood?

LAURS: Acceptance

This is about accepting the other person's reality, being open minded and having a non-judgemental attitude; this can enhance their feelings of autonomy and control. It may be useful to think about there being three 'realities' in any situation:

- *The first reality*: This is our own reality and it is shaped by our individual conditioning, life experiences, education and deeply held belief systems. It is sometimes hard to remember that people do not necessarily relate to our reality and that their experience of what is happening is very different from ours.
- *The second reality*: This is another person's reality and is often characterised by a strong emotional attachment to a belief. This can be hard to accept if it seems illogical or even stupid to us. Discordance between our different realities can lead to miscommunication and conflict.
- *The third reality*: This is the reality outside our own experience and perceptions and those of the person we are engaging with. Where there is no common ground in an interaction, an outside reality can provide a wavelength at which communication can take place.

LAURS: Utilisation

If you are familiar with strengths-based approaches to care, you will recognise the idea of helping people to draw on (utilise) the strengths and abilities that they have used in previous experiences when facing new challenges. Utilisation may also involve using the sensory language of the other person – visual, auditory or kinaesthetic – to aid communication. Some examples of sensory language responses are:

- *Visual*: You can *look* forward to each contraction bringing you closer to *seeing* your baby.
- *Auditory*: It *sounds* as though you are clear about what you want.
- *Kinaesthetic*: It may *feel* like a numbing sensation.

LAURS: Reframing

Sometimes a thought, perception or behaviour that is potentially unhelpful can be reframed into something positive or helpful. An example might involve explaining the nature of contractions to someone who says that they have a low pain threshold (see Chapter 2), perhaps suggesting how, in an uncomplicated labour, most women will describe the pain as 'a different sort of pain' from the pain of injury (see Chapter 2).

LAURS: Suggestion

Suggestions are verbal or non-verbal communications that can be received in a subconscious way and lead to potential changes in mood, perception or behaviours that are non-volitional (not part of a person's conscious control). A heightened awareness of suggestion enables us to use verbal or non-verbal cues that are likely to elicit subconscious, positive responses in others (placebo); we can also avoid communication and behaviours that are likely to elicit negative or harmful (nocebo) responses.

The power of suggestion

Whenever we interact with others, communication takes place through multiple layers of conscious and subconscious awareness for all involved. Most of us are probably aware of theories related to conscious communication, such as listening skills and body language; however, even when we are functioning in a conscious state, we are also operating using our subconscious. Examples might include when we employ 'intuition' or when we are alerted to a niggling anxiety prompted by previous experiences that are not specifically recalled. We invite you to consider how suggestion plays an important role in your practice through the intricate interaction of body and mind – some would add 'and spirit'.

Suggestibility and communication with pregnant women

Suggestibility refers to the ability of people to respond subconsciously to verbal or nonverbal cues. It increases when people are highly anxious, distressed, in pain or in hypnosis. In our everyday life, however, we operate at a subconscious level most of the time, for example when we are 'daydreaming'; this is something that is exploited by consumerism and advertising. A more positive aspect of this way of being in the world, though, is that our subconscious renders us able to engage fully, on many levels, with creative arts since the language of the subconscious is contained in imagery, metaphor, symbolism and suggestion.

As a result of neuro-hormonal changes, women in late pregnancy operate at a 'daydream-ing', subconscious level a lot of the time and are thus highly susceptible to suggestion (Alexander *et al.*, 2009). Similarly, in response to both stress and the physiology of labour, women tend to dissociate from external stimuli and retreat into what midwives tend to refer to as 'the zone'; this altered state of consciousness heightens the woman's responsiveness to suggestion (Alexander *et al.*, 2009; Tiba, 1990).

Many (probably most) of the messages – or suggestions – that pregnant and labour-ing women receive from midwives and other birth workers are processed involuntarily at a subconscious level. This creates the potential for positive influences like confidence building and reducing anxiety, even when, at a conscious level, negativity and doubts prevail. Obviously, the reverse is also true; words and behaviours can have either placebo or nocebo effects, depending on the actual words that are used, but also the midwife's demeanour, posture, attitude, the tone of her voice and the emphasis she puts on certain words.

Box 5.3   Reflective Activity: Suggestibility and the effect of tone and emphasis in communication

Andrea Robertson (2007, p.16) suggests the following activity for exploring the effect of tone and emphasis. (For full effect, we suggest that you try this activ-ity *in pairs*, so that you say the phrases out loud, hear them from someone else and have a chance to discuss how emphasis and tone change the message that might be received.)

*   *Tone*: Try saying, 'She's the woman who wants an active birth' with excitement. Now try saying it with a sneer, as though you disapprove.
*   *Emphasis*: Imagine saying this sentence several times with the emphasis on a dif-ferent word each time:

    *   '**She** wants a vaginal birth after a previous caesarean section.'
    *   'She **wants** a vaginal birth after a previous caesarean section.'
    *   'She wants a **vaginal** birth after a previous caesarean section.'
    *   'She wants a vaginal birth after a **previous caesarean section**.'

The language of positive suggestion

When we are engaging with a pregnant woman, certain phrases are likely to stimulate positive motivation and useful responses, even when the woman's conscious thoughts are focused on anxiety-related issues, for example: 'Your baby is a perfect size'; 'You're doing so well'. In Box 5.4 we have placed some examples of different ways in which we might use positive suggestion, drawing on the work of Cyna *et al.* (2011). You can add to these with examples from your own practice.

Box 5.4   The language of positive suggestion: definitions and examples

Direct suggestion

A comment that suggests that something will happen, or a recommendation: 'You will find that . . . You will be able to . . .' or 'You may be surprised to find that . . .'.

Indirect suggestion

A very powerful suggestion: through implying that, if others have experienced something, there is a high likelihood that the woman will have the same experience: 'Most women find that . . . I was with someone only last week who . . .'.

Positive reinforcement

A comment that reinforces the woman's wisdom, knowledge, understanding and abilities: 'You've obviously thought a lot about that. . . . It's great the way you . . .'.

Embedded suggestion

A suggestion is embedded in the conversation in a way that is seamless and doesn't draw attention to the fact that a suggestion is being made: 'The stronger the contraction is, the more effective it is so you can respond by moving around and finding the best positions as your body tells you what to do'.

Repetition

Repetition using a variety of phrases that mean the same thing can help women retain important information both consciously and subconsciously: [after a contraction as the woman exhales] 'Well done, that was great, you're doing really well'.

The language of encouragement as 'persuasion'

Words of encouragement that are used by midwives and birth workers are steeped in positive suggestion, for example:

- 'Your body will tell you what to do – trust your body.'
- 'Each contraction brings you one step closer to meeting your baby.'
- 'Between each contraction you can have a rest.'
- 'The uterus is the strongest working muscle in the human body – it's a wonderful, powerful organ.'
- 'You will find an inner strength that you didn't know you had.'

When we think about these phrases we can see that they are direct suggestions and have a deliberate persuasive intent. These phrases are quite different in style to a lot of our conversations with women where we are attempting to promote 'informed choice'. It is easy to underestimate the influence of the person who is doing the 'informing' on 'choice' (Leap and Edwards, 2006) but, in all of our interactions, there is a fine line between influencing and what we shall call the 'gentle art of persuasion' (Leap, 2005).

Box 5.5   Reflective Activity: Exploring the role of persuasion in practice

James Herrick (2001, p.3) talks about 'the pervasiveness of persuasiveness' and suggests that we are 'perpetual persuaders' in our personal, occupational and social interactions in everyday life – this in spite of the fact that we are 'leery of persuasion'.

In pairs or small groups:
• Discuss the role of 'persuasion' in terms of the messages that women receive from multiple sources. How does the word 'persuasion' make you feel in relation to your practice of encouraging pregnant women and their supporters?

Placebo and the power of suggestion

In order to understand the power of suggestion further we shall have a brief look at the curious world of 'placebo'. If anyone feels sceptical about the power of placebo they would do well to consider Allan Cyna's words:

> Half of all drugs that fail in late-stage trials drop out of the pipeline due to their inability to beat sugar pills.
>> (Allan Cyna: Birth International workshop presentation for midwives, 2013)

In a summary of studies, Allan Cyna (2013) shows that sugar pills (placebo) are more effective in the following circumstances:

• It helps if the pills have an official-looking code engraved on them.
• Placebos stamped or packaged with widely recognised trademarks are more effective than 'generic' placebos.
• Placebos taken four times a day deliver greater relief than those taken twice daily, and if the placebo is injected it is even more effective.
• A more expensive placebo can create the impression that it is of higher value: a pill identified as costing $2.50 works better than one identified as costing 10c.
• The colour of the pills will alter how effective they are for specific treatments: red for stimulation; white for soothing digestion; green for reducing anxiety; yellow as the most effective anti-depressant.
>> (Allan Cyna: Birth International workshop presentation for midwives, 2013)

Box 5.6   Reflective Activity: Discussing homeopathy – contested opinions

Given the chemical 'nil-potency' of homeopathic remedies, homeopathy is often explained by sceptics as a belief-system based on placebo effect. The discussion in this systematic review by Ernst (2010) provides us with a resource to think about this:

Ernst, E. (2010). Homeopathy: what does the 'best' evidence tell us? A systematic review. *Medical Journal of Australia*, *192*(8), 458–460.

In pairs or small groups:
- Discuss the following questions:

  - Are you convinced by this article that homeopathy works on a placebo basis?
  - Why do you think that observational studies of homeopathy might produce different results?
  - As midwives and birth workers, how do you think we should respond when a woman who uses homeopathy regularly asks us what our opinion is about the use of homeopathic remedies in pregnancy and labour?

'Nocebo' and the power of suggestion – when words hurt

For some time there has been evidence that warning patients that a potentially painful procedure – such as cannula insertion – might hurt (using negatively loaded words like, 'little sting' and 'sharp scratch') increases their anticipatory pain and anxiety (Cyna, 2019; Cyna and Lang, 2011; Dutt-Gupta *et al.*, 2007; Lang *et al.*, 2005; Varelmann *et al.*, 2010). The person's subconscious hears 'STING' or 'SHARP SCRATCH' and that is exactly how the subsequent procedure is experienced. (An alternative is to talk about 'numbing' the skin.)

Advances in magnetic imaging are contributing to neuroanatomical and neurochemical explanations of the effect of language on anticipatory pain and anxiety (Benedetti *et al.*, 2007). This emerging theory helps us to interpret research findings, such as those in the study in the following research briefing.

Box 5.7   Research Briefing: The power of suggestion – placebo and nocebo effects

Chooi, C.S.L., White, A.M., Tan, S.G.M., Dowling, K. and Cyna, A.M. (2013). Pain vs comfort scores after caesarean section: a randomized trial. *British Journal of Anaesthesia*, *110*(5), 780–787. doi:10.1093/bja/aes517.

Following caesarean section, women who were asked questions related to their levels of pain were more likely to describe pain and request extra analgesia than women who were asked questions about their levels of comfort.

Sabotage: the failure words 'try' and 'not'

Negative suggestions include using the failure words 'try' and 'not'. 'Try' implies a likelihood of failure. If you tell someone to 'try not' to do something they are likely to do it as the subconscious does not hear the word 'not' (Cyna and Lang, 2011). For example, telling a woman in labour not to 'worry' tells her subconscious that there is something to worry about.

'Vomit' can be a sabotage word when a woman is in labour; even producing a bowl with or without the verbal message, 'in case you need to vomit', can set up an involuntary response so that the woman feels like vomiting. This might make sense if you think about what happens to your salivary glands when someone talks about eating a lemon!

Concentrated attention: countering nocebo effects

When someone concentrates on an image or experience over and over again, it tends to realise itself through subconscious reinforcement. This is worth considering in relation to the negative effect of repeatedly asking a woman in labour if they want pain relief (Cyna and Lang, 2011). Another example is when a woman in labour is struggling and repeatedly says, 'I can't do this'. Suggesting that, instead, she says, '*I can* do this' repeatedly, often means that concentrated attention can be used with positive effect.

Metaphor and meaning

The subconscious thrives on making connections through metaphor. As George Eliot so aptly pointed out in the novel *The Mill on the Floss* (Book 2, Chapter 1):

> Intelligence so rarely shows itself in speech without metaphor . . . we can so seldom declare what a thing is, except by saying it is something else.

The word 'metaphor' comes from the Greek word 'matapherein', which means 'to transfer'. A metaphor is a figure of speech in which a comparison is made between two unlike objects; the aim is to illuminate similarities, shedding light on the essence of one or both objects. Words or stories can convey meaning without using literal words.

As we have already seen in the work of Karlsdottir *et al.* (2014), it is not unusual for women to describe the continuum from pregnancy through to new motherhood as a 'journey'. Some have suggested that accompanying women on this journey speaks to the meaning of the midwife–woman relationship (Leap, 2010; Thompson, 2004). When we talk in this way about a 'journey' we are using a metaphor to highlight meaning.

Box 5.8   Reflective Activity: A journey metaphor for childbirth

In pairs:

- Using creative art forms tell a story about going on a journey as a metaphor for an individual woman's experience of pregnancy, labour and birth, and new motherhood – including the support and influences from others in preparation, along the way and in the sequel to the journey.
- Present or perform what you have created to others in the wider group.

Metaphors evoking sporting activities are often used to convey endurance and triumph when facing the physical and mental challenges of labour (Dempsey, 2013; Lowe, 2002; Reiger and Dempsey, 2006). There are, however, reasons to think carefully about using sporting activities as a metaphor for labour, not least that this might alienate or worry women who do not see their bodies as 'sporty'. Also, although we often hear people talking about labour being like running a marathon, Michel Odent (1994; Odent and Odent, 2015) suggests that it is inappropriate and potentially dangerous to draw such parallels: unlike advice given to marathon runners, the promotion of birth physiology should involve the avoidance of sugar and carbohydrate intake and the conservation of muscular energy in order to reduce the antagonism of oxytocin by adrenaline.

When we use metaphors, we need to be careful about the potential impact for individual women; for example, the idea of 'waves' might be useful for a woman who loves surfing but counterproductive for a woman who has a fear of being dunked and rendered out of control by the force of waves. In a similar vein, the force described by this childbirth educator could be scary for some women, particularly those who are worried about losing control in labour:

> Each of these waves brings the tide in, but before it finally comes in it's often experienced as a storm, and you feel at one with nature, that this great contraction is like mountains building. You can only really take analogies from the natural world, there's nothing else like it, and your body is part of this; the power of creation is sweeping through your body.
> (Childbirth educator/birth supporter, Sandall *et al.*, 2010, unpublished data)

Metaphor to convey meaning about labour in creative writing

Mixed metaphors involving the natural world are also used in the following excerpts from various sections of Enid Bagnold's semi-autobiographical novel, *The Squire* (first published in 1938 and republished in 2013 by Persephone Books). The central character describes her reflections as she approaches the birth of her fifth child and then gives birth at home, with a midwife and GP in attendance.

Box 5.9 Metaphor and meaning: excerpts from *The Squire* (2013) by Enid Bagnold* originally published in 1938 (recommended reading)

Pain is but a branch of sensation. Perhaps childbirth turns into pain only when it is fought and resisted?

There comes a time, after the first pains have passed, when you swim down a silver river running like a torrent, with the convulsive, corkscrew movements of a great fish, threshing from its neck to its tail. And if you can marry the movements, go with them, turn like a screw in the river and swim on, then the pain . . . then I believe the pain . . . becomes a flame that doesn't burn you . . . It's not awful, the thing's progressive. And when you are right *in* the river to marry the pain requires tremendous determination, and will, and self-belief. You have to rush ahead into it, not pull back against it. It's very hard to do.

The monk and nun [GP and midwife in attendance] were about her bed, acutely directed on her, tuned to her every manifestation. With eyes fast shut she lent herself to their quiet directions, clinging to the memory of her resolve that when the river began to pull she would swim down with it, clutching at no banks. . . .

Her mind went down and lived in her body, ran out of her brain and lived in her flesh. She had eyes and nose and ears and senses in her body, in her backbone, living like a spiny woodlouse, doubled in a ball, having no beginning and no end. Now the first twisting spate of pain began, swim then, swim with it for your life. If you resist, horror and impediment! If you swim, not pain but sensation! Who knows the heart of pain, the silver, whistling hub of pain, the central bellows of childbirth, which expels one being from another? None knows it who, in disbelief and dread has drawn back to the periphery, contradicting the will of pain, braking against inexorable movements. Keep abreast of it, rush together, you and the violence which is also you! Wild movements, hallucinated swimming! Other things exist than pain!

It is hard to gauge pain. By her movements, by her exclamations, she would have struck horror into anyone but her monk and nun. She would have seemed tortured, tossing, crying, muttering, grunting. She was not unconscious but she had left external life. She was blind and deaf to world surface. Every sense she had was down in Earth to which she belonged, fighting to maintain a hold on the pain, to keep pace with it, not to take an ounce of will from her assent to its passage. It was as though the dark river rushed her to a glossy arch. A little more, a little more, a little longer. She was not in torture, she was in labour; she had been thus before and knew her way.

*Reproduced with permission, Nicola Beauman, Persephone Books: www.persephonebooks. co.uk.

**Box 5.10   Reflective Activity: Metaphor promoting meaning
in *The Squire***

In pairs or small groups:
* Discuss the personal impact of the excerpts from *The Squire* in Box 5.9 and the ways in which metaphor tends to convey meaning for you.
* There are a series of different metaphors used in these passages. Make a list of these and discuss the meaning they convey in terms of how we conceptualise pain and support.

The power of words

Words are powerful (Leap, 2012). The way they are used needs care and awareness, as the celebrated author and poet Maya Angelou cautions:

> Words are things. You must be careful, careful about calling people out of their names, using racial pejoratives and sexual pejoratives and all that ignorance. Don't do that. Some day we'll be able to measure the power of words. I think they are things. They get on the walls. They get in your wallpaper. They get into your rugs, in your upholstery, and your clothes, and finally into you.
>
> (Maya Angelou: The Power of Words. YouTube film clip)

Over the years there have been a plethora of articles in the midwifery and medical press about the potential for the words we use to have a disempowering effect on childbearing women (see some examples in the articles in Box 5.11). These words tend to reflect, perpetuate and reinforce a culture in maternity service provision where the language of 'managing', 'allowing', 'conducting', 'delivering' and 'risk' reflects who has the power in any given situation (Leap, 2012).

**Box 5.11   Research Briefing: Language, communication
and power dynamics – a sample of articles in
the midwifery press**

Hastie, C. (2005). How understanding semantics helps us be 'with women'. *MIDIRS Midwifery Digest*, *15(4)*, 475–477.

Hunter, L. (2006). Women give birth and pizzas are delivered: language and Western childbirth paradigms. *Journal of Midwifery and Women's Health*, *51(2)*, 119–124.

Leap, N. (2012) The power of words revisited. *Essentially MIDIRS*, *3(1)*, 17–21.

Mander, R. (1997). What are we called? Words that colleagues use. *British Journal of Midwifery*, *5(7)*, 406.

Wickham, S. (2005). Language of the complicated. *Practising Midwife*, *8(9)*, 33.

Box 5.12   Reflective Activity: Language, communication and power dynamics

Group activity, in pairs or small groups:

- Choose one of the articles in Box 5.11 and create a script for a short sketch around the words that are highlighted in the article.
- After everyone has performed their sketches, a facilitated discussion in the wider group can address the following questions:

  - What are the advantages of finding alternatives to these words when talking to pregnant women about labour and birth?
  - What are the social pressures within the maternity care environment to continue using these words?

Andrea Robertson (2007) suggests that the acceptance and use of one word in particular – 'delivery' – sidesteps power away from women:

> Just eliminating that one word from your daily conversations with women will help them feel more positive about what they will be doing and remind you of your position as an assistant in the process. . . . Once we have substituted 'birth' for every example of 'delivery' in our conversations, written works and medical records, we will have made some very basic progress towards normalising birth.
>
> (pp.16, 17)

Box 5.13   Reflective Activity: The 'delivery' word

- Discuss how you might substitute 'birth' for 'delivery' in the following phrases in ways that might make a difference to workplace culture and how pregnant women/new mothers feel:

  - 'She had a wonderful delivery last night.'
  - 'I had a wonderful delivery last night.'
  - 'In the Delivery Suite our forceps delivery rate is going down as we do more ventouse deliveries.'
  - 'She was delivered by caesarean section in the end.'
  - 'The normal delivery rate is very high where I work.'
  - 'Since qualifying I've delivered over 500 babies.'

How might you respond to a colleague who says, 'It's all just semantics. And anyway, when they have an instrumental delivery or caesarean section, they're not giving birth, we *are* delivering the baby for them.'

Some midwives refer to 'catching babies' as a way of avoiding the 'delivery' word. What do you think about this?

Pains, contractions, surges or rushes?

Talking about 'pain' when a woman is in labour is probably the most common example of sabotage language. Asking a woman in labour about 'pain relief' at regular intervals or asking her to complete a 'pain score' (advocated in some units) has obvious repercussions in the sensitive world of the subconscious, beyond the obvious undermining of her confidence. We explore this further in Chapter 6.

Some people think that we should not use the word 'pain' when talking to pregnant women in preparation for labour and that the word 'contraction' is also a negative suggestion. For example, in *Spiritual Midwifery* Ina May Gaskin (2002) refers to contractions as 'rushes' and, in hypnobirthing, the words, 'surges' or 'waves' are often used as an alternative to 'contractions'. Ruth Sanders (2015) proposes that this likens the experience of contractions to external forces imposed on women; while the intention is supportive, women cannot be in control of external environmental forces and there is the possibility of this metaphor distancing them from what is occurring in their bodies. She also makes the case for isolating the 'functional discomfort' associated with normal labour from the pathological pain paradigm that permeates cultural representations of birth and the language of midwifery practice.

Like Ruth Sanders (2015), childbirth educator and birth supporter Rhea Dempsey (2013) suggests that pregnant women are preoccupied by how they will cope with pain in labour; it is therefore important to invite conversations about reframing the word 'pain' within a philosophy of working with physiological pain in labour:

> Getting hung up on the idea that labour shouldn't be painful or that, with the right technique and control, it will be painless, is a capacity-limiting viewpoint . . . the birthing woman runs the risk of having nowhere to go when it all begins to crumble.
>
> (Dempsey, 2013, p.59)

Box 5.14   Reflective Activity: The words we use for contractions

If you search the Internet using the words 'reframing contractions as surges', you will find plenty of postings from women about this issue: some explaining why they thought this reframing of the word 'contraction' was useful, others suggesting that this masks the reality that contractions are painful, thus doing a disservice to women.

Individual activity:

- Discuss this issue with: women who have experienced labour; women who have practised hypnobirthing; colleagues who have experience of working with women using hypnobirthing techniques; and practitioners who prefer to use alternative words to describe 'contractions'.
- Decide on the words that you will choose to use and whether there are circumstances when this might change, for example in the context of preparation for birth or during a woman's labour. Share your thoughts about these issues with colleagues.

The language of 'normal birth'

When thinking about the words that we use in our speaking and writing, we may do well to consider the 'normal birth' debate (Downe and Byrom, 2019; Feeley *et al.*, 2020; Lynch, 2020). The phrase 'normal birth' has become a 'code' for something we think we all understand; it is embedded in the documentation and discourses that shape and reflect contemporary maternity service provision. But the notion is fraught with difficulty, not least finding a consensus on what we mean by 'normal birth' (Darra, 2009; Gould, 2000). The complex process of an interdisciplinary attempt to arrive at a consensus definition for normal labour and birth, one that involves women and measures the process of labour, rather than outcomes, is discussed in *Making Normal Birth a Reality* (Maternity Care Working Party, 2007).

The word 'normal' is hardly in keeping with the midwifery philosophy of embracing the concept of each woman's birth being seen by her as quintessentially unique and 'special' (Darra and Murphy, 2016; Downe, 2006; Kennedy and Shannon, 2004). Women will sometimes talk about 'natural birth' but, as with 'normal birth', we are left questioning the binaries of 'normal/abnormal' and 'natural/unnatural'. What do these phrases mean in situations where the majority of women have some form of intervention and in countries where increasing numbers of women are choosing elective caesarean birth?

The potential for the majority of women to feel marginalised if birth is only seen as meaningful when it is 'normal' concerns all of us (Lyerly, 2012). Perhaps this thinking informed a paper published in the *British Journal of Obstetrics and Gynaecology* (Smith *et al.*, 2008), where the authors (obstetricians) chose the title: 'The natural caesarean section: a woman-centred technique' in advocating a 'natural approach that mimics the situation at vaginal birth' (p.1037). Whilst welcoming the suggestion of improving women's experiences of caesarean birth, birth activist Lareen Newman and midwife Heather Hancock (2009) expressed concerns about the use of the phrase 'natural caesarean' in their critique of the article by Smith *et al.* (2008).

In most Western countries, women are still having to negotiate their pregnancies through systems dominated by risk management and will end up being labelled in relation to notions of risk status. If normal birth is for 'low risk' women and some midwives provide care to 'all risk' women, does this mean that there is no such thing as 'no risk', and that risk is always lurking in the wings to justify those who persist in saying, 'Birth is only normal in retrospect'?

The phrase 'physiological birth' is sometimes chosen as an alternative to 'normal birth' but this is not a phrase that many women or maternity care providers would use or consider appropriate. Furthermore, computerised summaries identifying birth as 'normal' may include a range of non-physiological processes, for example acceleration with synthetic oxytocin and episiotomy.

As an attempt to avoid this difficult territory, the term 'straightforward labour and birth' is often used in the UK (for example in NCT publications) and there is a tendency to refer to 'labour and birth with complications' to avoid the term 'abnormal'. Not everyone is happy with the idea of 'straightforward' though, given the variations and meanderings of women's individual labours where physiological processes prevail.

There is a move afoot in the USA to talk about: 'optimal birth: the maximum perinatal outcome with minimal intervention placed against the context of the woman's social, medical and obstetrical [sic] history' (Kennedy, 2006, p.763). An Optimality Index scoring tool has been devised to assess optimality of care and outcomes for individual women. The paper describing this contains some stimulating discussion about the biomedical prioritising of risk and technology in maternity care (Cragin and Kennedy, 2006).

Box 5.15   Reflective Activity: The problem with 'normal'

In pairs or small groups:
- Discuss the following questions:

  - In thinking about the language that you use in your practice, which words to describe normal birth do you use? Can you think of any reason why you might consider changing these in particular situations? If so, what might be the effect on others and yourself?
  - What do you think are the potential benefits and pitfalls associated with the terminology and use of the concept of 'optimal' birth and how might this approach affect women?
  - The article written by obstetricians: 'The natural caesarean section: a woman-centred technique' (Smith *et al.*, 2008) raises issues about promoting the very best experience for women and babies who experience caesarean birth. After studying this article and the critique by Newman and Hancock (2009), discuss the issues these articles raise for you, particularly in relation to the use of language?

The effect of environment and models of care on communication

---

Box 5.16   Research Briefing: Communication in antenatal 'booking' visits

McCourt, C. (2006). Supporting choice and control? Communication and interaction between midwives and women at the antenatal booking visit. *Social Science & Medicine, 62,* 1307–1318.

This article describes how different models of care and settings influenced styles and patterns of communication between midwives and women in antenatal booking visits.

Communication and continuity of care: addressing the needs of women who are most at risk of poor outcomes

Effective communication lies at the heart of supporting women who are socially disadvantaged and most at risk of poor birth outcomes and experiences, in particular, Australian Indigenous women (Australian Institute of Health and Welfare, 2020) and, in the UK, women from Black, Asian and minority ethnic (BAME) groups (Knight *et al.*, 2020). Policy documents aiming to improve communication with women in these groups identify practical initiatives, such as providing interpreter services and information systems for women facing the myriad of difficulties associated with resettlement and language barriers. Increasingly, though, policy documents are proposing midwifery continuity of care as the most important public health strategy to help improve outcomes and experiences for the most vulnerable mothers and babies (Australian Government Department of Health, 2019;

NHS, 2019). Midwifery continuity of care enables adequate time to build trusting relationships and explore with the woman what her individual needs are, including access to other health and support services (Allen *et al.*, 2016; Corcoran *et al.*, 2017; McCourt and Pearce, 2000; Odentourt and Pearce, 2000; Rayment Jones *et al.*, 2019). We offer a chance to explore this in the following Reflective Activity.

Box 5.17   Reflective Activity: Enhancing communication through midwifery continuity of care

Group activity, in pairs or small groups:
Create a table demonstrating which features of each of the midwifery continuity of care projects described in these articles may have enhanced communication with women and others, thus improving outcomes.

Homer, C.S.E., Foureur, M., Allende, T., Pekin, F., Caplice, S. and Catling-Paull, C. (2012). 'It's more than just having a baby' women's experiences of a maternity service for Australian Aboriginal and Torres Strait Islander families. *Midwifery, 28*, e509–e513.

Homer, C.S.E., Leap, N., Edwards, N. and Sandall, J. (2017). Midwifery continuity of carer in an area of high socio-economic disadvantage in London: a retrospective analysis of Albany Midwifery Practice outcomes using routine data (1997–2009). *Midwifery, 48*, 1–10.

Rayment-Jones, H., Murrells, T. and Sandall, J. (2015). An investigation of the relationship between the caseload model of midwifery for socially disadvantaged women and childbirth outcomes using routine data – a retrospective, observational study. *Midwifery, 31*(4), 409–417.

Communication when we don't warm to the woman or her birth companions

Inevitably there will be times when we are caring for a woman in labour who has different values to ours and whom we don't warm to. Establishing rapport with a woman we like is easy but managing to achieve this with someone we do not warm to requires concentration on our non-verbal as well as verbal skills (Robertson, 2007). For all caregivers there are times when we find it hard to communicate well with women, as this midwife discusses:

> It's hard sometimes. The other day when a very large woman refused the meal we got for her in a long labour and her husband came in with huge quantities of burgers, chips and pizza – I had to work at containing my disapproval! He's the manager of a McDonald's and there she was with her epidural complaining about this being the worst day of her life. Lots of things that were said that made me think, 'Let this be over'. And she had her bottles of formula ready to feed her baby.
>
> I find it really difficult not to be judgemental sometimes. What I'm often seeing is that an epidural goes in and it seems like nothing's happening and so the phones come out. He'll sit over here on his phone and she'll sit over there on her phone, there's no talking, no nothing other than communication with the outside world. And the number of people who are putting things on Facebook while they're in labour, even during and immediately after the birth – I can't believe it!
>
> The other day I took over from a midwife who told me the young woman had done really well and ended up having a lovely water birth. The woman was a teenager. She told me the midwife had denied her her right to have an epidural; she was really disgruntled. It reminded me that you have to go with their agenda, not yours.
>
> (Midwife, Leap, 2015, unpublished data)

**Box 5.18   Reflective Activity: When personal values get in
the way of rapport**

In pairs or small groups:

- Discuss the quotation above with reference to your own experiences and identify some strategies for providing supportive care in such situations. Think of how you might handle other situations where you might feel judgemental when supporting someone in labour, for example if someone is making racist or sexist comments.
- Share a story of a situation that you have been in where personal values made it hard for you to develop positive communication with a pregnant woman and/or her supporters. How did it feel at the time? How do you feel about it now? What did you learn? What will you do next time you're in a similar situation?

Communication and thoughtful encouragement: a student assignment

Drawing on all of the issues we have discussed in this chapter, we end with a suggestion for a written assignment that we have used in university programmes for midwives. This assignment offers students an opportunity to explore how the language and phraseology we use when talking with a pregnant woman might promote her confidence to embrace physiological labour and birth.

Reading in preparation for the assignment

Cutajar, L., Steen, M., Fleet, J-A. and Cyna, A.M. (2020). Language used during antenatal education for labour and birth: a literature review. *Evidence Based Midwifery*, *30(3)*, 307–318.

Within this review are useful examples of the use of positive and negative suggestions and the potential use of the LAURS framework for effective communication.

Cutajar, L., Miu, M., Fleet, J-A., Cyna, A.M. and Steen, M. (2020). Antenatal education for childbirth: labour and birth. *European Journal of Midwifery*, *4*, 11. doi:10.18332/ejm/120002.

This paper reports on research that analysed language and phraseology used in antenatal education according to pre-determined categories of language techniques related to positive and negative suggestions.

Instructions: Your task is to write a script – similar to that which would be written for a play (with stage directions) – for an interaction between a pregnant woman and midwife in an antenatal clinic. The midwife will use language and phrases that have the potential to encourage the woman's confidence in her identified wish to have a normal birth. You will identify and categorise these types of verbal communication using a template.

Start your script by copying the following headings and words, which explain the setting, characters and initial interactions:

The setting: A midwife-led antenatal clinic at Lucina Hospital, where women have 20-minute appointments.

The characters: Samantha is a healthy 38-year-old woman having her first baby. Her pregnancy has been straightforward and she has good support from her partner, Tony. Today her 36-week antenatal appointment is with Eileen, whom she has not met before. Eileen has been a midwife for ten years at Lucina Hospital.

The initial interaction: Eileen has checked that all is well with Samantha's health and her baby is active and growing well. They start discussing Samantha's hopes for her labour.

SAMANTHA (looking anxious): 'I'd really like to have a normal birth with no interventions or drugs but my Mum says I'm going to need to have an epidural because I've got a really low pain threshold . . .'.

What happens next: Continue to write the script in the style identified in the example (no more than five minutes of conversation, 1,000–1,500 words), including stage directions. Drawing on your prior reading, identify in the script (in brackets) as many examples as you like of each of the types of communication outlined in the template below.

Example:

EILEEN: 'Yes (Listening attentively and nodding) . . . When your mother says that it must make you feel a bit unsure (Acceptance) but it sounds as though you're very clear about why you want to avoid an epidural (Positive reinforcement) . . . You know, many women find that labour is a different sort of pain from the pain of injury (Indirect suggestion) . . .

What you need to submit: Place one example of each type of verbal communication in the third column of the template and submit this with your script. Also submit an annotated bibliography* identifying 5–10 publications and/or resources that you have found useful when completing this assignment.

* A short paragraph giving a synopsis of the resources you have listed (to share with colleagues)

Table 5.1 Template for analysing a conversation with a pregnant woman

Type of verbal communication	Definitions	Example from the script
Listening	Listening, observing, checking in that the woman knows she has been heard/understood	
Acceptance	Appreciating different realities, the woman's, the midwife's own, that of others	
Reframing	Reframing the woman's concerns in a way that generates a helpful thought, perception or behaviour	
Sharing information	The woman and/or midwife shares ideas or information	
Command	Instruction/s are given to the woman	
Direct suggestion	A comment that suggests something will happen or a recommendation	
Indirect suggestion	A recommendation or comment that implies a recommendation	
Positive reinforcement	Reinforcing and complimenting the woman's wisdom, knowledge, understanding, hopes and wishes	
Positive suggestion	A statement or language that potentially stimulates positive motivation and useful subconscious responses	
Embedded suggestion	Suggestions embedded in the conversation without making it obvious that a suggestion is being made	
Metaphor	Imagery and imaginative comparisons to encourage subconscious responses and facilitate meaning	
Research evidence	Drawing on relevant research in the discussion	

Source: Adapted from Cyna, A.M., Andrew, M.I., Tan, S.G.M. and Smith, A.F. (eds). (2011). *Handbook of Communication in Anaesthesia and Critical Care: A Practical Guide to Exploring the Art.* Oxford: Oxford University Press.

Table 5.2 Assessment criteria: Communication and thoughtful encouragement student assignment

The analysis of a conversation with a pregnant woman will demonstrate evidence of	*Possible marks*
A written script of a conversation lasting no more than five minutes (1,000–1,500 words) containing types of verbal communication that potentially encourage pregnant women's confidence and promote physiological birth	30
Use of a template to analyse and identify the script for types of verbal communication	40
Arguments/ideas/concepts supported by an annotated bibliography: 5–10 resources that relate to exemplary communication in midwifery	30

Communication skills training

Finally, we suggest that, however experienced we are, there is always value in engaging in communication skills training.

Box 5.19   Research Briefing: Communication skills training

Škodová, Z. (2016). Communication and interpersonal skills enhancement in midwifery: review. *Central European Journal of Nursing and Midwifery, 7(3)*, 504–510.

This review identified positive effects of communication training methods in midwifery education and practice in terms of participants' self-confidence, self-awareness, subjective feelings of competency and communication within the team. The majority of the nine studies took place in midwifery education settings.

Chang, Y-S., Coxon, K., Portela, A.G., Furuta, M. and Bick, D. (2018). Interventions to support effective communication between maternity care staff and women in labour: a mixed-methods systematic review. *Midwifery, 59*, 4–16.

The introduction to this article provides a useful overview of publications and policy directives linking effective communication to improving experiences and outcomes for pregnant women. However, only two studies were identified in this review. The authors concluded that there is an urgent need for research to identify the characteristics of interventions that support effective communication in maternity care, including how organisations prepare, monitor and sustain communication interventions to reflect outcomes of priority for women, local culture and birth care.

The studies in Box 5.19 suggest that opportunities to engage in organised communication skills training for maternity care staff may be limited. We offer a list of topics that might be found in training courses if you are keen to hone your communication skills as part of your continuing personal and professional development:

- Group facilitation
- Motivational interviewing
- Assertiveness skills
- Leadership
- Clinical supervision
- Conflict resolution
- Neuro linguistic programming (NLP)
- 'Dealing with difficult people'
- Giving and receiving feedback

We shall be exploring communication further in the next two chapters, where we look at how we support women during labour.

Addendum to Chapter 5

Communication while wearing masks and PPE

As we write this 2nd edition, the global Covid pandemic is challenging how we all communicate in multiple ways, not least how health practitioners communicate while wearing PPE. In Box 5.20 we have reproduced a section of a document that you can download from the website of the stillbirth and neonatal death charity (Sands) and share as a leaflet or poster. The document acknowledges the barriers to building trusting relationships, particularly by the wearing of facemasks, but reinforces the important message that applies to all situations involving loss:

> Compassionate communication can positively influence how parents and families experience their care even when the worst happens . . . Good communication can't take away the pain parents and families feel, but it can reduce the impact of trauma, both in the short and long term.
>
> (Sands, 2020)

Box 5.20   Communication while wearing PPE

Carry a photograph of yourself

- without a mask and share when appropriate, or display staff photographs in a public area.

Introduce yourself clearly

- have your name badge visible and gesture to it as you make your introductions.

Acknowledge the difficulties

- explain why you can't shake hands or make physical contact and that the situation is difficult.

Use eye contact and smile,

- even if they can't see your mouth, people will be able to see a smile in your eyes.

Consider your tone of voice

- ensure you can be heard, but be gentle, kind and honest.

Support understanding,

- by using hand gestures.

Take your time

- don't talk too fast, check back for understanding, use written prompts if necessary.

Say things in a different way

- if you have not been understood.

Think about the physical environment,

- face parents, try to stand still when speaking, try not to stand with light or a window behind you.

Adapted from: Sands. (2020). Communication while wearing PPE. Available at: https://www.sands.org.uk/sites/default/files/Communication%20with%20PPE.pdf.

Postscript

The postscript to this chapter is a story written by Meg Hitchick in 2014, following her first experience of attending a birth as a student midwife. It is a perfect example of the value of storytelling to promote reflection. The story has the potential to stimulate a wealth of discussion about the communication skills of midwives in supporting women in labour whom they have not met before, whilst also supporting students. It also speaks volumes about how much we can learn about birth through the sensual responses and fresh perspectives of student midwives.

Reflection by Meg Hitchick

A baby boy was born last night. Not my baby, but almost as momentous – it is my first birth, as a student midwife. Quick! Pay attention! Take notes!

> Multip, G2P1. Attempted VBAC. Induction for post-dates by Foleys, Syntocinon. Foetal distress, worrying CTG, CS indicated. Fast second stage. Vacuum. VD. Second-degree tear. Meconium in liquor. APGARS 8 & 9. Active third stage. Mother and baby doing well.

It's becoming simple enough to describe what happened in this code, this language of midwifery that I am learning to speak, but these abbreviations and technical terms, they don't tell the full story. Not even the half of it. There's no abbreviation for 'afraid', 'uncertain' or 'tired' or 'anxious'. There's no mention in the notes of 'that look that just passed between midwife and expectant dad', nor of 'the way that five minutes felt like forever'. There's no shorthand for 'trust between mother and midwife established at x time'.

There is the real story, and then there's the one you'll read in the notes after.

Birth. A strange and heady mix of high drama and the rhythms of the everyday – a heart beating, breaths being drawn in, the swift and sure movements of calm hands. As a brand new baby midwife, I so admire those hands, moving with steady purpose, performing a hundred tiny tasks as though on autopilot. Gloves on, gloves off. Pen scribbling a note. A gentle touch. A swift tug. Plastic being unwrapped. Membranes being stretched and prodded. It is a ballet, full of complex and perfect manoeuvres, made to look effortless through the sheer polish of having been performed by those hands a hundred, a thousand times before. My own hands feel sluggish and uncertain by comparison, and seem to hover a lot, at a loss. Am I doing it right? Why won't my fingers work like they normally do? Come on, surely I can get a blood pressure cuff on faster than this, now!

For this one, there were three midwives, three sets of hands, from start to 'finish'. I know why they call it a 'handover'. But it is not the impression of hands that most remains with me.

Instead, it's all in the eyes.

There's the eyes of my woman, half closed in tiredness, squeezed shut with determination, lit up with new love. And all the while, searching, searching for what she wants to find in the faces of those around her. 'Do you care for me? Will you be with me through whatever happens? Can you be gentle with me? Will I get through this?'

The eyes of the dad-to-be, creased with concern, flicking with distraction, to the phone, to his partner, to the funny, beeping medical equipment. To the staff who come and go. Always on the look out for signs. 'Is it alright? Is this normal? Do you all know what you're doing? Do I need to panic yet?!'

The eyes of the tiny newborn boy, blearily gazing around him, an exhausted triumph. And the eyes of the midwives.

A midwife is capable of saying a thousand things with her eyes. When there isn't time for words, this is a handy skill. She can say 'I'm here, he's okay, you're going to be okay, I'm competent, I care about you, you're in safe hands, and you're wonderful' all at once. At the same time, if she is really skilled, she can hide things so they don't show in her eyes – 'I'm tired, I missed a tea break, there's a baby in the next room not doing so well, this is going to take a while, and I have a gut feeling this one will end up as a C-section. I don't like the look of that trace'. If she doesn't want you to know, you'll never know.

The first midwife, I think she knows that she won't be seeing this baby born on her watch. Her eyes, they've seen this before, and even as she's saying the obvious, that nobody has a crystal ball, that birth is unpredictable, I can sense that she's preparing my woman for that moment at which she'll have to go, and the next midwife will be along to take over. I've only just arrived, and I'm somewhere in between 'staff' and 'clueless bystander', but oh, I'm thankful for this one. She speaks to me as if I'm part of the team. When she ducks out quickly, she doesn't see the flash of dismay in my woman's eyes – the one that says 'Oh no. We can't keep her. She's so lovely and we can't keep her as long as we need her for. How will we go on without her?' And I am left wondering, how did she do that? Such trust, built so quickly. How will I ever do that?

The second midwife arrives, and her eyes take everything in, the woman on the bed, the weary partner, the trace folding slowly onto the floor. The drip flowing steadily into an arm. She looks to the woman, really looks at her. Speaks a few calm words, asks a gentle question. I wonder if she notices the woman's body relaxing, melting back on to the bed as she responds, the look of relief – this isn't a stranger after all. She's one of us. She's on our team. It's magic. Our new midwife leaves the room, but she's still 'with' us.

'We're in such good hands', smiles my woman to her partner and me. But she doesn't really mean the hands. She means the eyes. She knows just how the look in those eyes made her feel, and it's all she wants to feel now. She feels safe.

Later, when big calls have to be made, action has to be decided on, it's those eyes my woman searches out. 'You're my midwife', she says pleadingly. 'What should I do? And I know that she's trying to read 'the answer' in her midwife's eyes. We are here in this big hospital, in the province of medicine and doctors and shifts and procedures, but what she really wants to know is 'what would YOU have me do? Because I trust you.'

The third midwife, the one who will eventually 'catch' the baby, she has a lot on her plate. There's a trace that now has more steep drops than the Grand Canyon. There's a doctor calling for a section – NOW – and a surgical team that aren't ready, an OR still in use. There's a dad looking very green around the gills. There's a woman in transition, shaking and calling for a sick bag and wanting to push and there's a baby with his own agenda who is inching slowly but surely down the birth canal, low heart rate notwithstanding.

And yet somehow within ten minutes of this ridiculously dramatic situation unfolding, midwife and mum are smiling together over the face of this brand new person, and they've never met each other before this day, but right now, they are two of the closest people in the world. This midwife, she's nailed it. She has spent only an hour, with someone who was basically out of their right mind, during one of the most momentous challenges life has to offer, and yet somehow, there's a relationship there. As the woman grins and strokes the little head and repeatedly thanks the midwife, me, her partner and anyone else who comes within earshot, I wonder how I will ever remember what to say to a woman at such an occasion, let alone what to do.

We do the newborn check. 'Hallo, little guy', says the midwife cheerfully, as she points out all the features we are looking for. Somehow after all that has transpired, she is still taking time to be friendly with me, to be patient with my complete ignorance, to treat me as an equal. I realise: she does this, all the time, it's the DNA of her job. To climb into the passenger seat alongside people who are mere tourists to this, her realm, and allow them to 'drive'.

That night, it takes me hours to get to sleep. It's a lot to take in, to process. The 'technical skills' of birth – I'm reasonably sure I'll figure those out given enough time to practise. But how will I become capable of being 'with woman'? Outside of the delivery room, it's much easier to be relaxed, to create a rapport, to encourage and compliment and do all those other things that are 'social lubricant' for forging relationships, but inside? There's only being real, being gentle, being the rock in the turbulent unknown, being YOU.

Midwives, on behalf of all midwifery students we want to say thank you for helping us learn to be 'with woman'. We students are watching your hands, yes. But it's the use of our eyes, our smiles, and our words, which we really need to learn. By your compassion to us, your patience with us, your 'letting us drive' you are being 'with student'. Thank you for giving us our 'safe landing' into practice as authentic, with-woman midwives.

References

Alexander, B., Turnbull, D. and Cyna, A.M. (2009). The effect of pregnancy on hypnotizability. *American Journal of Clinical Hypnosis, 52(1)*, 13–22.

Allen, J., Kildea, S. and Stapleton, H. (2016). How optimal caseload midwifery can modify predictors for preterm birth in young women: integrated findings from a mixed methods study. *Midwifery, 41*, 30–38.

Australian Government Department of Health. (2019). *Clinical Practice Guidelines. Pregnancy Care.* Canberra: Australian Government.

Australian Institute of Health and Welfare. (2020). *Health across Socioeconomic Groups.* Canberra: Australian Government.

Bagnold, E. (2013). *The Squire.* Originally published by Heinemann in 1938. Republished by Virago in 1987. London: Persephone Books.

Benedetti, F., Lanotte, M., Lopiano, L. and Colloca, L. (2007). When words are painful: unraveling the mechanisms of the nocebo effect. *Neuroscience, 147*, 260–271.

Bewley, C. (2000). Feelings and experiences of midwives who do not have children about caring for childbearing women. *Midwifery, 16(2)*, 135–144.

Bewley, C. (2010). Midwives' personal experiences and their relationships with women: midwives without children and midwives who have experienced pregnancy loss. In Mavis Kirkham (ed.), *The Midwife–Mother Relationship*, 2nd edn (pp.190–207). Basingstoke: Macmillan.

Callister, L.C. (2004). Making meaning: women's birth narratives. *Journal of Obstetric, Gynecologic and Neonatal Nursing, 33(4)*, 508–518.

Chang, Y.-S., Coxon, K., Portela, A.G., Furuta, M. and Bick, D. (2018). Interventions to support effective communication between maternity care staff and women in labour: a mixed-methods systematic review. *Midwifery, 59*, 4–16.

Chooi, C.S.L., White, A.M., Tan, S.G.M., Dowling, K. and Cyna, A.M. (2013). Pain vs comfort scores after caesarean section: a randomized trial. *British Journal of Anaesthesia, 110(5)*, 780–787. doi:10.1093/bja/aes517.

Corcoran, P.M., Catling, C. and Homer, C.S.E. (2017). Models of midwifery care for Indigenous women and babies: a metasynthesis. *Women and Birth, 30*, 77–86.

Cragin, L. and Kennedy, H.P. (2006). Linking obstetric and midwifery practice with optimal outcomes. *JOGNN Clinical Issues, 35(6)*, 779–785.

Cutajar, L., and Cyna, A.M. (2018). Antenatal education for childbirth – epidural analgesia. *Midwifery, 64*, 48–52.

Cutajar, L., Miu, M., Fleet, J-A., Cyna A.M. and Steen, M. (2020). Antenatal education for childbirth: labour and birth. *European Journal of Midwiery, 4*, 11.

Cutajar, L., Steen, M., Fleet, J-A. and Cyna, A.M. (2020). Language used during antenatal education for labour and birth: a literature review. *Evidence Based Midwifery, 30(3)*, 307–318.

Cyna A.M. (2019). The LAURS of hypnotic communication and the 'lived in imagination' technique in medical practice. *International Journal of Clinical and Experimental Hypnosis, 67(3)*, 247–261.

Cyna, A.M., Andrew, M. and Tan, S.G.M. (2011). Structures. Chapter 2 in A.M. Cyna, M.I. Andrew, S.G.M. Tan and A.F. Smith (eds), *Handbook of Communication in Anaesthesia and Critical Care. A Practical Guide to Exploring the Art* (pp.17–29). Oxford: Oxford University Press.

Cyna A.M. and Lang, E.V. (2011). How words hurt. In A.M Cyna, M.I Andrew, S.G.M Tan and A.F. Smith (eds), *Handbook of Communication in Anaesthesia and Critical Care* (pp.30–37). Oxford: Oxford University Press.

Dahlen, H., Kumar-Hazard, B. and Schmied, V. (eds). (2020). *Birthing Outside the System: The Canary in the Coal Mine*. Abingdon-on-Thames, Oxfordshire: Taylor & Francis.

Darra, S. (2009). 'Normal', 'natural', 'good' or 'good-enough' birth: examining the concepts. *Nursing Inquiry, 16(4)*, 297–305.

Darra, S. and Murphy, M. (2016). Coping and help in birth: an investigation into 'normal' childbirth as described by new mothers and their attending midwives. *Midwifery, 40*, 18–25.

Dempsey, R. (2013). *Birth with Confidence. Savvy Choices for Normal Birth*. Fairfield, Australia: Boathouse Press.

Deprez-Sims, A-S. and Morris, S.B. (2010). Accents in the workplace: their effects during a job interview. *International Journal of Psychology, 45(6)*, 417–426.

Downe, S. (2006). Engaging with the concept of unique normality in childbirth. *British Journal of Midwifery, 14*, 352–357.

Downe, S. and Byrom, S. (eds). (2019). *Squaring the Circle: Normal Birth Research, Theory and Practice in a Technological Age*. London: Pinter & Martin.

Dutt-Gupta, J., Brown, T. and Cyna, A.M. (2007). Effect of communication on pain during intravenous cannulation: a randomized controlled trial. *British Journal of Anaesthesia, 99(6)*, 871–875.

Ernst, E. (2010). Homeopathy: what does the 'best' evidence tell us? A systematic review. *Medical Journal of Australia, 192(8)*, 458–460.

Feeley, C., Byrom, A., Byrom, S. and Tizard, H. (2020). Normal Birth: position statement. *The Practising Midwife, 23(1)*, 34.

Gaskin, I.M. (2002). *Spiritual Midwifery*, 4th edn. Summertown, TN: Book Publishing Company.

Gilron, R. and Gutchess, A.H. (2009). Remembering first impressions: effects of intentionality and diagnosticity on subsequent memory. *Cognitive, Affective and Behavioral Neuroscience, 12*, 85–98.

Gould, D. (2000). Normal labour: a concept analysis. *Journal of Advanced Nursing, 31(2)*, 418–427.

Hastie, C. (2005). How understanding semantics helps us be 'with women'. *MIDIRS Midwifery Digest, 15(4)*, 475–477.

Herrick, J.A. (2001). *The History and Theory of Rhetoric: An Introduction*, 2nd edn. Needham Heights, MA: Allyn & Bacon.

Homer, C.S.E., Foureur, M., Allende, T., Pekin, F., Caplice, S. and Catling-Paull, C. (2012). 'It's more than just having a baby' women's experiences of a maternity service for Australian Aboriginal and Torres Strait Islander families. *Midwifery, 28*, e509–e513.

Homer, C.S.E., Leap, N., Brodie, P. and Sandall, J. (eds). (2019). *Midwifery Continuity of Care*, 2nd edn. Chatswood, NSW: Elsevier Australia.

Homer, C.S.E., Leap, N., Edwards, N. and Sandall, J. (2017). Midwifery continuity of carer in an area of high socio-economic disadvantage in London: a retrospective analysis of Albany Midwifery Practice outcomes using routine data (1997–2009). *Midwifery, 48*, 1–10.

Hu, Y., Parde, C.J., Hill, M.Q., Mahmood, N. and O'Toole, A.J. (2018). First impressions of personality traits from body shapes. *Psychological Science, 29(12)*, 1969–1983.

Hunter, L. (2006). Women give birth and pizzas are delivered: language and Western childbirth paradigms. *Journal of Midwifery and Women's Health, 51(2)*, 119–124.

Karlsdottir, S.I, Halldorsdottir, S. and Lundgren, I. (2014). The third paradigm in labour pain preparation and management: the childbearing woman's paradigm. *Scandinavian Journal of Caring Sciences*, *28*, 315–327.

Kay, L., Downe, S., Thompson, G. and Finlayson, K. (2017). Engaging with birth stories in pregnancy: a hermeneutic phenomenological study of women's experiences across two generations. *BMC Pregnancy and Childbirth*, *17*, 283.

Kennedy, H.P. (2006). A concept analysis of 'optimality' in peri-natal health. *Journal of Obstetric, Gynecologic and Neonatal Nursing*, *35*, 763–769.

Kennedy, H.P and Shannon, M.T. (2004). Keeping birth normal: research findings on midwifery care during labour. *Journal of Obstetric Gynecologic and Neonatal Nursing*, *33(5)*, 554–560.

Kirkham, M. (1997). Stories and childbirth. In M.J. Kirkham and E.R. Perkins (eds), *Reflections on Midwifery* (pp.183–204). London: Bailliere Tindall.

Knight, M., Bunch, K., Tuffnell, D., Shakespeare, J., Kotnis, R., Kenyon, S., *et al.* (eds). (2020). *Saving Lives, Improving Mothers' Care – Lessons Learned to Inform Maternity Care from the UK and Ireland Confidential Enquiries into Maternal Deaths and Morbidity 2016–18*. Oxford: National Perinatal Epidemiology Unit, University of Oxford.

Lang, E.V, Hatsiopoulou, O., Koch, T., Berbaum, K., Lutgendorf, S., Kettenmann, E., Logan, H. and Kaptchuk, T.J. (2005). Can words hurt? Patient–provider interactions during invasive procedures. *Pain. Journal of the International Association for the Study of Pain*, *114*, 303–309.

Leap, N. (2005). Rhetoric and reality: narrowing the gap in Australian midwifery. Professional doctorate in midwifery. http://hdl.handle.net/2100/265.

Leap, N. (2010). The less we do the more we give. Chapter 2 in M. Kirkham (ed.), *The Midwife–Mother Relationship*, 2nd edn (pp.17–35). London: Palgrave Macmillan.

Leap, N. (2012). The power of words re-visited. MIDIRS Focus. *Essentially MIDIRS*, *3(1)*, 17–21.

Leap, N. (2015, unpublished data). Identifying the experiences of receiving and providing support in labour.

Leap, N. and Edwards, N. (2006). The politics of involving women in decision making. Chapter 5 in L.A. Page and R. Campbell (eds), *The New Midwifery: Science and Sensitivity in Practice*, 2nd edn. London: Churchill Livingstone/Elsevier.

Leap, N., Sandall, J., Buckland, S. and Huber, U. (2010). Journey to confidence: women's experiences of pain in labour and relational continuity of care. *Journal of Midwifery and Women's Health*, *55(3)*, 235–242.

Lowe, N.K. (2002). The nature of labor pain. *American Journal of Obstetrics and Gynecology*, *186(5)*, S16–S24.

Lyerly, A.D. (2012). Ethics and 'normal birth'. *Birth*, *39(4)*, 315–317.

Lynch, E. (2020). Normal birth 1: contention and debate in the UK. *The Practising Midwife*, *23(8)*, 19.

Mander, R. (1997). What are we called? Words that colleagues use. *British Journal of Midwifery*, *5(7)*, 406.

Maternity Care Working Party. (2007). Making normal birth a reality: consensus statement from the Maternity Care Working Party – our shared views about the need to recognise, facilitate and audit normal birth. London: NCT/RCM/RCOG. http://bhpelopartonormal.pbh.gov.br/estudos_cientificos/arquivos/normal_birth_consensus.pdf.

McCourt, C. (2006). Supporting choice and control? Communication and interaction between midwives and women at the antenatal booking visit. *Social Science & Medicine*, *62*, 1307–1318.

McCourt, C. and Pearce, A. (2000). Does continuity of carer matter to women from minority ethnic groups? *Midwifery*, *16*, 145–154.

Naumann, L.P., Vazire, S., Rentfrow, P.J. and Gosling, S.D. (2009). Personality judgments based on physical appearance. *Personality and Social Psychology Bulletin*, *35(12)*, 1661–1671.

Newman, L. and Hancock, H. (2009). How natural can major surgery really be? A critique of 'the natural caesarean' technique. *Birth*, *36(2)*, 168–170.

NHS. (2019). *The NHS Long Term Plan*. www.longtermplan.nhs.uk.

Odent, M. (1994). Laboring women are not marathon runners. *Midwifery Today*, *31*, 23–26.

Odent, M. and Odent, P. (2015). Essay: From homo superpredator to homo ecologicus. *WombEcology.com*. https://www.wombecology.com/home/from-homo-superpredator-to-homo-ecologicus.

Prineas, S., Smith, A.F. and Tan, S.G.M. (2011). To begin . . . Chapter 1 in A.M. Cyna, M.I. Andrew, S.G.M. Tan and A.F. Smith (eds), *Handbook of Communication in Anaesthesia and Critical Care. A Practical Guide to Exploring the Art* (pp.3–16). Oxford: Oxford University Press.

Rayment-Jones, H., Harris, J., Harden, A., Khan, Z. and Sandall, J. (2019). How do women with social risk factors experience United Kingdom maternity care? A realist synthesis. *Birth*, *46*(*3*), 461–463.

Rayment-Jones, H., Murrells, T. and Sandall, J. (2015). An investigation of the relationship between the caseload model of midwifery for socially disadvantaged women and childbirth outcomes using routine data – a retrospective, observational study. *Midwifery*, *31*(*4*), 409–417.

Reiger, K. and Dempsey, R. (2006). Performing birth in a culture of fear: an embodied crisis of late modernity. *Health Sociology Review*, *15*(*4*), 364–373.

Robertson, A. (2007). *The Midwife Companion: The Art of Support during Birth*, 2nd edn. Sydney: Birth International.

Sandall, J., Leap, N., Grant, J. and Bastos, M.H. (2010). Supporting women to have a normal birth: development and field testing of a learning package for maternity staff. Health and Social Care Research Division, King's College London.

Sanders, R. (2015). Midwifery facilitation: exploring the functionality of labor discomfort. Commentary. *Birth*, *42*(*3*), 202–205.

Sands. (2020). Communication while wearing PPE. https://www.sands.org.uk/sites/default/files/Communication%20with%20PPE.pdf.

Škodová, Z. (2016). Communication and interpersonal skills enhancement in midwifery: review. *Central European Journal of Nursing and Midwifery*, *7*(*3*), 504–510.

Smith, J., Plaat, F. and Fisk, N.M. (2008). The natural caesarean: a woman-centred technique. *British Journal of Obstetrics and Gynaecology*, *115*, 1037–1042. doi:10.1111/j.1471-0528.2008.01777.x.

Thompson, F.E. (2004). *Mothers and Midwives: The Ethical Journey*. Edinburgh: Books for Midwives.

Tiba, J. (1990). Clinical, research and organisational aspects of preparation for childbirth and the psychological diminution of pain during labour and delivery. *British Journal of Experimental and Clinical Hypnosis*, *7*, 61–64.

Varelmann, D., Pancaro, C., Cappiello, E. and Camann, W. (2010). Nocebo-induced hyperalgesia during local anesthetic injection. *Anesthesia and Analgesia*, *110*(*3*), 868–870.

Wickham, S. (2005). Language of the complicated. *Practising Midwife*, *8*(*9*), 33.

Willis, J. and Todorov, A. (2006). First impressions. Making up your mind after a 100-ms exposure to a face. *Psychological Science*, *17*(*7*), 592–598.

Yu, M., Saleem, M. and Gonzalez, C. (2014). Developing trust: first impressions and experience. *Journal of Economic Psychology*, *43*, 16–29.

6   Supporting women for normal birth

Introduction

Labour and birth present complex, highly intimate, physical and emotional challenges for women; interpersonal relationships with professionals can have a profound effect on how they cope with the potential loneliness, fear and vulnerability of the experience (Van der Gucht and Lewis, 2015). These effects can last a lifetime:

> The way a woman is treated by the professional on whom she depends may largely determine how she feels about the experience for the rest of her life.
>
> (Simkin, 1991, p.210)

As we discussed in Chapter 1, the resounding message from women is that they value continuous support during labour to increase their comfort and help them feel safe and secure in the unfolding ebb and flow of their emotional needs (Downe *et al.*, 2018; Olza *et al.*, 2018; Ross-Davie and Cheyne, 2014). The next three chapters can be viewed as a trilogy addressing how we respond to that message from women.

In this chapter we explore how we might support women who have uncomplicated pregnancies, who start labour spontaneously and who hope to have a normal birth. We build on this in Chapter 7 by looking at the practicalities of labour support – the 'toolkit' of support measures that we can draw on when supporting women in labour. In Chapter 8, we then look at some of the variations in the way we can support women when they have the extra challenges of using epidurals or are experiencing complications that require help from obstetricians or other health practitioners.

Across the world, the majority of women want to have a physiological birth, with practical and emotional support from birth companions and reassurance from competent, kind caregivers (Downe *et al.*, 2018). This chapter draws on research findings and the experiences of women, midwives and other birth workers, to explore some principles for promoting physiological birth (which we shall refer to as 'normal birth', since this is the commonly used term). We shall also consider the potential impact of the environment on the quality of support we offer.

First, though, we quote some words of advice from the late Brian Pridmore, an experienced and much-loved South Australian obstetrician. When asked to address the first cohort of three-year Bachelor of Midwifery students on their graduation day, he said, 'I have only two words of advice to guide you as you embark on your midwifery careers and they are: "Assume nothing"'. This mantra is a theme that runs throughout this chapter, especially when we consider the diversity and characteristics of effective support for labour and birth.

DOI: 10.4324/9781003092520-7

Some key texts to inform this chapter

Box 6.1   Recommended Resources: Supporting women for normal birth

Buckley, S.J. (2015). *Hormonal Physiology of Childbearing: Evidence and Implications for Women, Babies, and Maternity Care*. Washington, DC: Childbirth Connection Programs, National Partnership for Women and Families. https://www.nationalpartnership.org/our-work/resources/health-care/maternity/hormonal-physiology-of-childbearing.pdf.

Downe, S. and Byrom, S. (eds). (2019). *Squaring the Circle: Normal Birth Research, Theory and Practice in a Technological Age*. London: Pinter & Martin.

Robertson, A. (2007). *The Midwife Companion: The Art of Support During Birth*, 2nd edn. Sydney: Birth International.

Simkin, P. with Rohs, K. (2018). *The Birth Partner: A Complete Guide to Childbirth for Dads, Doulas, and All Other Labor Companions*, 5th edn. Boston, MA: Harvard Common Press.

Walsh, D. (2012). *Evidence and Skills for Normal Labour and Birth*, 2nd edn. London: Routledge.

Walsh, D. and Downe, S. (eds). (2010). *Essential Midwifery Practice: Intrapartum Care*. Chichester: Wiley-Blackwell.

Supporting women to have a 'normal' labour and birth

The ways that midwives support women who want to have a normal labour and birth are universal and embedded in the midwifery philosophy of woman centred care (Leap, 2009). The organisation of care and the preferences of healthcare providers will, however, have a profound effect on how this support is enacted. The article profiled in Box 6.2 is a study of the experiences of promoting normal birth as described by midwives in British Columbia, Canada. The strategies identified by the midwives are congruent with the issues that we shall discuss in this chapter.

Box 6.2   Research Briefing. Strategies that midwives use to promote normal birth

Butler, M.M. (2017). Exploring the strategies that midwives in British Columbia use to promote normal birth. *BMC Pregnancy and Childbirth, 17*, 168.

The midwives in this study identified how providing continuity of care enabled them to work closely with women from early pregnancy to facilitate informed choice and prepare for a normal birth. They described a range of approaches as 'instruments of care', including: managing early labour, an appropriate, low-tech environment that promotes privacy; careful watching and waiting; support from a partner, friend or doula; helping the woman to prepare and cope with labour; and 'tools in the toolkit' for responding to different scenarios.

Concerted global efforts to define, measure and promote normal birth

For several decades, the issue of 'normal birth' and how it can be defined, measured and promoted has been debated by maternity care professionals and policy makers. Global concerns about the erosion of normal birth began to be voiced by the World Health Organization (WHO) in 1985 following a conference in Brazil entitled, 'Appropriate Technology for Birth'. Recommendations arising from this conference and published in the *Lancet* (WHO, 1985) included statements that there is no justification for any region to have a caesarean section rate higher than 10–15 per cent; that VBAC should be encouraged where emergency surgical intervention is available, and that until research shows any benefits for continuous electronic fetal monitoring in labour, 'national health services should refrain from purchasing new equipment' (p.437). The WHO published *Care in Normal Birth: A Practical Guide* in 1996, with an overtly identified message in the summary of that document that, 'in normal birth there should be a valid reason to interfere with the natural process' (WHO, 1996, p.4). This statement was justified by drawing on the ongoing publication of evidence from the Oxford Database of Perinatal Trials (forerunner of Cochrane) and published initially in the groundbreaking *Effective Care in Pregnancy and Childbirth* (Chalmers *et al.*, 1989; Enkin, 2006).

The following decade saw a spate of consensus statements defining 'normal birth' in high-income countries. In attempts to standardise a collection of statistics for research purposes, normal birth definitions included interventions such as augmentation of labour, artificial rupture of membranes, pharmacological pain relief, continuous electronic fetal monitoring and managed third stage of labour (Young, 2009). Debates continue about whether such inclusions are justified and the limiting use of the word 'normal' in data collection.

Concerns about the emotional and psychological effects on women of using the word 'normal' as the yard stick to define their experiences of birth has led to a shift towards talking about promoting positive experiences, rather than promoting normal birth, for example, the 1996 WHO document *Care in Normal Labour: A Practical Guide* was succeeded by *Intrapartum Care for a Positive Childbirth Experience* in 2018. In a maternity service culture where epidurals and interventions are the norm (Newnham *et al.*, 2017, 2018), the term 'physiological birth' is often favoured by midwives; 'normal birth', however, continues to be used by women and the media as a broad term that does not include caesarean section or birth assisted by forceps or ventouse.

Box 6.3　Reflective Activity: Concerted efforts to define, measure and promote normal birth

Individually, in pairs or in small groups:

In preparation for this activity, read the following articles:

Enkin, M. (2006). Guest editorial. Beyond evidence: the complexity of maternity care. *Birth*, *22(4)*, 265–269.
Romano, A.M. and Lothian, J.A. (2008). Promoting, protecting, and supporting normal birth: a look at the evidence. *Journal of Obstetric, Gynecologic and Neonatal Nursing*, *37(1)*, 94–104.
Young, D. (March 2009). What is normal childbirth and do we need more statements about it? Editorial. *Birth*, *36*, 1–3.
Newnham, E., McKellar, L. and Pincombe, J. (2015). Documenting risk: a comparison of policy and information pamphlets for using epidural or water in labour. *Women and Birth*, *28*, 221–227.
Feeley, C., Byrom, A., Byrom, S. and Tizard, H. (2020). Normal birth: position statement. *The Practising Midwife*, *23(1)*, 34.
Lynch, E. (2020). Normal birth 1: contention and debate in the UK. *The Practising Midwife*, *23(8)*, 19.

In different ways, each of these articles addresses complex issues about how evidence has been used to define, measure and promote normal birth.

- Discuss how these issues relate to your own experiences of how normal birth is defined, measured and promoted, including how evidence is used in these contexts. Consider this in relation to the policy documents, guidelines and practices that you are familiar with.
- Make notes about four main issues arising from your discussion to share with the wider group.

The changing face of labour support

As can be seen in Box 6.3, our efforts to promote physiological birth occur within a culture of increasing acceptance of obstetric interventions and epidurals.

Box 6.4　Research Briefing: Women's acceptance of obstetric interventions

Green, J.M. and Baston, H.A. (2007). Have women become more willing to accept obstetric interventions and does this relate to mode of birth? Data from a prospective study. *Birth*, *34(1)*, 6–13.

This paper identifies that women are more prepared to accept obstetric interventions and epidurals than they were 20 years ago, when researchers carried out a similar large survey in England.

Women with high willingness to accept interventions, in particular epidurals, had a two-fold increase in the chance of having an instrumental or operative birth. Conversely, a low willingness to use epidurals had a protective effect.

The researchers suggest that women who favour epidurals may not be aware of the implications and that explanations about this should include support and encouragement to use other coping strategies.

As we discussed in Chapter 4, the concept of developing skills in 'getting women through' labour that was prevalent decades ago has given way to a focus on responding to women's choices, particularly around epidural use. This can mean that midwives are vulnerable to criticism when we engage in conversations with women about the increased likelihood of interventions if they opt for epidurals, as recommended by the researchers profiled in Box 6.4 Denis Walsh (2010b, p.xi) suggests that there is 'a sense of crisis confronting advocates of physiological birth . . . and a marginalisation of the low-tech non-hospital birth'. Where such a culture prevails, it is increasingly important that we are able to articulate why normal birth matters.

Box 6.5   Reflective Activity: Why normal birth matters

In small groups:
- Take ten minutes to make a list identifying why you think it matters to promote normal birth. Read your list out loud to the larger group and compare your ideas. Engage in a facilitated discussion about everyone's ideas and the implications for how we support women in labour.

Supporting women in labour: some basic principles

Having considered why the promotion of normal birth matters, we now explore some principles concerning how we provide individualised support to women in labour.

Trusting women to find their way

In her books for midwives and childbirth educators, the late Andrea Robertson (2006, 2007) describes the art of labour support in terms of observing and responding to individual women and providing them with peace, privacy, a permissive, accepting atmosphere and protective surroundings. She describes how, through attending births as a support person over many years, she learnt to trust women's innate ability to find their way in labour:

> Women know how to give birth. A woman who is encouraged to be instinctive and tune into her body during labour can discover exactly what she needs to do to make labour easier for herself and her baby . . . provided [she] is willing to explore her hidden capabilities, and if she is provided with an environment conducive to this exploration.
> (Robertson, 2006, p.101)

The skill of being alongside women and trusting them to find their way in normal labour has been described by Sheila Kitzinger (1988, p.18) as 'patience and the willingness to wait for the unfolding of life'. These skills are vividly described by this midwife:

> I think, left alone, women are completely able to do it themselves and go right into their own depth of resources. And they don't look out at all, except to open their eyes and plead for a caesarean or something in a panic moment when they're desperate in transition. But I think in a woman who's not desperate and who's coping, she'll disappear completely from connection with you, her environment and from whoever is supporting her, and she's in her own little space. It's like being in a bubble really . . . and you as the midwife can only sit and watch and really admire, I suppose, how it works and what's going on.
> (Midwife, Leap, 1996, p.45)

As we explored in Chapter 1, the underlying philosophies of such approaches are associated with a universal safety net in the form of watchful anticipation:

> I remember seeing that film – I think it was in a remote area of South America – where all the women supporting the mother get up and dance when the baby is born. The nuggety old midwife continues to sit there, calmly concentrating on the woman. After the woman has delivered her placenta and it's clear that she's not bleeding excessively, the midwife springs up with a big beam on her face and joins in with the dancing women [laughter!].
>
> (Midwife, Leap, 2015, unpublished data)

Words of encouragement: midwifery muttering

Women have described the importance of their midwives' repetitive use of encouraging words throughout their labours, often quietly voiced after each contraction. This 'midwifery muttering' (Leap, 2010) can be particularly useful during moments of self-doubt:

> The whole time during my labour they kept saying, 'You're fantastic, you're brilliant, you're doing absolutely great', and I just thought, 'Oh well, actually I must be doing fine, I must be doing something right.' So that was really positive.
>
> (Mother, Sandall *et al.*, 2010, p.38)

'Midwifery muttering' has been likened to the 'whispered words of wisdom' of 'letting it be' (Kennedy *et al.*, 2010), immortalised by Lennon and McCartney (1970). For many women, repeated, quiet reminders from the midwives that they are doing well and that 'this is normal' have a steadying effect:

> All the midwives just seem so calm around you, and they just keep reminding you that this is normal, and just by the way they behave and the calm in the room . . . it just all seemed like the most natural, normal thing, my labour, although it was long and hard.
>
> (Mother, Sandall *et al.*, 2010, unpublished data)

For women's partners, this sense of calm can be particularly important if a woman's way of managing her labour is to roar and make dramatic rhythmic movements, as was the case described by this father:

> I remember thinking at the time, gosh she [the midwife] seems so relaxed it's amazing, she's not panicking at all . . . I kind of felt like it grounded me at least to see her just being quite, you know, 'Oh this is really great. . . .' And just, yes, she was very calm.
>
> (Father, Sandall *et al.*, 2010, unpublished data)

Sending women messages of encouragement requires the midwife to believe that the woman will be able to get through her labour with support:

> You can't pretend really, you have to feel it, and it is hard work and it is incredibly tiring, but you have to be genuine about it. And I think if you're up there, you pull them up with you, and they stay there. The minute you feel, 'Oh God, this isn't working is it?' they, you know . . . [deflating sound] they're back down to the ground again and then they lose it completely.
>
> (Midwife, Sandall *et al.*, 2010, p.45)

Trusting women to give us feedback

If you are worried about annoying a woman with your 'midwifery muttering' or anything else you are doing to support her, you can rest assured that she will let you know. Women often get very monosyllabic as labour intensifies and they tell us in no uncertain terms if they don't like what we are doing or saying. It is not unusual to hear women say, with an urgent tone, things like: 'Be quiet', 'Don't press like that', 'Rub here, not there', 'Don't call me Blossom'; or, responding to the heightened sense of smell that women have in labour: 'Your breath smells of coffee/cigarettes'. (Recommending that birth companions have a toothbrush handy is a good idea, as is remembering to tell everyone that the woman may react negatively to perfume, aftershave, incense or aromatherapy.)

There is no room for politeness when a woman is consumed with concentrating on her labour. This can be challenging for women's partners and other birth companions, who may need reassurance that we often see this sort of thing in normal labour:

> I remember a woman I was looking after who thought before labour that what she'd want was people rubbing her back and talking to her, all that sort of thing. For some reason she ended up using the gas and at the start of each contraction she'd say, 'Shut up, shut up, shut up . . . stop talking . . . don't touch me . . .' with great urgency! I do talk about that – the fact that you don't always know what's going to work for you in labour. You might like this – but you might hate it too. Only the woman will know at the time. And she will tell you.
>
> (Midwife, Leap, unpublished data, 2015)

Midwifery reassurance: the concept of 'knitting' in the corner

As we saw in the diary of the eighteenth-century midwife Martha Ballard in the Prologue (Ulrich, 1990), there is a time-honoured tradition of midwives sitting in a corner and knitting while waiting for a woman's labour to unfold. This concept is sometimes flagged as a metaphor for 'presence' – midwives giving quiet reassurance through their body language; a message that all is well; and that there is no need for concern. Although we have heard contemporary stories of midwives being banned from knitting in some maternity units, it was not uncommon in the UK in the 1970s when we were both student midwives:

> On night duty, if you had difficulties with your knitting, you went and found Sister Huckle. She only had one eye but there was nothing she didn't know about knitting. And nothing she didn't know about how to get women through labour when they didn't believe they could do it.
>
> (Midwife, Leap, 2015, unpublished data)

In our experience, it is not unusual for midwives to knit in a corner when women are giving birth at home. In a study involving videotaped narratives about midwifery practice (Kennedy and Shannon, 2004), experienced American midwives described how they consciously created a reassuring presence as they learnt to 'sit' with a labouring woman while knitting:

> I knit with women in labor. It's my way . . . of telling everyone who is willing to pay attention, that labor is normal . . . everyone thinks, OK, she's knitting, things have to be OK, otherwise she'd be doing. So I sit and knit.
>
> (p.557)

Knitting – crocheting, tatting, embroidery or any other needlework – can also have a calming effect on the midwife. Her hands are occupied in a rhythmic activity that is known to have meditative qualities. She can keep a quiet eye on what is unfolding without having to gaze at the woman (a type of surveillance that women often find unnerving).

We cannot leave the concept of knitting without a word of caution about the effect that knitting can have on some people. Those of us who knit are well aware that the image of Madame Defarge and her friends knitting at the guillotine in Charles Dickens's *A Tale of Two Cities* (1859) can provoke conscious and subconscious associations and reactions:

> My sister had a midwife (36 years ago) who knitted during her many, many hours of obstructed labour that ended in a caesarean section – she was horrified by the whole experience and the image she has stuck in her mind is of women knitting at the guillotine.
>
> (Midwife, Leap, 2015, unpublished data)

Box 6.6 Reflective Activity: 'Midwifery muttering'

Classroom or workshop activity, *in small groups:*
- Make a list of the sort of phrases that you might use to encourage a woman (quietly) after each contraction if you were sitting in the corner of the room, perhaps knitting. Practise saying these phrases out loud and notice the tone of voice you use.

- 'Homework' – in preparation for a presentation with the larger group:

  - Find colleagues or friends who speak another language and ask them if you can audio-record them saying the same words in their language – as if they were gently encouraging a woman in labour after a contraction.
  - Combine your audio recordings in different languages and superimpose them onto a slide show of images depicting women in labour.

- After your presentation, lead a group discussion on what you learnt about 'midwifery muttering' and labour support with reference to the impact of the slide show presentations.

Midwifery presence: being in the room

During informal conversations, some midwives have told us that they see the concept of knitting in the corner of the room as 'unprofessional'. In some cases, this perception can extend to seeing the very act of sitting in a relaxed way as 'unprofessional':

> I'm not comfortable about sitting down and being seen as not working. You wouldn't want to be caught sitting in the support person's easy chair because it's just not professional. The only professional seating you can have is the little round stool, the one that's used for suturing.
>
> (Midwife in Hammond *et al.*, 2014b, unpublished data)

The above quote raises important issues about professionalism and how the design and culture of birth in institutions affects how we are able to be in the room and provide emotionally sensitive care and support for women in labour (Hammond *et al.*, 2014a). We shall return to this later when considering how we promote a supportive environment for birth.

Being in the room: addressing documentation and other tasks

The lack of a suitable place in the birthing room to sit alongside women and their birth supporters was identified as an important issue in the study by Hammond *et al.* (2014a); sometimes this resulted in midwives leaving the room, especially when they needed to complete documentation. Whilst encouraging midwives to find a way to stay in the room when writing their notes, we are aware that, whatever the setting, some women find it disconcerting when the midwife is obviously writing things down about them; again, this can feel like surveillance:

> I said to the midwife, 'What are you writing about me?' I must have sounded very suspicious because after that she involved me in what she was writing and quietly told me and my partner what she was recording. Then it became reassuring.
>
> (Mother, Leap, 2015, unpublished data)

The same sort of explanations can be important if we are entering information on a computer in the room or when we have to concentrate on a task, as this midwife explains:

> If I have to concentrate on writing in the notes or doing something, I say to them, 'I'm not talking to you right now because I'm concentrating on doing this . . . whatever it is'. That way they're not left wondering if my silence is something to worry about. The same applies if I'm explaining something to a student. I check out with them that it's OK to do that. Generally women and their partners really like hearing all of that, especially when you're telling the student to notice how well the woman is managing her labour – but I wouldn't do that if the woman's in the zone and needs a quiet space. You have to think hard about all of these things.
>
> (Midwife, Leap, 2015, unpublished data)

The 'thinking hard' that this midwife refers to means responding with all of our senses in order to find the most appropriate way to 'be' alongside a labouring woman as she responds to the evolving nature of her experiences. It means being brave about changing tack if we seem to be getting it wrong.

> You have to modify your behaviours to suit hers. If she's not saying much, you don't say much. If her eyes are closed, don't ask her a question so she's got to look at you. You have to play it by ear.
>
> (Childbirth educator/birth supporter, Leap, 2015, unpublished data)

Reassuring women: avoiding assumptions

When a woman appears to be managing well in labour, it is easy to assume that she knows this; we might underestimate how much she appreciates reassurance:

> A woman told me once that she only had positive feedback indirectly when a doctor came into the room and the midwife said to the doctor, 'She's doing really well', . . . it was the end of the first stage, she was really struggling because it was full on, and

the midwife was offering her choices, she wasn't saying, 'You're doing beautifully', she was saying, 'Do you want to move position? Do you want some pain relief?' and the mother interpreted that as the midwife saying, 'You're not coping with this very well'.

(Childbirth educator/birth supporter, Sandall *et al.*, 2010, unpublished data)

In a similar vein, we should not assume that, because a woman appears to be getting good support from one of her birth companions, she therefore does not need midwifery reassurance. This is particularly so if we are with a woman whose language we do not speak:

I was with a woman once and she appeared to be getting good support from her mother, who was rubbing her back and murmuring to her. As I didn't speak their language, I withdrew and left them to it, just going in to check every 15 minutes or so. I was surprised when her labour stalled and she ended up having Syntocinon and a forceps. I went to see her a few days later on the postnatal ward and she told me that her mother had been telling her repeatedly that it was taking too long, that her own births were faster, that there must be something wrong. I misinterpreted what was going on. I learnt from that not to assume that what I'm seeing is necessarily what's going on for the woman.

(Midwife, Leap, 2015, unpublished data)

This story reminds us to be alert to how we might make assumptions based on our perceptions of other people's cultures. In our efforts to work in a way that is culturally competent we need to be mindful of the differences within, between and among cultures and that we might not be able to pick up cues about what is going on for others (Purnell, 2000).

Addressing the fallacy of prediction

Experienced midwives know the importance of avoiding assumptions and predictions about how a woman will or will not manage her labour:

They do surprise themselves, they do. I always think that instinctive midwives can predict but I don't know that I can myself. I think that I can sometimes, but then quite often I'm wrong. Women constantly shock me and I think I've learnt from those women. You could sit there and think, 'She's a hopeless case, she said her pain threshold's really low' – and all you've got to do is tell her she's doing well, that it's normal and allow her to get on with it in her own way, and I think she will.

(Midwife, Leap, 1996, p.49)

Being tolerant for wide variations in how a normal labour might unfold and a willingness to keep an open mind have been described as important midwifery skills (Kennedy and Shannon, 2004; Kennedy *et al.*, 2004). Sometimes, this means being open to the idea of supporting a woman whose labour has stalled while she works through psychological, rather than physiological challenges (Dempsey, 2020; Kennedy and Shannon, 2004). An example of this is presented in the following activity, drawing on a story from an Australian home birth midwife.

Box 6.7   Reflective Activity: 'I just want to talk. And I want you to listen'

Individually or in pairs or small groups:

- Discuss the issues that this story raises for you and what we can learn from it:

I was with a woman recently. She had had two babies at home in the UK with NHS midwives. She had quite fast labours. With the second one, the midwives hadn't made it to that birth. So we were all expecting a really quick birth.

When I arrived at her home she was clearly transitional. And then everything just stopped. She didn't get another contraction. Nothing. I couldn't work out was going on. This seemed like more than a 'rest and be thankful' phase of labour, which we often see, don't we, just before they go into second stage.

Anyway, she asked everyone to leave the room except for me – the husband and the two little girls. She said, 'I just want to try something.' So they all left. She said, 'I just want to talk. And I want you to listen.' So basically she divulged that she'd been sexually abused as a child by several men in her family and she'd never told anyone, not even her husband.

With the first two babies, each time she had found out in pregnancy that she was having a girl. The fear that was coming up for her this time was that she didn't know the sex of this baby and she was so frightened that it might be a boy. She was scared that there was something genetic in males in the family that would 'create a monster' as she called it.

We spent about 20 minutes and she was just talking and crying in the pool and then very slowly the contractions started coming back. I was just sitting there listening and she said, 'Can I be on my own for a little while?' I walked out of the room and heard her roar: 'Aaaaaaaargh!' And then we heard, 'Waa, Waa [baby noises]'. We came back in the room and she was holding a baby boy who she'd lifted out of the water. And she's madly in love with him.

But when everything stops, I don't think we should always assume something psychological is going on. We can get caught up in all that and miss other things that are going on.

(Midwife, Leap, 2015, unpublished data)

Several authors have warned against midwives trying to engage in predicting underlying psychological problems that might have physiological consequences for childbearing women, citing the potentially disempowering effect that this might have on women (Gosden, 1996; Gosden and Saul, 1999; Oakley, 1980). Engaging in such predictions can also change the dynamic of the midwifery relationship:

Yes, I'm au fait with popular psychologising, but that's not terribly helpful with a process that's so b_____ complicated. I make a conscious effort – which sometimes works and sometimes doesn't – to put that prediction stuff to one side, because it gets in the way. If I'm engaging in that process, I'm not with her.

(Midwife, Leap, 1996, p.49)

Midwives have described a maternity service culture where predictions about how women will cope are a regular feature of informal discussions, often dominated by value judgements and stereotyping:

> At the desk, you hear things like, 'We'll see where those hypnobirthing classes get her once she's in proper labour.' It's almost as if they get some warped pleasure out of seeing women turn to epidurals when they had planned otherwise.
>
> (Midwife, Leap, 2015, unpublished data)

Box 6.8   Reflective Activity: Confronting the stereotyping of labouring women

Green, J.M., Kitzinger, J. and Coupland, V. (1990). Stereotypes of childbearing women – a look at some of the evidence. *Midwifery*, *6*, 125–132.

Two commonly observed stereotypes are challenged in this paper: 'the well-educated, middle class woman who has obsessive, fixed ideas and unrealistically high hopes about what she wants in labour', and 'the uneducated working class woman who is thoroughly unprepared, abdicates all responsibility to staff and has no aspirations for the type of birth she'd like'. These caricatures were not supported: women of different levels of education were equally likely to subscribe to the ideal of avoiding drugs in labour. It was more likely to be the less educated women who had the highest expectations for a fulfilling birth experience and who did not want to hand over all control to the staff.

In pairs or small groups:
- After studying this article, discuss situations that you have been in where you have heard these stereotypes (or others, for example, race and ethnicity, age, sexuality) being used.
- It can often be difficult for us to challenge these stereotypes and prejudices in the moment. Practising responses can be useful, so that they feel familiar and 'do-able'. Write a script for possible responses and practise saying these to each other out loud.
- Discuss how you might overcome barriers to challenging such stereotyping and why you think it matters.

Supporting the supporters for labour and birth

Women often worry about their partners or other chosen birth companions during labour, potentially resulting in their 'worry brains' inhibiting the swirling hormonal cascades of physiology (Buckley, 2015). Where midwives, doulas or other birth workers take on the role of supporting the support team, this can put the woman's mind at ease, releasing her to withdraw into the sensations of labour (Robertson, 2007). This may mean simple things like making sure the supporters have access to hot drinks, snacks and a place to rest or sleep. The following story is an example of this:

Box 6.9   Reflective Activity: 'Looking after Auntie'

Individually or in pairs or small groups:
- Discuss the issues that this story raises for you and the implications for practice:

A woman from Sierra Leone came into the unit in the night. She'd had two normal births before and she thought her waters had gone. In fact they hadn't but then she was seen by someone and it was understood that she was more than 42 weeks. And that's of course a definite no-no and she'd apparently somehow slipped through the net and not been induced. So we didn't let her go home and she had to go to the antenatal ward and someone gave her some Prostin. In the morning she came back up to the labour ward, contracting strongly; her cervix wasn't very far dilated – but she was labouring.

She was very tired; she'd had no sleep at all. She was probably contracting two in ten and between contractions she was snoring her head off. With her was her aunt – quite an elderly lady, who was also very tired. She'd been with her for two days and had had no sleep. So I put a mattress on the ensuite bathroom floor, gave the aunt some sheets and pillows and she had a couple of hours' sleep in there. After that she was much refreshed and able to be more supportive.

The woman got into the bath at about lunchtime to help her with the pain – she was still very tired and was lying in the bath, snoring her head off between contractions. She decided she wanted to get out of the bath so I was there in the room trying to support her when her aunt said, 'Ooh, I really feel like having a bath too.' So I said, 'OK, I'll get you a couple of towels' and so off she went to have a bath.

And in the middle of the aunt having her bath in came the whole medical team and I was just praying that she wouldn't wander out with a towel wrapped round her, this elderly woman. But she heard them and stayed in the bathroom.

In the afternoon the woman got a strong urge to push and out came this beautiful baby – completely covered in vernix, not 42 weeks at all. But everything was fine. Typically, as soon as the baby was out the woman was completely alert and absolutely delighted. They were ringing family in Sierra Leone, all completely overwhelmed with joy. It was gorgeous.

(Midwife, Leap, 2015, unpublished data)

Supporting partners for labour and birth

It appears that there is an association between men's distress about their experiences of labour and women's subsequent symptoms of post-traumatic stress; women's dissatisfaction with partner support in labour is also associated with an increase in post-traumatic stress and postnatal depression (Iles *et al.*, 2011). If we also consider suggestions that the most positive experiences of labour for fathers occur when their partners have an epidural (Capogna *et al.*, 2007), we have to think very carefully about how we can support women's partners in labour, particularly when the woman hopes to labour without an epidural. It should go without saying that these considerations apply equally when the woman is in a lesbian relationship, where the couple may be facing the extra challenges of homophobic reactions on their journey to becoming new parents (Chapman *et al.*, 2012).

Simple reassurance can go a long way to alleviating partners' distress:

> Often the most useful thing we can say to a woman's birth companions is, 'If you're worried, look at me; if I'm not looking worried you can assume that all is well. I will tell you if I'm worried about anything – so if I look calm you can feel reassured that this is all normal.'
>
> (Midwife, Leap, 2015, unpublished data)

The following activity draws on a story from an experienced birth centre midwife who explains how she supports partners:

Box 6.10   Reflective Activity: Supporting partners to provide labour support

Individually or in pairs or small groups:

*   Discuss the issues that this story raises for you with reference to your own experience of supporting labour support partners.

> I often tell the partner that they don't need to ask her anything – they don't need to ask her if she wants a drink – that it's better just to offer things. So: 'Here's a drink', or get a cloth and wipe her brow. If she doesn't want it she'll tell you. But if you're asking questions you're bringing her back the whole time, activating that frontal cortex that can get in the way of her going into her body and getting on with labour.
>
> I think very often when they don't know what to say you hear the partners say, 'Are you all right?' But of course they're not 'all right' and women often tell them so in no uncertain words. So I try to give partners different words to say to encourage the woman rather than keep asking her if she's all right! Like, 'You're doing well', or, 'Keep concentrating on breathing out.' I talk to the partners about 'encouraging' rather than 'feeling sorry' for the woman. I suggest it's like if someone's running a marathon and their partner says, 'I'm proud of you and I know you can do it', then you can do it better.
>
> Partners can do 'midwifery muttering' too. I was once with a couple who had done hypnobirthing preparation and after every contraction he said (very quietly so as not to disturb her) all the things that midwives say, 'Well done . . . that was great . . . you're doing so well. . . .' It was lovely to watch. He did it all the way through a long labour. He'd been taught that. She said afterwards that even though she was deeply in her own space she could hear those words of encouragement and they steadied her.
>
> It's one thing sitting next to her if she's on a bed, mopping her brow – that's what they tend to see on reality TV shows – but if a woman is roaming around it's a different sort of role, especially if women are 'in the zone'. They don't want to be touched; they don't want to be coached; they don't want anyone near them. That can be hard for partners to deal with so I explain to them that this is what she needs – to be quietly encouraged between contractions but to move around with free will. That's why the shower or birth pool or sitting on the loo is often so good for women – it gives them a space where people can't get close and disturb their concentration, a good barrier that gives them privacy.
>
> If the woman has to be monitored or has a drip in place, one of the things I say to the partners is that inevitably there may be times when they feel in the way with all those machines that go 'ping': no matter where they sit people will be asking them to move when they need to get in there and do something. I try and reassure them and suggest that they try and keep close to her in all of that and not move right away.
>
> (Midwife, Leap, 2015, unpublished data)

It is easy for partners to feel inhibited by the expertise of the midwife or doula. Awareness of this should be uppermost in our minds as we provide support, as this doula explains:

> I always work hard at not getting in the way between the woman and her partner. So if, for example, she needs a drink, I pass it to the partner to give to her. Sometimes I'll start doing something and invite them to take over. For example, the other day, a woman I was with was doing a little labour dance. Her partner watched me doing it with her for a couple of contractions and then he took over and I stepped back.
>
> (Doula, Leap, 2015, unpublished data)

Supporting partners who are finding it hard to be supportive

We have probably all been in situations where we think that a father is finding it hard to be with his partner in labour and may be present because of social pressure:

> Some are really brilliant but occasionally you get this feeling that they're only there under pressure and it's pretty miserable for them. I was with one the other day who, as the head came on view, suddenly had to go to the toilet. And he was in the toilet when the baby was born! I think he escaped because he couldn't cope. He didn't seem that disappointed when he returned.
>
> (Midwife, Leap, 2015, unpublished data)

In such circumstances, we have to curb any value judgements arising from our own interpretations of how a couple are interacting (Robertson, 2007). It can be tricky working out whether we should encourage the father to be involved or avoid asking him to do things out of respect for the dynamic that exists between the couple:

> Some couples are so close that you feel like you're intruding – the guy is right there with her and knows exactly what she needs. But then there are other guys who have no idea and don't seem to know the woman very well. You can often tell if their relationship is very new or under a lot of strain.
>
> (Midwife, Leap, 2015, unpublished data)

As we explored in Chapter 1, doulas can play an important role in supporting the woman's partner. This is particularly relevant in the absence of midwifery continuity of care, where the doula, rather than the midwife, has been able to develop a trusting relationship with the couple.

When there are relationship problems

Sadly, even when there are no physical problems with labour, birth is not always welcome or joyous. It is always important to be alert to the potential that the woman may be in an abusive relationship. Women experiencing intimate partner violence (IPV) during pregnancy have an increased risk of pre-term birth, and having a baby who is low birth weight or small for gestational age (Donovan *et al.*, 2016). They may also find labour and birth very challenging, especially if the partner is their only birth companion (Dempsey, 2020). It is important that midwives, students and all health professionals know the signs of IPV to look out for, including any hints of physical and emotional abuse. After the birth, midwives need to feel confident about initiating and engaging in an individualised conversation, responding appropriately when a woman discloses IPV; this includes being aware of local support and referral policies (Smith *et al.*, 2018).

The following story from a UK community midwife provides us with an opportunity to discuss ways of being with women in labour when the couple have complex relationship difficulties.

Box 6.11   Reflective Activity: When midwives need to step in with support

Individually or in pairs or small groups:
- Discuss the issues that this story raises for you and what we can learn from it.
- How might you initiate a conversation with the woman in the postnatal period?
- What resources are you aware of in your local area that you would discuss with the woman?

I really think the back rubbing and massage, wet flannels, mopping the brow and holding the hand things should be the partner's role, not mine. But sometimes you have to step in.

I was with a woman who was needing very intense labour support. I hadn't met her before, but I knew from colleagues who had seen her antenatally that there were concerns about their relationship and his control over her. So there had been all sorts of concerns about them from a social point of view.

In labour, the partner was sort of doing his own thing, didn't seem very supportive or present and was very much leaving her to it. He kept himself very separate. She totally needed support and he wasn't giving it. So that was the total extreme of labour support where you think, 'Well he's not going to give her labour support and she actually doesn't want it from him either'. So as a midwife you then have to fill that little gap.

She was in the pool and we had real trouble getting the water hot enough so he did actually respond to my requests and boiled kettles and helped to get the pool warmer. But she had hold of me on my arm, pretty much constantly, having to have me almost embracing her and then her friend giving her pressure on her back. She was saying, 'No, no, you can't listen to the baby now, I need you, you have to hold onto me.' So I had to ring the bell to get another midwife to come in and listen to the baby's heartbeat.

Now we found out later that there were issues about that baby not being planned or wanted because from her point of view it was tying her to him. She had been planning to leave him before this pregnancy and now this meant she couldn't leave. So she really didn't want the baby and I think that was maybe why she found that labour so hard, besides the fact that this was a bigger baby and maybe in an awkward position.

In transition, she said she really needed something else – she was using gas and air and she hadn't needed it for the first labour – so I agreed to get her half a dose of Diamorphine and asked someone else to go and get it, hoping that during that time she would get there, which she did. She was pushing by the time that Diamorphine arrived so she never had it.

The baby was born and she didn't really want to do anything with the baby and so I think the baby went to the friend initially. The dad did hold the baby for a while. The woman appeared really traumatised by the whole experience.

At some point I said, 'Would it be all right for the baby to lie next to you? So you don't have to hold the baby yet but she can lie next to you?' The mum was crying a lot, obviously feeling rotten about the whole thing, knowing that she should be bonding with her baby but didn't want to do it. And then at some point she said would I help her breastfeed.

Recently I saw her when the baby was eight weeks old and I had lunch with her. And she was saying that she was starting to like the baby more and even love the baby. I reassured her that sometimes other women say that it takes time.

(Leap, 2015, unpublished data)

Supporting children at birth

If you place 'siblings at birth' in your Internet browser you will access a wealth of articles and some very positive stories about children being present at the birth of their baby brother or sister. You will also find articles highlighting what parents need to think about, if this is what they want. From our own experience in this area we suggest that the following considerations are important:

*   A child should only be present if they want to be and throughout the experience there should be an open-door policy so that they can leave or come and go as they please.
*   Someone who is not the mother or father, but who knows the child well, should be assigned the role of being with the child throughout the labour, whether or not the child wants to be in the same room as the woman in labour.
*   Preparation with visual images and simulated potential noises and behaviours helps the child know what to expect.
*   If the birth is not taking place at home, there may need to be negotiations and plans put in position well before the labour.

When there's a crowd in the birthing space

Usually, women giving birth at home have a lot more control over who they want in the room at different stages of their labour; for example, women often withdraw into fast labour the minute someone has responded to their request for their toddler to be taken off for a walk. In hospital settings, where the woman often feels less in control of the space, it can be hard for the midwife to work out whether the presence of family and friends is enhancing or inhibiting the woman's ability to feel safe enough to concentrate on her labour. This can be particularly confronting if the woman seems happy with the presence of her chosen supporters, but the midwife feels they are providing little or inadequate support, as is discussed in the article in Box 6.12.

Box 6.12   Reflective Activity: Interactions with birth support people

Maher, J. (2004). Midwife interactions with birth support people in Melbourne, Australia. *Midwifery*, *20*, 273–280.

Individually, in pairs or small groups:
*   Discuss the issues that this paper raises in relation to your own experience of supporting a woman in labour when she has several support people in attendance.

Facilitating a supportive environment for labour and birth

The word 'environment' in the context of labour and birth encompasses the culture of the space in which birth is enacted and the philosophical beliefs of the people involved, as well as the physical space.

> The birth environment powerfully shapes and impacts on the birth experience of women and carers. There is nothing neutral in this context with environment, attitudes and relationships all contributing in an enabling or disabling way.
>
> (Walsh, 2010a, p.57)

It is probably no surprise that, when midwives have had experiences of attending women who give birth at home and in midwifery-led units, they are more likely to feel confident about their skills in supporting normal birth in hospital settings where the dominant culture is one of obstetric intervention (Zinsser *et al.*, 2016).

In order to acknowledge how issues of power and control in birthing environments impact on both women's and midwives' experiences, the term 'birth territory' has been used to describe the environment for birth. Within this territory, 'midwifery guardianship' is linked to the protection of all the intricacies of psychological, spiritual and neuro-hormonal processes that promote straightforward, undisturbed birth (Fahy and Parrat, 2006; Fahy *et al.*, 2008).

'Holding the space': creating a safe and supportive environment

Another word that is sometimes used to describe the birth environment in a multidimensional way is the word 'space' (Hammond *et al.*, 2013). We often talk about 'holding the space' when describing labour support. This philosophical concept encompasses providing a steady presence that is totally focused on the woman, including making sure that the environment feels safe for her, described here by a woman when telling the story of her labour:

> What I loved the most was my midwives not telling me what to do. They were just there, 'holding a safe space'. When I was struggling I knew to look up and you see a face that's calm and you can go back into it knowing that there's someone else on top of what's going on, checking everything's OK and safe.
>
> (Mother, Leap, 2015, unpublished data)

'Holding the space' in a woman's home

The woman in the quote above was talking about the sort of support she received when giving birth to her first baby at home. An ever-increasing body of literature identifies the value of encouraging the majority of healthy women to consider giving birth at home (Hutton, *et al.*, 2019; Reitsma *et al.*, 2020).

Box 6.13   Research Briefing: Clinical outcomes for women with healthy pregnancies who intend to give birth at home

Reitsma, A., Simioni, J., Brunton, G., Kaufman, K. and Hutton, E.K. (2020). Maternal outcomes and birth interventions among women who begin labour intending to give birth at home compared to women of low obstetrical risk who intend to give birth in hospital: a systematic review and meta-analyses. *EClinicalMedicine*, 100039.

This review included 16 studies identifying outcomes for 500,000 women who intended to give birth at home at the start of labour. Among women with healthy pregnancies, those intending to birth at home experienced fewer birth interventions and untoward maternal outcomes.

Hutton, E.K., Reitsma, A., Simioni, J., Brunton, G. and Kaufman, K. (2019). Perinatal or neonatal mortality among women who intend at the onset of labour to give birth at home compared to women of low obstetrical risk who intend to give birth in hospital: a systematic review and meta-analyses. *EClinicalMedicine*, *14*, 59–70.

The 14 studies eligible for meta-analysis included 500,000 intended home births. The risk of perinatal or neonatal mortality was not different when birth was intended to take place either at home or in hospital.

Box 6.14   Reflective Activity: Changing the culture to promote home birth

Homer, C.S.E, Leap, N., Edwards, N. and Sandall, J. (2017). Midwifery continuity of carer in an area of high socio-economic disadvantage in London: a retrospective analysis of Albany Midwifery Practice outcomes using routine data (1997–2009). *Midwifery*, *48*, 1–10.

Reed, B. (2015). Changing a birthing culture: Becky Reed explores why so many women with the Albany Midwifery Practice had home births. *AIMS Journal*, *27(4)*, 6–7.

In pairs or small groups:

- After studying these two articles, make a list of all the factors that you think may have contributed to 43.5 per cent of women booked with the Albany Midwifery Practice choosing to give birth at home when the UK home birth rate 'remains stubbornly below three per cent' (Reed, 2015, p.7).
- Discuss the implications for promoting positive experiences for all women, babies and their families, given the outcomes demonstrated by this midwifery group practice, which operated in an inner-city area of high socioeconomic disadvantage.

Supporting women who choose to give birth outside of the system

Across the world, women are choosing to give birth outside of the system, either when homebirth attended by a midwife is not an available option in mainstream maternity care or in situations where they are rejecting medical advice or are themselves being rejected by maternity care systems. Often this decision is a reaction to previous distressing experiences of institutionalised childbirth. The recommended resource in Box 6.15 explores this phenomenon, bringing research, legal and ethical perspectives to bear on why women choose to reject medical advice, including those who choose to give birth at home with an unregulated care provider or without assistance (freebirth).

Box 6.15   Recommended Resource

Dahlen, H., Kumar-Hazard, B. and Schmied, V. (eds). (2020). *Birthing Outside the System: The Canary in the Coal Mine*. London: Routledge.

The reviews on the Routledge website tell an important story; global leaders in maternity care describe this book as a 'wake-up call' to address the urgent need for reform in maternity service provision and the way women are treated in childbirth as a human rights issue. https://www.routledge.com/Birthing-Outside-the-System-The-Canary-in-the-Coal-Mine/Dahlen-Kumar-Hazard-Schmied/p/book/9781138592704.

The Reflective Activity in Box 6.16 allows us to think about how we respond to situations where women are thinking about choosing to 'freebirth' without midwifery support, with or without attendance of a doula at their birth.

Box 6.16 Reflective Activity: Conversations with women contemplating 'freebirthing'

Dahlen, H., Jackson, M. and Stevens, J. (2011). Homebirth, freebirth and doulas: casualty and consequences of a broken maternity system. *Women and Birth, 24*, 47–50.

Feeley, C. and Thomson, G. (2016). Tensions and conflicts in 'choice': women's experiences of freebirthing in the UK. *Midwifery, 41*, 16–21.

Jackson, M., Dahlen, H. and Schmied, V. (2012). Birthing outside the system: perceptions of risk amongst Australian women who have freebirths and high risk homebirths. *Midwifery, 28*, 561–567.

McKenzie, G., Robert, G. and Montgomery, E. (2020). Exploring the conceptualisation and study of freebirthing as a historical and social phenomenon: a meta-narrative review of diverse research traditions. *Medical Humanities, 46*, 512–524.

Norton, J. (2020). Why women freebirth: a modified systematic review. *MIDIRS Midwifery Digest, 30(4)*, 509–513.

In preparation for this activity study these five articles.

In pairs:

- Discuss how your personal attitudes to freebirthing might influence the conversations you would have with a woman who wishes to freebirth with the support of a doula. She tells you that this decision was influenced by a previous traumatic birth in hospital that ended in a caesarean.
- Practise variations in these conversations, taking it in turn to be the woman and the midwife, doula or other birth worker.
- Discuss what you learnt from this activity.

'Holding the space' in birth centres

The chances of women having a normal birth with positive outcomes are considerably higher when they plan to give birth in a midwifery-led unit (Birthplace in England Collaborative Group, 2011; Hodnett *et al.*, 2012; Homer *et al.*, 2019). Midwives find it easier to initiate all the labour support practices that we describe in the next chapter when they are working in out-of-hospital settings (Zinsser *et al.*, 2016). Denis Walsh (2006b) suggests that this is not simply that the practicalities of promoting normal birth are easier to initiate outside of technocratic institutions. In an ethnographic study to explore the culture, beliefs, values, customs and practices around birth within a free-standing birth centre in the UK, he showed how the environment elicited nurturing behaviours from both women and staff. He challenges us to review our conceptualisation of 'safety' and the nature of relationship as we provide support for women progressing through labour to new motherhood.

Box 6.17 Research Briefing: Creating a safe and nurturing space for birth

Walsh, D. (2006). 'Nesting' and 'matrescence' as distinctive features of a free-standing birth centre in the UK. *Midwifery, 22(3)*, 289–239.

The Serenity Birth Centre (BC) is a midwifery-led unit that is the default option for all women with uncomplicated pregnancies booked in an inner-city maternity service in Birmingham, UK. It is held up as an example of an initiative that made dramatic changes to the culture, practices, experiences and outcomes by creating an environment specifically designed to enable midwives to 'hold the space' for women and promote normal birth. (Beech *et al.*, 2015; Gutteridge, 2013, 2015).

Box 6.18   Reflective Activity: Supporting women in birth centres

In preparation for this activity study the following papers:

Walsh, D. and Gutteridge, K. (2011). Using the birth environment to increase women's potential in labour. *MIDIRS Midwifery Digest, 21*(2), 143–147.

Gutteridge, K. (2015). Midwifery-led care for a low-risk cohort – a clinical outcomes overview: over a three year period in a multicultural setting. *MIDIRS Midwifery Digest, 25*(2), 178–185.

Walsh, D., Spiby, H., McCourt, C., Grigg, C., Coleby, D., Bishop, S., . . . Thornton, J. (2020). Factors influencing the utilisation of free-standing and alongside midwifery units in England: a qualitative research study. *BMJ Open Access, 10*(2), e033895.

Individually, in pairs or in small groups:
- Make a list of all the factors that may have contributed to supporting women to have a positive experience of physiological birth in the Serenity and Halcyon Birth Centres (papers 1 and 2)
- Discuss which of these features currently exist – or that you would be able to implement – in the environment in which you practise.
- Search for research papers identifying outcomes related to birth centres/midwifery-led units internationally and in your own country. Discuss the barriers to the wide-spread utilisation of these units, drawing on paper 3.

Birth space and neuroscience

Emerging theory based in neuroscience explores how birth unit design can affect the culture, practices and experiences of birth, suggesting that the physical environment can promote neurobiological responses in both women and their birth attendants. On the one hand, hormones related to stress can inhibit both the physiology of labour and the quality of communication (Foureur *et al.*, 2010; Stenglin and Foureur, 2013); on the other hand, the birth environment may enhance the orchestration and interaction of hormonal processes that are important for both the mother and her baby (Buckley, 2015). In particular, oxytocin can play a critical role in reducing stress, increasing trust and heightening empathy, reciprocity and generosity, thereby promoting both the physiology of labour and the provision of quality midwifery care and support (Hammond *et al.*, 2013). The papers highlighted in Box 6.19 explore these issues further.

Box 6.19   Research Briefing and Reflective Activity: Thinking about how birth unit design affects supportive care in labour

Bowden, C., Sheehan, A. and Foureur, M. (2016). Birth room images: what they tell us about childbirth. A discourse analysis of birth rooms in developed countries. *Midwifery, 35*, 71–77.

Hammond, A., Foureur, M. and Homer, C.S.E. (2014a). The hardware and software implications of hospital birth room design: a midwifery perspective. *Midwifery, 30*, 825–830.

Hammond, A., Foureur, M., Homer, C.S.E. and Davis, D. (2013). Space, place and the midwife: exploring the relationship between the birth environment, neurobiology and midwifery practice. *Women and Birth, 26*, 277–281.

Symon, A., Paul, J., Butchart, M., Carr, V. and Dugard, P. (2008). Maternity unit design study part 3: environmental comfort and control. *British Journal of Midwifery, 16(3)*, 167–171.

Gould, D. (2002). Subliminal medicalisation. *British Journal of Midwifery, 10(7)*, 418.

In pairs or small groups:

- After reading these five articles draw a mind map reflecting the ways in which the features of your working environment impact positively and negatively on your ability to provide supportive care for women in labour.
- NICE guidelines (2014, p.23) suggest that we should 'encourage the woman to adapt the environment to meet her individual needs'. Identify on your mind map the sort of adaptations that are possible in the environment/s in which you work and who has the power to make these happen.
- Share your mind maps in the larger group and discuss what you learnt through engaging in this activity. Discuss the complexity of identifying and responding to individual women's needs in relation to adapting different birthing environments.

Creating a supportive environment for birth: avoiding assumptions

When we think about creating a supportive environment for birth, we may have preconceptions about what this will look like:

> I'll never forget this. I was in the Birth Centre waiting for a woman to come in. So I got the place ready: lights off, mat down on the floor, bean bag to lean over. And she said it felt like walking into a cave – a really private, peaceful space – and that was really important to her. So it's important to set the scene if you're there before the woman arrives.
>
> (Midwife, Leap, 2015, unpublished data)

While preparing the labour room in this way is laudable, we feel obliged to point out that not everyone thinks of a cave as a beautiful private space. We can remember situations in some homes where such cave-enhancing efforts have been overturned impatiently by women re-entering the room and switching back on all the lights and the focal TV screen, with its blaring commercial breaks. One woman's oxytocin-enhancing cave might be another woman's adrenaline-provoking nightmare! Once again, we should be careful not to make assumptions. Women will show us what feels right for them if they have a sense of control over their surroundings and if we are open to helping them create the 'right' space for them.

Promoting and facilitating normal birth: responding to global imperatives

The Normal Birth Position Statement published by All4Maternity (Feeley *et al.*, 2020) identifies global attention on the need to reduce caesarean section rates; it highlights the imperative for *all* midwives to have the skills and knowledge to support women in ways that will facilitate the physiological processes of childbirth. The ten-part series on normal birth published by All4Maternity in *The Practising Midwife* in 2020 and 2021 showcases articles applying evidence for the promotion of normal birth in everyday practice situations. This series provides a useful resource for all birth workers and forms the basis of the activity in Box 6.20.

Box 6.20   Reflective Activity: Facilitating normal birth in practice

A large group activity
- After a short presentation based on the principles discussed in this chapter, the facilitator explains the activity and divides the large group into smaller working groups.
- Each group is allocated one article from the ten-part series on normal birth published in *The Practising Midwife* in 2020 and 2021 and given an allocated time to summarise the article (not more than ten dot points) and discuss the issues it raises, drawing on stories of experiences.
- One member of each small group presents their dot-point summary of the article to the whole group and, in turn, each of the other members of the small group tells a relevant short story relating to the issues that were discussed.
- The facilitator leads a final discussion with the whole group about the experience of engaging in this activity and the implications for learning and practice.
- This activity could be adapted to form a student assignment.

The principles we have explored in this chapter underpin the practicalities of labour support that we shall explore in the next chapter. We leave the chapter with a postscript that encapsulates the sense of triumph that women often display when giving birth has been an empowering experience.

Postscript: greeting Maisie (firstborn baby of Sara and Jon)*

* recorded verbatim

1.30 am
Sara is in the birthing pool at home; Jon, Sara's sisters – Claire and Ella – and midwives Cathy and Nicky are in attendance. The baby's head has been born and everyone is waiting with huge anticipation.

Cathy: Sara, with the next contraction your baby will be here. Let your baby out.
Sara: It *will* come out.
            Doing good baby.
            Has it restituted? [Sara is a newly qualified midwife].
            Will it do that soon?
Cathy: It may not have to . . .

1.38 am

Cathy: We may have to get you up a bit.
Sara: Are you worried about the shoulders?
Cathy: A little bit.
Sara: It's because I haven't had another strong contraction. If I could have a strong contraction it would come.
Cathy: OK, let's wait for one of those.

1.45 am
Sara has her big contraction and Maisie slithers out into the water. Sara and Cathy lift her out of the water. She snuffles on Sara's abdomen.

Sara: I knew it! Baby GIRL!
            I love you!
            A baby girl!
            I love you!
            A baby girl – I knew it!
            I'm so glad you're here!
            I've been dreaming of you!
            You're so beautiful!
            And that's your Daddy! Just there!
            You're so clever!
            Oh I love you!
            We're going to have fun together!
            You're so pretty!
            I love you!
            You're such a clever girl!
            You're so clever!

Sara and Jon pore over their baby daughter, exclaiming at every detail of her wriggling features.

Sara: You have a little Filipino nose like your Dad! And your crazy Uncle Marco! I'm so proud of you! I'm so proud of you! I'm so proud of you! You're beautiful! You're beautiful! You're beautiful! I'm so glad you're here! You don't understand how glad I am! You've got a little Filipino nose! That's the funniest thing ever! Look at your vernix! You've got so much hair!

Jon: She's got a bigger little toenail than yours Sara!

Ella: That's the best thing I've ever seen!

Sara: That's your Dad! I LOVE YOU JON!

Jon kisses their daughter who is pink and calm, snuggling into Sara's body, licking, exploring, eyes wide open.

Sara: Thanks girls!
          Thanks Cathy!
          I can't believe it's over!
          WOOOOOOOOOGH! [fist in the air]

Sara turns to Hermie [the cat] who is sitting nearby, calmly taking it all in.

Sara: This is the pudding I was telling you about Hermie.
          Hermie was great! He kept me company.
          I LOVE CATS!

Sara: [to everyone] I'm so glad you're all here!
          I was worried that it would be too much – but it wasn't!
          I HAD A BABY!
          My vagina opened up!
          I've so wanted for this!
          I didn't know if I'd ever have one of these!
          Pretty girl!
          Pretty girl!
          Pretty girl!
          Pretty girl!
          Pretty girl!
          Pretty girl!

          Here, look, it's your Aunties!
          F___ING HELL WE DID IT! [Fist in the air and laughter]
          I was a bit scared . . .
          Cathy – you were great!
          I DID IT!

Sara turns to Cathy:

          When you put your hand on me in the bedroom it was such a relief!
          You were so important for me!
          Jon you were good too.
          You were all great.

Nicky stops taking notes and asks Sara if she would like her to use the video camera as they had planned. The rest of the greeting and phoning time is on film.

***

A few years later, Nicky recalled this profound account and contacted 'Sara' to ask permission to use it in this book. The transcript of that email discussion is provided here to show how women continue to reflect on their birth experiences (Simkin, 1991, 1992).

Email from Sara (who is now a midwife practising in a large maternity unit) to Nicky:

> Regarding that file – of course you can use it! I would like you to change our names, because quite frankly I sound a little bit demented which of course I am (but don't like to publically [sic] admit that too often). I'm so glad you wrote it all down – it brings that amazing moment in my life all back. I have to say I haven't seen many women going on the way I did!!! Ella and I were just laughing at Christmas time about the cats [sic] comment. . . . She brings it up at random times to various people and I try not to look embarrassed.
>
> The thing is I still do love cats :).

Email from Nicky to Sara:

> I'm really interested that you say you don't see women carrying on like that. We see it a lot in home birth situations. It's useful to think that students don't see that often in hospitals. . . . And you really don't sound demented. It's a wonderful outpouring of triumph and joy. In my practice in London the second midwife always wrote down what women said around birth – as a gift for them. Similar ecstatic outpourings – and all really moving.

Email from Sara to Nicky:

> I'm glad you see many women behaving the way I did. I still wonder about a lot of the practices I see in hospitals and how it affects the experience of birth. . . . I often wonder too about the freedom and security of home birth and how it affects women's ability to give birth and to experience the magic and internal power of it (having only been at one other home birth).

Email from Nicky to Sara:

> Thank you Sara. This is a real gift – to me and to anyone who will read the book.

References

Beech, B., Edwards, N. and Leap, N. (2015). Serenity. *AIMS Journal, 27(4)*, 14–16.

Birthplace in England Collaborative Group (2011). Perinatal and maternal outcomes by planned place of birth for healthy women with low risk pregnancies: the Birthplace in England national prospective cohort study. *BMJ Open Access* (published 24 November, 2011), 343, d7400.

Bowden, C., Sheehan, A. and Foureur, M. (2016). Birth room images: what they tell us about childbirth. A discourse analysis of birth rooms in developed countries. *Midwifery, 35*, 71–77.

Buckley, S.J. (2015). *Hormonal Physiology of Childbearing: Evidence and Implications for Women, Babies, and Maternity Care*. Washington, DC: Childbirth Connection Programs, National Partnership for Women and Families.

Butler, M.M. (2017). Exploring the strategies that midwives in British Columbia use to promote normal birth. *BMC Pregnancy and Childbirth, 17*, 168.

Capogna, G., Camorcia, M. and Stirparo, S. (2007). Expectant fathers' experience during labor with or without epidural analgesia. *International Journal of Obstetric Anaesthesia, 16(2)*, 110–115.

Chalmers, I., Enkin, M. and Keirse, M.J.N.C. (eds). (1989). *Effective Care in Pregnancy and Childbirth*. Oxford: Oxford University Press.

Chapman, R., Wardrop, J., Zappia, T., Watkins, R. and Shields, L. (2012). The experiences of Australian lesbian couples becoming parents: deciding, searching and birthing. *Journal of Clinical Nursing, 21*, 1878–1885. doi:10.1111/j.1365-2702.2011.04007.x.

Dahlen, H.G., Jackson, M. and Stevens, J. (2011). Homebirth, freebirth and doulas: casualty and consequences of a broken maternity system. *Women and Birth, 24*, 47–50.

Dahlen, H., Kumar-Hazard, B. and Schmied, V. (eds). (2020). *Birthing Outside the System: The Canary in the Coal Mine*. Abingdon-on-Thames: Taylor & Francis.

Dempsey, R. (2020). *Beyond the Birth Plan: Getting Real about Pain and Power*. Fairfield, Victoria, Australia: Boathouse Press.

Donovan, B.M., Spracklen, C.N., Schweizer, M.L., Ryckman, K.K. and Saftlasa, A.F. (2016). Intimate partner violence during pregnancy and the risk for adverse infant outcomes: a systematic review and meta-analysis. *British Journal of Obstetrics and Gynaecology, 123*, 1289–1299.

Downe, S. and Byrom, S. (eds). (2019). *Squaring the Circle: Normal Birth Research, Theory and Practice in a Technological Age*. London: Pinter & Martin.

Downe, S., Finlayson, K., Oladapo, O.T., Bonet, M. and Gülmezoglu, A.M. (2018). What matters to women during childbirth: a systematic qualitative review. *PLoS ONE, 13*(4), e0194906.

Enkin, M. (2006). Guest editorial. Beyond evidence: the complexity of maternity care. *Birth, 22*(4), 265–269.

Fahy, K., Foureur, M. and Hastie, C. (2008). *Birth Territory and Midwifery Guardianship: Theory for Practice, Education and Research*. Oxford: Elsevier.

Fahy, K. and Parrat, J.A. (2006). Birth territory: a theory for midwifery practice. *Women and Birth, 19*, 45–50.

Feeley, C. and Thomson, G. (2016). Tensions and conflicts in 'choice': women's experiences of freebirthing in the UK. *Midwifery*, 41, 16–21.

Feeley, C., Byrom, A., Byrom, S. and Tizard, H. (2020). Normal birth: position statement. *The Practising Midwife, 23*(1), 34.

Foureur, M., Davis, D.L., Fenwick, J., Leap, N., Iedema, R., Forbes, I.F. and Homer, C.S.E. (2010). The relationship between birth unit design and safe, satisfying birth: developing a hypothetical model. *Midwifery, 26*(5), 520–525.

Gosden, D. (1996). Dissenting voices: conflict and complexity in the home birth movement in Australia. MA honours thesis. Anthropology Dept., Maquarie University, Sydney.

Gosden, D. and Saul, A. (1999). Reflections on the use of psychotherapy in midwifery. *British Journal of Midwifery*.

Gould, D. (2002). Subliminal medicalisation. *British Journal of Midwifery, 10*(7), 418.

Green, J.M. and Baston, H.A. (2007). Have women become more willing to accept obstetric interventions and does this relate to mode of birth? data from a prospective study. *Birth, 34*(1), 6–13.

Green, J.M., Kitzinger, J. and Coupland, V. (1990). Stereotypes of childbearing women – a look at some of the evidence. *Midwifery*, 6, 125–132.

Gutteridge, K. (2013). From Serenity to Halcyon Birth Centre. *The Practising Midwife, 16*(1), 33–36.

Gutteridge, K. (2015). Midwifery-led care for a low-risk cohort – a clinical outcomes overview: over a three year period in a multicultural setting. *MIDIRS Midwifery Digest, 25*(2), 178–185.

Hammond, A., Foureur, M. and Homer, C.S.E. (2014a). The hardware and software implications of hospital birth room design: a midwifery perspective. *Midwifery*, 30, 825–830.

Hammond, A., Foureur, M. and Homer, C.S.E. (2014b, unpublished data). Exploring the impacts of physical and aesthetic design of hospital birth rooms on midwives. Birth Unit Design (BUD) project.

Hammond, A., Foureur, M., Homer, C.S.E. and Davis, D. (2013). Space, place and the midwife: exploring the relationship between the birth environment, neurobiology and midwifery practice. *Women and Birth, 26*, 277–281.

Hodnett, E.D., Downe, S. and Walsh, D. (2012). Alternative versus conventional institutional settings for birth. *Cochrane Database of Systematic Reviews*, Issue 8. Art. No.: CD000012. doi:10.1002/14651858.CD000012.pub4.

Homer, C.S.E., Cheah, S.L., Rossiter, C., Dahlen, H., Ellwood, D., Foureur, M., . . . Scarff, V.L. (2019). Maternal and perinatal outcomes by planned place of birth in Australia 2000–2012: a linked population data study. *BMJ Open Access*, *9*, e029192. doi:10.1136/bmjopen-2019-029192.

Homer, C.S.E., Leap, N., Edwards, N. and Sandall, J. (2017). Midwifery continuity of carer in an area of high socio-economic disadvantage in London: a retrospective analysis of Albany Midwifery Practice outcomes using routine data (1997–2009). *Midwifery*, *48*, 1–10.

Hutton, E., Reitsma, A., Simioni, J., Brunton, G. and Kaufman, K. (2019). Perinatal or neonatal mortality among women who intend at the onset of labour to give birth at home compared to women of low obstetrical risk who intend to give birth in hospital: a systematic review and meta-analyses. *EClinicalMedicine*, *14*, 59–70.

Iles, J., Slade, P. and Spiby, H. (2011). Posttraumatic stress symptoms and postpartum depression in couples after childbirth: the role of partner support and attachment. *Journal of Anxiety Disorders*, *25*, 520–530.

Jackson, M., Dahlen, H. and Schmied, V. (2012). Birthing outside the system: perceptions of risk amongst Australian women who have freebirths and high risk homebirths. *Midwifery*, *28*, 561–567.

Kennedy, H.P, Anderson, T. and Leap, N. (2010). Midwifery presence: philosophy, science and art. Chapter 7 in D. Walsh and S. Downe (eds), *Essential Midwifery Practice: Intrapartum Care* (pp.105–124). Chichester: Wiley-Blackwell.

Kennedy, H.P and Shannon, M.T. (2004). Keeping birth normal: research findings on midwifery care during labour. *Journal of Obstetric Gynecologic and Neonatal Nursing*, *33*(5), 554–560.

Kennedy, H.P., Shannon, M.T., Chuahorm, U. and Kravetz, M.K. (2004). The landscape of caring for women: a narrative study of midwifery practice. *Journal of Midwifery and Women's Health*, *49*(1), 14–23.

Kitzinger, S (ed.). (1988). *The Midwife Challenge*. London: Pandora.

Leap, N. (1996). A midwifery perspective on pain in labour. Unpublished MSc dissertation, South Bank University, London. Available on request from nickyleap@me.com.

Leap, N. (2009). Woman centred care or women centred care: Does it matter? *British Journal of Midwifery*, *17*(1), 12–16.

Leap, N. (2010). The less we do the more we give. Chapter 2 in M. Kirkham (ed.), *The Midwife–Mother Relationship*, 2nd edn (pp.17–35). London: Palgrave Macmillan.

Leap, N. (2015, unpublished data). Identifying the experiences of receiving and providing support in labour.

Lennon, J. and McCartney, P. (1970). 'Let it Be' (lyrics). London: Northern Songs.

Lynch, E. (2020). Normal birth 1: contention and debate in the UK. *The Practising Midwife*, *23*(8), 19.

Maher, J. (2004). Midwife interactions with birth support people in Melbourne, Australia. *Midwifery*, *20*, 273–280.

McKenzie, G., Robert, G. and Montgomery, E. (2020). Exploring the conceptualisation and study of freebirthing as a historical and social phenomenon: a meta-narrative review of diverse research traditions. *Medical Humanities*, *46*, 512–524.

Newnham, E., McKellar, L. and Pincombe, J. (2015). Documenting risk: a comparison of policy and information pamphlets for using epidural or water in labour. *Women and Birth*, *28*, 221–227.

Newnham, E., McKellar, L. and Pincombe, J. (2017). Paradox of the institution: findings from a hospital labour ward ethnography. *BMC Pregnancy and Childbirth*, *17*, 2.

Newnham, E., McKellar, L. and Pincombe, J. (2018) *Towards the Humanisation of Birth: A Study of Epidural Analgesia and Hospital Birth Culture*. London: Palgrave Macmillan.

NICE. (2014). Intrapartum care: care of healthy women and their babies during childbirth. Clinical guideline 190. National Collaborating Centre for Women's and Children's Health UK. Commissioned by the National Institute for Health and Care Excellence (NICE): www.nice.org.uk/guidance/cg190.

Norton, J. (2020). Why women freebirth: a modified systematic review. *MIDIRS Midwifery Digest*, *30*(4), 509–513.

Oakley, A. (1980). *Women Confined: Towards a Sociology of Childbirth*. Oxford: Martin Robertson.

Olza, I., Leahy-Warren, P., Benyamini, Y., Kazmierczak, M., Karlsdottir, S.I., Spyridou, A., . . . Nieuwenhuijze, M.J. (2018). Women's psychological experiences of physiological childbirth: a metasynthesis. *BMJ Open Access*, *8*, e020347.

Purnell, L. (2000). A description of the Purnell Model for cultural competence. *Journal of Transcultural Nursing*, *11(1)*, 40–46.

Reed, B. (2015). Changing a birthing culture: Becky Reed explores why so many women with the Albany midwifery practice had home births. *AIMS Journal*, *27(4)*, 6–7.

Reitsma, A., Simioni, J., Brunton, G., Kaufman, K. and Hutton, E.K. (2020). Maternal outcomes and birth interventions among women who begin labour intending to give birth at home compared to women of low obstetrical risk who intend to give birth in hospital: a systematic review and meta-analyses. *EClinicalMedicine*, 100039.

Robertson, A. (2006). *Empowering Women: Teaching Active Birth*. Sydney: Birth International.

Robertson, A. (2007). *The Midwife Companion: The Art of Support during Birth*, 2nd edn. Sydney: Birth International.

Romano, A.M. and Lothian, J.A. (2008). Promoting, protecting, and supporting normal birth: a look at the evidence. *Journal of Obstetric, Gynecologic and Neonatal Nursing*, *37(1)*, 94–104.

Ross-Davie, M.C. and Cheyne, H. (2014). Intrapartum support: what do women want? A literature review to identify how far the nature of labour support shapes women's assessment of their birth experiences. *Evidence Based Midwifery*, *12(2)*, 52–58.

Sandall, J., Leap, N., Grant, J. and Bastos, M.H. (2010). Supporting women to have a normal birth: development and field testing of a learning package for maternity staff. Health and Social Care Research Division, King's College London.

Simkin, P. (1991). Just another day in a woman's life? Women's long term perceptions of their first birth experience. Part 1. *Birth*, *18*, 203–210.

Simkin, P. (1992). Just another day in a woman's life? Women's long term perceptions of their first birth experience. Part II: Nature and consistency of women's long term memories of their first birth experience. *Birth*, *19*, 64–68.

Simkin, P. with Rohs, K. (2018). *The Birth Partner: A Complete Guide to Childbirth for Dads, Doulas, and All Other Labor Companions*, 5th edn. Boston, MA: Harvard Common Press.

Smith, C.A., Levett, K.M., Collins, C.T. and Crowther, C.A. (2018). Relaxation techniques for pain management in labour. *Cochrane Database of Systematic Reviews*, Issue 3. Art. No.: CD009514. doi:10.1002/14651858.CD009514.pub2.

Stenglin, M. and Foureur, M. (2013). Designing out the fear cascade to increase the likelihood of normal birth. *Midwifery*, *29*, 819–825.

Symon, A., Paul, J., Butchart, M., Carr, V. and Dugard, P. (2008). Maternity unit design study part 3: environmental comfort and control. *British Journal of Midwifery*, *16(3)*, 167–171.

Ulrich, L.T. (1990). *A Midwife's Tale: The life of Martha Ballard, based on her diary 1785–1812*. New York: Vintage Books.

Van der Gucht, N. and Lewis, K. (2015). Women's experiences of coping with pain during childbirth: a critical review of qualitative research. *Midwifery*, *31*, 349–358.

Walsh, D. (2006). 'Nesting' and 'matrescence' as distinctive features of a free-standing birth centre in the UK. *Midwifery*, *22(3)*, 289–239.

Walsh, D. (2010a). Birth environment. Chapter 4 in D. Walsh and S. Downe (eds), *Essential Midwifery Practice: Intrapartum Care* (pp.45–62). Chichester: Wiley-Blackwell.

Walsh, D. (2010b). Introduction. In D. Walsh and S. Downe (eds), *Essential Midwifery Practice: Intrapartum Care* (pp.xi–xiii). Chichester: Wiley-Blackwell.

Walsh, D. (2012). *Evidence and Skills for Normal Labour and Birth*, 2nd edn. London: Routledge.

Walsh, D. and Downe, S. (eds). (2010). *Essential Midwifery Practice: Intrapartum Care*. Chichester: Wiley-Blackwell.

Walsh, D. and Gutteridge, K. (2011). Using the birth environment to increase women's potential in labour. *MIDIRS Midwifery Digest*, *21(2)*, 143–147.

Walsh, D., Spiby, H., McCourt, C., Grigg, C., Coleby, D., Bishop, S., . . . Thornton, J. (2020). Factors influencing the utilisation of free-standing and alongside midwifery units in England: a qualitative research study. *BMJ Open Access, 10(2)*, e033895.

WHO. (1985). Appropriate technology for birth. *Lancet, 326(8452)*, 436–437.

WHO. (1996). *Care in Normal Birth: A Practical Guide.* Geneva: Department of Reproductive Health and Research. World Health Organization. https://cdn1.sph.harvard.edu/wpcontent/uploads/sites/2413/2014/08/WHO_FRH_MSM_96.24.pdf.

Young, D. (March 2009). What is normal childbirth and do we need more statements about it? Editorial. *Birth, 36*, 1–3.

Zinsser, L.A., Stoll, K. and Gross, M.M. (2016). Midwives' attitudes towards supporting normal labour and birth – a cross-sectional study in South Germany. *Midwifery, 39*, 98–102.

7 Supporting women in labour
Practicalities

Introduction

In this chapter we look at some practical ways to support women during labour and birth, bearing in mind the issues we explored about approaches to pain in labour in Chapter 2 and the principles of promoting physiological birth that we discussed in Chapter 6. We explore ways of supporting women through the progressive continuum of rhythms, emotions and behaviours that characterise individual women's labours (Dixon *et al.*, 2013a, 2013b, 2014; Gould, 2000; Walsh, 2001, 2010), bearing in mind that many of these support measures can be useful at any point in a woman's journey through labour. First, though, we look at some of the resources we might draw on in providing individualised support for women in labour.

Labour support resources

The art of labour support includes having a 'toolkit' of ideas and resources that we can offer to women as things that might help. These are often referred to as 'comfort measures', and if you search the Internet using this phrase you will find a wealth of information, including some useful videos on YouTube.

Many of these resources relate to the original work of Penny Simkin, whose books on labour support we highly recommend, in particular *The Birth Partner: A Complete Guide to Childbirth for Dads, Doulas, and All Other Labor Companions* (Simkin, 2018) and the midwives' 'bible', co-authored with Ruth Anchetta and recently with Lisa Hanson: *The Labor Progress Handbook: Early Interventions to Prevent and Treat Dystocia* (Simkin *et al.*, 2017). For quick reference, two articles by Penny Simkin are highlighted in Box 7.1; these are available online and contain a comprehensive overview of practical support strategies, enhanced with descriptive line drawings.

Box 7.1   Recommended Resources: Support in labour – comfort measures

Simkin, P. (2002). Supportive care during labor: a guide for busy nurses. *JOGNN*, *31*(6), 721–732. doi:10.1177/0884217502239208.

Simkin, P. (2007). *Comfort in Labour: How You Can Help Yourself to a Normal Satisfying Childbirth*. Childbirth Connection. https://www.nationalpartnership.org/our-work/resources/health-care/maternity/comfort-in-labor-simkin.pdf.

DOI: 10.4324/9781003092520-8

Labour support: identifying skills, knowledge and learning needs

The activity in Box 7.2 enables us to consider the skills and knowledge that we already have in supporting women in labour as well as the resources that we might access in order to identify our individual learning.

Box 7.2   Reflective Activity: Supportive strategies in labour – identifying individual competency and learning needs

Walsh, D. (2012). Pain in labour. Chapter 7 in D. Walsh (ed.), *Evidence and Skills for Normal Labour and Birth*, 2nd edn (pp.82–100). London: Routledge.

Simkin, P. and Bolding, A. (2004). Update on nonpharmacologic approaches to relieve labor pain and prevent suffering. *Journal of Midwifery and Women's Health*, *49*(*6*), 489–504.

Individually or in pairs:

• Drawing on these texts and the Cochrane review of pain management for women in labour (Jones *et al.*, 2012), make a list of all the practical methods for supporting women that are mentioned in these articles and any others you can think of that are not mentioned.

• Complete a table or 'inventory' identifying your skills, knowledge and learning needs for each item using the format in Box 7.3 below.

• Discuss your inventory with a colleague. Consider whether this activity might contribute to your professional portfolio.

Box 7.3   Example of format for a skills, knowledge and learning needs inventory

Support measure	*How I achieved skills and knowledge in this area*	*How I will address my learning needs in this area*
Active Birth techniques	Birth International workshop (date)	Find a Robozo workshop Identify YouTube resources
Sterile water injections for back pain relief in labour	Knowledge of evidence (list of articles accessed with notes)	N/A at my unit
Supporting women in the effective use of Entonox	Everyday practice knowledge, reflection on experience	Literature search to explore issues and latest evidence

---

Supporting women who want to use complementary therapies for managing pain in labour

Women who want to avoid interventions and pharmacological pain relief in labour are increasingly turning to complementary therapies and mind–body methods, such as mindfulness and hypnobirthing (Walker *et al.*, 2009). During pregnancy, they engage in courses with their birth supporters to learn about ways of promoting normal birth physiology, using methods such as: acupuncture, acupressure, breathing techniques, 'calm birth', mindfulness, music, relaxation, self-hypnosis, visualisation and yoga (Levett *et al.*, 2016). In Chapter 4, we explored evidence related to women's experiences of labour and birth having attended such courses. We shall now focus on some of the practicalities of supporting women who want to use complementary therapies in labour.

Box 7.4   Reflective Activity: Supporting women who want to use complementary therapies in labour

Levett, K.M., Smith, C.A., Bensoussan, A. and Dahlen, H.G. (2016). Complementary therapies for labour and birth study: a randomised controlled trial of antenatal integrative medicine for pain management in labour. *BMJ Open Access, 6.* doi:10.1136/ bmjopen-2015-010691.

Levett, K.M., Smith, C.A., Dahlen, H.G. and Bensoussan, A. (2014). Acupuncture and acupressure for pain management in labour and birth: a critical narrative review of current systematic review evidence. *Complementary Therapies in Medicine, 22,* 523–540.

Smith, C.A., Levett, K.M., Collins, C.T. and Jones, L. (2012). Massage, reflexology and other manual methods for pain management in labour. *Cochrane Database of Systematic Reviews 2012,* Issue 2. Art. No.: CD009290. doi:10.1002/14651858.CD009290.pub2.

Smith, C.A., Levett, K.M., Collins, C.T. and Crowther, C.A. (2018). Relaxation techniques for pain management in labour. *Cochrane Database of Systematic Reviews,* Issue 3. Art. No.: CD009514. doi:10.1002/14651858.CD009514.pub2.

Individually, in pairs or small groups:

• After studying these articles make a list of the methods that are mentioned and discuss what you learnt about the issues of supporting women who choose to use each one of these in labour.

• Discuss the potential dilemmas that you – or pregnant women – might face in light of the NICE (2014) guidelines: 'Do not offer acupuncture, acupressure or hypnosis, but do not prevent women who wish to use these techniques from doing so' (p.35).

Supporting women who use self-hypnosis in labour

The paper profiled in Box 7.5 offers useful insights to promote discussion about supporting the increasing number of women who have prepared for labour using self-hypnosis, often referred to as 'hypnobirthing'.

Box 7.5   Research Briefing: Women's experiences of using self-hypnosis in labour

Finlayson, K., Downe, S. and Hinder, S. (2015). Unexpected consequences: women's experiences of a self-hypnosis intervention to help with pain in labour. *BMC Pregnancy and Childbirth, 15,* 229.

An important finding of the research by Finlayson and colleagues (2015) was that staff misinterpreted signs of labour progress due to the relaxed state of women using self-hypnosis techniques. The 'cues' that we discuss later in this chapter were not apparent, something that this midwife describes:

> Some of the clues of labour can be masked when a woman has prepared using hypnotherapy – for the woman, but also for the midwife. I feel at sea when with a woman who is hypnobirthing. I almost have to do VEs more because I really can't tell and there might be someone who is looking really calm and she could be about to push her baby out or, alternatively, not yet in strong labour.
>
> (Midwife, Leap, 2015, unpublished data)

Another issue that we may need to consider is that our behaviours and language might conflict with the approach the woman has been taught in hypnobirthing classes, impacting negatively on her experience. The following story enables us to reflect on this issue.

Box 7.6   Reflective Activity: Supporting women who have prepared for labour using self-hypnosis techniques

The first time I looked after a woman who had done hypnobirthing classes I felt really uncomfortable. I didn't know much about it and it was in the early days of hypnobirthing. The woman was having her second baby at home.

We were given the book to read as we walked through the door and it was very much like, 'You're not to say this . . . you're not to get her to push . . . you're not to say "pain" or "contraction . . .".' We were told to use the word 'surge' or something. There were real scripts about what words to use so all the patter that you have, where you think you're quite good at making this a normal life event thing, you had to re-adjust and I felt really quite out of my depth. So I was quickly reading the book and then trying to give the right sort of comments and understanding.

Since then I've very much wanted to find a balance between the women being in control through hypnobirthing and us being able to support them. For some pregnant women I'll say, 'It's great that you're doing hypnobirthing but if the midwife who attends you in labour doesn't know about it or isn't used to it, we'll have to make a plan for how she can best support you. And sometimes our skills are in helping you to be a bit more proactive in the labour, rather than just breathing with things.' I'll explain, for example, that sometimes it can be such hard work bringing a baby down and that you need to do more than just breathe, you actually need to put force behind what your body is doing to get a baby born.

(Midwife, Leap, 2015, unpublished data)

In pairs or small groups:
- Discuss how this story helps us identify our individual learning needs in order to support women who have prepared for labour using 'hypnobirthing' or similar approaches.

Supporting women through the continuum of labour

As we mentioned in Chapter 4, women tend to think of labour as a continuous process rather than something defined by stages and phases (Dixon *et al.*, 2013a). Textbook definitions of labour stages, with their contested acceptable durations (Albers, 1999; Neal *et al.*, 2010), are often unhelpful to us in supporting women through the variations in experiences and timings that constitute normal birth (Abalos *et al.*, 2018; Gould, 2000; Walsh, 2001). We shall therefore explore ways of supporting women using headings that might resonate more with the diversity of women's experiences and the phrases they tend to use: in early labour; when contractions are close together and strong; when contractions are expulsive ('pushing the baby out'); giving birth and immediately after giving birth.

Supporting women in early labour

The importance of supporting women in early labour begins with recognition that many women experience painful contractions during what is (unhelpfully) often defined as 'the latent phase of labour'; stories abound of women feeling crushed and dispirited when told that they're 'not really in labour yet':

> I thought, 'If this isn't real labour, I'm never going to cope with the real thing.' The midwife I saw later explained that your body gets used to the contractions as time goes on and that each one was doing good work and helping me get nearer to seeing the baby. That sort of changed my attitude and made me think I could do it after all. She gave me lots of ideas about things I could do to rest and save my energy and said, 'Call me if you need me.' So I just settled into it.
>
> (Mother, Leap, unpublished data, 2015)

The woman in the above quote benefited from having a midwife whom she knew and trusted, who was able to visit her at home. This type of caseload care has been associated with benefits, including later admissions to hospital and reduced caesarean section rates (Davey *et al.*, 2013). Even where midwives work in models of care which mean they are unable to provide this level of continuity, they can still play a crucial role in supporting women during this time; for example, a Cochrane systematic review concluded that women receiving advice and support at home in early labour were more likely to be satisfied with their care and less likely to end up having epidurals and augmentation of their labours with oxytocin, compared to women who were admitted immediately to hospital. The resources in Box 7.7 can aid discussion about these issues as well as some of the dilemmas that women, their labour supporters and midwives face when strong labour is slow to establish.

Box 7.7   Recommended Resources: Supporting women in early labour

Baxter, J. (2007). Care during the latent phase of labour: supporting normal birth. *British Journal of Midwifery*, *15(12)*, 765–767.

Beake, S., Chang, Y-S., Cheyne, H., Spiby, H., Sandall J. and Bick, D. (2017). Experiences of early labour management from perspectives of women, labour companions and health professionals: a systematic review of qualitative evidence *Midwifery*, *57*, 69–84.

Davies, L. (2011). Supporting women through a prolonged latent phase of labour. *Essentially MIDIRS*, *2(2)*, 38–42.

Eri, T.S., Blystad, A., Gjengedal, E. and Blaaka, G. (2011). 'Stay home for as long as possible': midwives' priorities and strategies in communicating with first-time mothers in early labour. *Midwifery*, e286–e292.

Spiby, H., Walsh, D., Green, J.M., Crompton, A. and Bugg, G. (2014). Midwives' beliefs and concerns about telephone conversations with women in early labour. *Midwifery*, *30*, 1036–1042.

Finding comfort in the home environment

Mary Nolan (2010) describes how she encourages parents to think about the decision of when to go to hospital based on an assessment of their individual physical and emotional comfort, rather than a decision based on cervical dilatation and the pattern of contractions. She suggests helping couples in antenatal groups to think about how they can use their home environment to promote comfort in early labour. This approach could be useful for midwives visiting women at home. You might like to think about how you could help a woman and her supporter to use comfort positions in their home, such as those illustrated in the line drawings in this chapter (Figures 7.1–7.7).

Figure 7.1 Finding comfort positions for labour at home

Conversations to support women in early labour

The way we communicate with women in early labour can have a profound effect on how they face the rest of their labour and remember their experiences. The use of words like 'only' and 'not yet' in phrases like, 'You are only in early labour, you are not yet in active labour' can cause women to think that midwives are more interested in plotting cervical dilatation than understanding the pain they are in and making encouraging suggestions (Borrelli *et al.*, 2018).

Finding the right language to use requires sensitivity in order to acknowledge what individual women are experiencing in a way that also enables them to pace themselves. Natalie Meddings, doula and Active Birth teacher, suggests to parents that they see early labour as: '. . . being in the first room . . . an anteroom – a separate place from labour where the body is readying and contractions are still coordinating'. She encourages parents to settle into this 'baby-having-ideas phase' and wait until they are in 'the second room' where labour is so intense and absorbing that there is no choice but to concentrate: 'So put that contraction app away and wait for when the change becomes obvious' (Meddings, 2017, pp.146–147).

The next activity enables us to explore the conversations we might have in the relatively common situation where a woman and her partner are feeling distressed because labour is slow to establish. When thinking about your discussion with colleagues, bear in mind the World Health Organization's recommendation that a healthy woman arriving at a hospital or birth centre should be admitted and supported appropriately when in early labour, unless her preference is to be at home, and that medical interventions to accelerate labour should be avoided if all appears well with the woman and her baby (WHO, 2018).

Box 7.8   Reflective Activity: Supporting women in early labour

In pairs or small groups:

- After studying the articles in Box 7.7 and reading Section 1.3 of the NICE (2014) guidelines regarding 'Latent first stage of labour', design some scripts for telephone conversations and/or face-to-face conversations you might have with women (and their support people) who are in early labour at home and needing emotional support and practical suggestions. Read or perform your scripts to the larger group before engaging in a facilitated discussion about how to support women at home in early labour.

- Discuss the following scenario:

  Sophie is booked for a home birth with your midwifery group practice. She has been having irregular, painful contractions at home off and on for two days. She is 41 weeks' pregnant. This is her first baby and she is very scared. You have visited her four times at her request and her cervix has not dilated past 1 centimetre. She is now saying that she wants to go to hospital for an epidural. Her husband Tom is not sure that that's a good idea. You call your colleague Jill who is due to take over being on call because you are about to have the weekend off.

- Practise and discuss the sort of conversations you might have with Sophie, Tom, Jill and Harry, the obstetrician on call, in order to provide the most supportive care for Sophie and Tom.

Meeting the woman for the first time when she is in labour

As we have discussed in previous chapters, the advantages of midwifery continuity of care in enabling a trusting relationship and positive experiences of labour are manifold (Dahlberg and Aune, 2013; Hunter *et al.*, 2008; Leap *et al.*, 2010; Sandall *et al.*, 2016). The majority of women, however, do not know the midwife who attends them in labour. Midwives who work in 'shifts' on the labour ward tend to have well developed skills in developing rapport quickly when meeting a woman for the first time when she is in labour; they also play an important role in supporting midwives who are providing continuity of care when they bring women into hospital (Gilkison *et al.*, 2017). In Box 7.9 an experienced midwife explains some of her ways of communicating with a woman when she takes over her care in a hospital setting:

Box 7.9   Meeting the woman for the first time when she is in labour

If I haven't met the woman before, I try to make some connection through talking about the midwife she's been seeing during her pregnancy: 'Oh I see you've had you're antenatal care with Susie. She's such a lovely midwife. And has she talked to you about 'hugs before drugs' because that's what Susie does with everyone? She talks about 'hugs before drugs'. And that makes a connection! I keep things light. I suss out what mood they're in quickly as a couple, and think about how to find a way in.

Straight away I try to connect to the partner as well – or to the woman's mother or whoever else is there. I really have to remember to include them sometimes because I tend to focus on the woman somewhat.

Sometimes the woman is out of it because she's had Diamorphine and some women are in a really bad mood by the time you get to look after them because they're just so fed up with the labour. So in that situation I'd initially connect with her birth supporters and then slowly connect with her.

If a woman comes in and makes it clear she'd like to avoid an epidural, I try to find out what they've thought about doing during this labour. I might tell her supporters how important it is to keep encouraging her, telling her she's doing a good job and that sort of thing.

I do explain that I won't be routinely offering drugs but that she can ask me if this is something she wants at any time. I say that if I do suggest an epidural it's because I think it would be a really good option. I explain to the partner and to students why I don't offer drugs routinely and make it clear that it's about not wanting to undermine her confidence or give her a message that we think she won't cope without them.

When contractions are close together and strong: responding to cues

In Chapter 2, we discussed the difficulties associated with understanding another person's experience of pain in labour. The skill of labour support rests in our ability to observe any given situation, using all of our senses, so that we know when to make suggestions, when to take action and, most importantly, when to withdraw into a corner or remove ourselves:

> This will include the conscious and subconscious 'knowing' that has been generated from our experience and learning. It also involves a 'cluefulness' as we respond to the overt and covert clues from women and their worlds.
>
> (Leap, 2010, p.22)

When women or their birth supporters phone to say that labour has started it is not uncommon for midwives to keep the conversation going until they can hear the sounds the woman makes during a contraction. Similarly, experienced birth workers are often able to predict that labour is established and progressing well by observing all the complex nuances of how an individual woman is behaving in labour. Synthesising these cues through drawing on our knowledge and experiences may be a conscious process; at a subconscious level it may result in what we tend to call 'intuition'. These observational skills are really important to develop if we are to minimise intrusion and disturbance and provide appropriate reassurance to women in labour.

Assessing labour progress

Women's responses to contractions when they are in drug-free labour can provide them and their midwives with a way of gauging how labour is progressing and the sort of support that they might need:

> The way women are behaving, the way they respond to contractions – that doesn't just mean the noise – will give us a good indication of where they are in labour. And later on, the way they behave between contractions, whether they're communicating, whether they've gone completely into themselves and need to focus deeply and intensely on what's happening – we never see that withdrawal at one or two centimetres. . . . If you're relying on un-drugged feedback from women, you get a very good input, don't you, as to what's going on.
>
> (Midwife, Leap, 1996, p.46)

Box 7.10   Reflective Activity: Behavioural clues

Cheyne, H. and Duff, M. (2019). Anatomy and physiology of labour and associated behavioural clues. Chapter 3 in S. Downe and S. Byrom (eds), *Squaring the Circle: Normal Birth Research, Theory and Practice in a Technological Age* (pp.32–46). London: Pinter & Martin.

- In preparation for this activity read the chapter by Helen Cheyne and Margie Duff.
- Individually or in pairs make a list of behavioural cues and map these against the physiological processes that are described in the chapter.
- Make another list of all the supportive strategies that are mentioned in the chapter (plus others that you know of) and discuss how you have seen these used in practice.

Minimising vaginal examinations

When a woman is having a normal labour, a midwife can 'read' behavioural clues and assess labour progress without needing to carry out routine vaginal examinations. Anecdotally, women tend to have negative memories of the midwife or doctor 'doing an internal' or vaginal examination. It is easy to understand why if we stop to think about the discomfort, sensitivities, intrusion and power dynamics associated with this intimate procedure (Bergstrom *et al.*, 1992).

A Cochrane systematic review questioned the effectiveness of routine VEs and identified an urgent need for research to validate other ways of assessing labour progress (Downe *et al.*, 2013). When a vaginal examination is necessary, however, one of the most important things that we can do is to minimise disruption to the way the woman is choosing positions and the support she is receiving from her birth companion/s. This often means learning to perform VEs when the woman is kneeling or on all fours so that she can remain in the position of her choice.

For students this may mean using simulation equipment in order to practise performing VEs when the woman is in positions other than semi-reclining. It may also mean practising the language and communication skills that we can employ to minimise distress when we have to perform a VE.

Figure 7.2 Minimising disruptions to comfort and support during a VE

The physicality of labour and procedures like VEs can stir up powerful feelings for women, particularly with associated links to childhood abuse, previous postnatal depression or post-traumatic stress (Swahnberg *et al.*, 2011). In advocating awareness about this, Jenny Kitzinger (1992) identifies that childbirth can also be 'an opportunity for women to relate to their bodies in new ways and experience them as powerful, competent and creative' (p.220). Some women she interviewed spoke positively of how the care and support they received during labour facilitated this:

> A gentle examination, a listening ear, and a respectful approach can all help women to overcome alienation from their bodies. Sensitivity on the part of staff who understood and validated their distress, provided information, and offered practical support was vital in helping women through such experiences.

> (Kitzinger, 1992, p.220)

The freedom to move around and adopt positions that feel right

Women in labour know instinctively the benefits of moving around and being able to get into positions that feel right. There is strong evidence that we should support them in this in order to promote physiology and positive experiences of labour; women who are able to move around are more likely to have shorter labours and experience less pain and fewer interventions (Lawrence *et al.*, 2013; Priddis *et al.*, 2012). As midwives have, no doubt, always known, moving around and adopting different positions enhances physiology and can be particularly important in helping a baby who is lying in a posterior position to rotate (Fumagalli *et al.*, 2020).

From our experience, we know that feeling free to make rhythmic noises during contractions also helps many women and that some may need 'permission' or encouragement to do this. Rhythmic noise and rhythmic movement tend to combine in the dance of labour that promotes the physiology of birth as women withdraw into an altered state of consciousness.

Being free to respond to 'whatever your body tells you to do' is the basic principle of what is generally referred to as 'Active Birth' (see Chapter 4). Whilst we might want to question the use of a word like 'mobilisation' to describe this (particularly when talking to women), there is strong evidence (Gupta *et al.*, 2017; Lawrence *et al.*, 2013) underpinning the NICE (2014) guidelines that we should: 'encourage and help the woman to move and adopt whatever positions she feels most comfortable with throughout labour' (p.23) and 'encourage women with regional analgesia to move and adopt whatever upright positions they find comfortable throughout labour' (p.37).

Simple measures can create space for women to move around in, and provide storage for personal possessions and equipment. Such changes are possible when maternity care staff join together in making a concerted effort to improve the environment in hospital rooms (Spillane, 2018). Re-designing spaces in this way also means thinking about comfortable resting spaces for women and those supporting them (including midwives):

> I had to learn that it's OK to sit in a comfy chair in the corner of the room when you're supporting a woman in labour and she's roaming around. I used to think it was unprofessional and that those comfy chairs were only for partners.
>
> (Midwife, Leap, 2015, unpublished data)

Box 7.11   Reflective Activity: Positions for labour and birth

Priddis, H., Dahlen, H.G. and Schmied, V. (2012). What are the facilitators, inhibitors, and implications of birth positioning? A review of the literature. *Women and Birth*, 25, 100–106.

Workshop or classroom activity; in pairs or small groups:
- Draw a mind map of all the factors that facilitate and inhibit women's ability to move around and adopt the positions of their choice in labour in the context in which you practise. Share your mind map with the wider group and make a list of recommendations arising from a facilitated discussion.

Equipment to promote freedom of movement in hospital settings

In the previous chapter we discussed the importance of facilitating a supportive environment for birth. In terms of practicalities, every birthing room in hospital settings should provide the basics of equipment to promote freedom of movement for women in labour: for example, mattresses on the floor, resting spaces, plenty of cushions or pillows, bean bags, birthing balls and slings or ropes suspended from the ceiling (RCM, 2018). Demonstrating how to use this equipment, explaining the benefits and displaying a large poster on the wall showing different positions for labour may encourage women and their birth supporters to engage in freedom of movement, particularly those who have not had the opportunity to learn about Active Birth (Jenkinson *et al.*, 2013).

In a study to inform the development of a learning package to promote normal birth (Sandall *et al.*, 2010), midwives described labour ward rooms as clinical and impersonal, communicating that birth is anything but normal. When reflecting on their attempts to make changes in the hospital environment, staff in a large inner-city maternity unit identified the need to change the message for midwives as well as for women. Birth balls and mattresses had been bought for every room, but these were usually left in a cupboard, the room arranged traditionally with the bed in the centre. One midwife in this study had posted a photo in every room to demonstrate how the bed should be moved to one side, with the ball and mattress placed centrally:

> It's a way of saying let's have it ready as part of the room so that when a woman comes in she doesn't just see that bed, she sees this. So she could actually just go and kneel and flop on the bean bag without anyone . . . it's about messages.
>
> (Sandall *et al.*, 2010, p.37)

Figure 7.3 Equipment to promote Active Birth and comfort

Improvising where there are mattresses on the floor

The bare minimum of equipment in a birthing room should be mattresses on the floor and chairs, which lend themselves to improvisation. This usually requires a proactive approach on the part of the midwife. The NICE guideline: 'Encourage the woman to adapt the environment to her individual needs' (NICE, 2014, p.23) is potentially overoptimistic given the level of assertion that the woman might need in order to do this.

> In our culture, when we go to somebody's house, we don't usually rearrange their rooms . . . And on the whole, I think people feel they're not sure what they're allowed to do, they are inhibited, they feel buttoned up, and they don't feel relaxed and able to go with the flow.
> (Childbirth educator/birth supporter, Sandall *et al.*, 2010, p.37)

Figure 7.4 Using a mattress on the floor to promote Active Birth and comfort

When there is no mattress on the floor

When a maternity unit does not provide mattresses on the floor, the creative use of pillows, chairs and 'the loo/toilet' can enable upright positions. Again, women and their partners might need encouragement to do this; in some units this means advance warning to the woman and her supporters to bring in extra pillows, which are often scarce items in hospital birthing areas.

Figure 7.5 Promoting Active Birth and comfort in the absence of a mattress on the floor

Rebozo to promote Active Birth and comfort

A technique that can be used in the presence or absence of equipment to promote Active Birth and comfort is the 'Rebozo' (Iversen *et al.*, 2016). There are some useful video clips on YouTube showing how a Rebozo – or similar-sized sarong, cloth or sheet – can be wrapped around a pregnant woman's body and used to help her relax during labour. By holding the ends of the cloth, a midwife, doula or support person can use a variety of gentle rhythmic techniques called 'sifting' to relax tight ligaments and encourage babies to rotate into an ideal position.

Writing about how she used ripped-up hospital sheets to perform Rebozo techniques in an NHS free-standing birth centre, Jude Davis (2014) encourages midwives and other birth workers to attend Rebozo workshops to add to their skills in supporting pregnant women. She adds a note of caution, though. Whilst it may be empowering to teach women and their birth partners skills that facilitate normal birth, midwives and other birth workers might have to remember to curb their enthusiasm when considering using new techniques in the birthing room:

> We need to remain aware that any intervention is an intervention. We need to keep our default position of guardians of normal birth as predominantly 'sitting on our hands' unless there is a good reason to be using those hands.

> (Davis, 2014, p.6)

Positions for massage

Helping a woman get into positions to enable massage or the application of hot, wet towels can be particularly useful if she is experiencing back pain. Again, partners or other birth supporters may need encouragement in doing this:

> I've noticed a lot of partners do that fluffy back massage that can really annoy women so if the woman's OK with it, I show them how to do it stronger. And I encourage the women to tell them if it's too strong or too light.

> (Midwife, Leap, 2015, unpublished data)

This type of physical support can be hard work and very tiring for the supporters. Often the midwife or doula needs to suggest that they take it in turns and have rests in between. Where a woman is wanting firm back pressure, we recommend trying the 'tennis balls in a sock' idea – she can lean back against a firm surface with the two tennis balls held in the sock, positioned on her lower back, usually either side of her spine.

Figure 7.6 Positions for comfort and massage

Promoting privacy: 'cocooning'

Figure 7.7 Cocooning

Women who are free to move around in labour often choose to bury their head in a pillow or their partner's lap. This instinctive behaviour is about shutting out the outside world and concentrating on the intense physicality of labour, as well as assisting the all-important rests between contractions. Cocooning also facilitates the woman having private space to labour undisturbed:

> It's a way of giving women private space and it's a good way of avoiding unwelcome visitors and people from talking to her. Because you won't talk to someone you can't see. In hot places you can just use a sarong but something with a bit of weight works well. Sometimes it works really well if someone's feeling a bit stuck. Cocooning helps her just get back into that head space of being in the moment. You're not distracted by anyone – you're just in that little private world of your own.
>
> (Doula, Leap, 2015, unpublished data)

Box 7.12   Reflective Activity: Facilitating Active Birth and privacy

In pairs or threes:

- In turn, practise getting into the positions that are illustrated in the line drawings (Figures 7.1–7.7). Discuss how you might suggest these positions to a labouring woman and her partner/birth supporters during labour in the context in which you practise.
- Write some scripts and practise saying the words out loud, adjusting the scripts until you are confident about the messages they give to a woman and her supporter/s.

Immersion in water for comfort in labour

Immersion in water for comfort in labour and birth has become an accepted choice in Western countries, and is recommended for all women deemed to be 'low risk' by NICE guidelines (NICE, 2014). The subject continues to attract considerable attention and research (Burns *et al.*, 2012; Clews *et al.*, 2020; Cluett *et al.*, 2018; Dahlen *et al.*, 2013; Feeley *et al.*, 2021; Menakaya *et al.*, 2013).

Box 7.13   Reflective Activity: Water to promote comfort in labour and birth

Burns, E., Boulton, M.G., Cluett, E.R., Cornelius, V.R. and Smith, L.A. (2012). Characteristics, interventions, and outcomes of women who used a birthing pool: a prospective observational study. *Birth*, *39(3)*, 192–201.

Clews, C., Church, S. and Ekberg, M. (2020). Women and waterbirth: a systematic metasynthesis of qualitative studies. *Women and Birth*, *33*, 566–573.

Feeley, C., Cooper, M. and Burns, E. (2021). A systematic meta-thematic synthesis to examine the views and experiences of women following water immersion during labour and waterbirth. *Journal of Advanced Nursing*. doi:10.1111/jan.14720.

Milosevic, S., Channon, S., Hunter, B., Nolan, M., Hughes, A., Barlow, C., . . . Sanders, J. (2019). Factors influencing the use of birth pools in the United Kingdom: perspectives of women, midwives and medical staff. *Midwifery*, *79*, 102554.

Milosevic, S., Channon, S., Hughes, J., Hunter, B., Nolan, M., Milton, R. and Sanders, J. (2020). Factors influencing water immersion during labour: qualitative case studies of six maternity units in the United Kingdom. *BMC Pregnancy and Childbirth*, *20*, 719.

Classroom activity; in pairs:

- After studying these papers, access videos and accounts from women about their experiences of using water in labour and birth. Choose one of these resources to present to the wider group (maximum five minutes). Then lead a discussion about how this resource relates to the research evidence about the use of water in labour and the factors that may facilitate or impede its use.

Positions when babies are born into water

If women are to be free to get into whatever position feels right for them to give birth, the birth pool needs to be deep enough for the woman to get into an all fours position if this is what she chooses. You will notice many birth videos where women are semi-reclining to give birth in water. In some cases this may be because the pool is not deep enough for the baby to emerge into water if the woman is on all fours; sometimes it is because midwives are not confident about all fours birth in water or how to pass the baby under water through the mother's legs so that she can bring her baby up out of the water herself.

Managing or struggling: identifying appropriate support

If we accept the highly individual and complex nature of women's responses to pain in labour, we have to question the use of the numeric pain scoring techniques that are often used in maternity units, particularly in the USA (Roberts *et al.*, 2010). Quite apart from the intrusion of such mechanisms and the potential for them to disturb a woman's rhythm and confidence, the reductionist nature of evaluating the intensity of contractions is unlikely to identify or address the intricate emotional, social and cultural aspects of what each woman is experiencing (Lowe, 2002).

Box 7.14   Research Briefing: The Coping with Labor Algorithm ©

Roberts, L., Gulliver, B., Fisher, J. and Cloyes, K.G. (2010). The Coping with Labor Algorithm: an alternate pain assessment tool for the laboring woman. *Journal of Midwifery & Women's Health*, 55(2), 107–116.

An alternative to the practice of asking women in labour to score their pain – on a scale with 0 being no pain and 10 being the worst possible pain – was developed by Dr Leissa Roberts and colleagues at the University of Utah College of Nursing and clinicians in the maternity unit at the University Hospital. Women in labour were expressing confusion and annoyance at the intrusion of regular requests to 'rate' their pain, particularly those who had identified that they wanted to give birth without pharmacological 'pain relief' and those who wanted to use self-hypnosis. A Coping with Labor Algorithm © was developed, which avoided the use of the word 'pain'. Starting with the simple question, 'How are you coping with your labour?', the algorithm identifies cues that clinicians might observe if the woman is either coping or struggling with her labour and potential practical and emotional supportive activities to consider (see Figure 7.8). The paper provides a summary of the evidence for these supportive activities and outlines the process of developing and evaluating the algorithm.

Dr Leissa Roberts kindly gave us permission to reproduce the Coping with Labor Algorithm © in this chapter. Leaving aside any differences in the use of language and context, we invite you to consider the value of a resource like this for promoting a consistent approach to supporting women in labour in hospital settings.

Figure 7.8 Coping with Labor Algorithm, Version 2 ©

Source: Reproduced with permission of Dr Leissa Roberts, University of Utah College of Nursing

Box 7.15   Reflective Activity: 'Cluefulness' and the Coping with Labor Algorithm ©

Classroom or workshop activity; instructions for facilitators:
- In preparation, using the cues in the algorithm, devise 'cue cards'. You will need as many cards as there are participants; on each card list a couple of either 'coping' or 'not coping' cues, for example:

Coping:
- moans or vocalises, relaxes between contractions;
- focuses inwards, rhythmic breathing;
- sways or rocks rhythmically during contractions, rests in between.

Not coping:
- worrying about how she'll cope with the next contraction;
- panicky, thrashing about on the bed;
- clawing and biting;
- crying and/or tense.

   Ask the group/class to study the paper by Roberts *et al.* (2010) before engaging in the activity, paying attention to the latest version of the algorithm*: the cues, and suggested care measures and changes to the environment that can help women who want to avoid pharmacological intervention. Allow an hour for the activity.

Setting up the activity (5 minutes)
- Divide the participants into *threes* and explain the activity, according to the following instructions:

Stage 1 (10 minutes)
- Decide who will be a labouring woman and who will be her two birth companions: midwife, doula, partner or family member – you can decide. (You will all get a chance to be the labouring woman.)
- Labouring woman: take a card from the pile of 'cue cards'. Without disclosing to the others what is written on the card, show these behaviours while simulating two contractions, 1 minute apart.
- Birth companions: observe closely and, after the second contraction, ask the woman: 'How are you coping with your labour?' Before the next contraction, suggest an action to the woman – this might be reinforcing her abilities to carry on as she is doing or it might be a suggestion for managing the next contraction and the rest in between.**

Stage 2 (5 minutes)
- Discuss the activity in your threes, starting with what it was like being the labouring women, then moving on to the cues noticed by the birth supporters and the measures they suggested: how it felt, what was useful.

Stage 3 (30 minutes)
- Change roles and repeat the activity (Stage 1 and Stage 2: 10 minutes each being the labouring woman, followed by 5 minutes' discussion).

Stage 4 De-briefing the activity (10 minutes)
- Finish by discussing with the whole group how they experienced the activity. Without naming names, highlight helpful behaviours and what was learnt.

Notes: * Version 2 of the Algorithm is updated from that in the article and has an evidence legend. We have reproduced Version 2 above.
** You could have cue cards available identifying support measures when an intervention is needed or leave it to the birth companions to decide a course of action.

Supporting women when they are in 'the zone'

When labour is progressing well, women tend to withdraw into an altered state of consciousness that we often call 'the zone': a state of deep inward mind–body concentration precipitated by the intricate interaction of the hormones of labour (Buckley, 2008, 2015):

> There's a kind of inward progression. Between contractions she never comes out of that internal space, she stays in there. There's an inability to communicate. And either that inwardness becomes quite contained so that the body really becomes quite still and she doesn't move much, or there's the other extreme where it's like the demons have been released. They're actually quite easily differentiated states. What it's about is the intensity of the contractions and the sounds become more and more spontaneous. It has an authenticity, which is some sort of signal.
>
> (Midwife, Leap, 1996, p.46)

When they are in this state of consciousness, women are highly suggestible (personal communication with Allan Cyna, 2014) and therefore respond well to quiet encouragement to stay in the moment. Women who have practised mindfulness and other mind–body techniques may well be at an advantage in responding to such familiar cues (Byrne *et al.*, 2014; Whitburn *et al.*, 2014):

> The key is that sort of letting go, withdrawal thing. You see it and immediately you think, 'Ah good . . .'.
>
> (Midwife, Leap, 1996, p.45)

The study we have profiled in Box 7.16 reminds us of the importance of practices that we have discussed in previous chapters: 'non-disturbance' of labour, holding the space, trusting women to find their way, and the quiet 'midwifery muttering' of reassurance and encouragement.

Box 7.16   Research Briefing: Supporting women to withdraw into 'their own world' during labour

Reed, R., Barnes, M. and Rowe, J. (2015). Women's experience of birth: childbirth as a rite of passage. *International Journal of Childbirth*, *5*, 46–56.

This study provides a powerful exploration of the deep significance of women withdrawing from the external world in labour. Women describe a progressive state of focusing inward as they enter 'their own world' and an altered state of consciousness in which they were seeking to minimise external and internal distractions. After giving birth, women emerged slowly from their own world, reintegrating with the outside world with new knowledge about themselves that they described as transformative and empowering.

Supporting women in 'transition'

Rhea Dempsey (2013) suggests that, at any time in labour, we need to be able to support women through a 'crisis of confidence: when self-belief crumbles' (p.127). In a normal labour, this is most likely to happen during the phase of labour that we call 'transition'. The sort of things that women say in transition are usually quite predictable, for example, 'I can't do this anymore'. Women at home often say, 'I want to go to hospital' and women in hospital, 'I want to go home'. We can both remember women who insisted on getting fully dressed in their outdoor clothes and who left the labour ward before turning round when the urgency of transition gave way to the more manageable urgency of expulsive contractions.

When a woman hits a crisis of confidence and despair in labour, it can be helpful for her midwife, doula or support person to engage in what Penny Simkin (2002, p.728) refers to as 'The Take Charge Routine': making eye contact, providing intense support with every breath and helping her get back into some sort of rhythmic activity or ritual during contractions.

When women say, 'I can't do this': some supportive approaches

Sometimes when a woman is repeatedly saying, 'I can't do this', it can help if we suggest that she says, 'I *can* do this' instead. By repeating, 'I can do this', she often starts to believe she can do it. Other women will find it helpful to visualise their cervix opening and rhythmically chant, 'Open, open, open'. Suggestions like this for trying things out can be invaluable during transition:

> I do distracting, 'Why don't we try this. . . . Before we do that it would be good to do a wee, let's walk to the loo . . . then we should do this . . . and then this.' I put a few hurdles in that mean she gets further than she thinks she will. Often it's just enough to get them through that difficult spot, what we call transition: when they don't believe in themselves any more.
>
> (Midwife, Leap, 2015, unpublished data)

Transition can be a time when a woman responds well to a strong message that her midwife and birth supporters believe in her capabilities, as this woman in Box 7.17 explains.

Box 7.17   Reflective Activity: 'She believed in me when I didn't believe in myself'

In pairs:

Using the following quote as a guide, take turns acting being the woman and her midwife in an exchange. Discuss how it felt being both the woman and the midwife when the midwife's response was, 'You can do this' and when it was, 'We can get you an epidural'. How might it feel for both the woman and the midwife if they had not met before?

> I turned to my primary midwife – I'd been thinking about this for about four hours and I was like, 'Do you know, I'm thinking, I think I need to have a Caesarean.' She said my name and she just said, 'You're not having a Caesarean.' And it was just what I needed, she just cut it off, just nipped it off in the bud . . . she did it in a very loving way: she had a twinkle in her eye but she was very firm. . . . And it was the best thing . . . because honestly . . . I was just afraid and I was just not feeling very confident in my ability to do it.
>
> She just said clearly, 'No. That's not happening.' And I actually went, 'All right then', [laughter] and then just carried on with my contractions. I thought, 'Well that means I can do it. What she's saying to me, in saying you're not having that, is 'You can do it.' Whereas if someone had said, 'You need to have an epidural', the message would have been very clear: 'You're not coping, you can't do it, you need to have this. . . . I felt that she really believed in me when I didn't believe in myself and that was wonderful.
>
> (Sandall *et al.*, 2010, unpublished data)

Reassuring partners during transition

Women can be very volatile during transition and sometimes their partners need reassurance when women's retorts are snappy or hostile. For example, as women withdraw into their own intense, body-besieged world, the baby tends to become a blurred reality; well-meaning comments that each contraction is 'one step nearer to having the baby in your arms' can be met with furious responses, such as, 'I don't want *a baby*, I want it to *stop, now* . . . I'm never doing this again' and various expletives around the theme of 'If men had to go through this . . .'.

Box 7.18   Reflective Activity: 'You can do it' – supporting women in transition

In preparation for this activity, ask the participants to read the accounts by the women and midwives in the section above ('Supporting women in 'transition') as well as the online resource by Penny Simkin:

> Comfort in labour: how you can help yourself to a normal, satisfying childbirth. www.childbirthconnection.org/pdfs/comfort-in-labor-simkin.pdf.

• Prepare a pack of six cards for each group identifying the characters in the scenario that they will develop – you will need enough packs for everyone in each group to have one of the six character cards.

Setting up the activity (5 minutes)

- Divide participants into groups of six.
- Each participant picks a card identifying the character they will play (same six characters for each group).
- Each group prepares a **5-minute** 'skit'/scenario to perform for the whole group.
- The skit has to start with Maria saying: 'I know I said I didn't want an epidural but now I really do'. Thereafter it is up to each group to develop the scenario and the characters in whatever way they wish.
- They will only have **15 minutes** to work out and practise how they are going to present the scenario – reassure them that you will time-keep and let them know when they have 5 minutes and 2 minutes left during this preparation time.
- Warn them that you will cut them off after **5 minutes** of their performance, regardless of what is happening in the scenario.
- Scenario presentations (5 minutes × the number of groups).
- Finish with a 15–20-minute group discussion about the issues that the activity raises in terms of practice.

Characters for 'You can do it' activity

Note: You can add characters: e.g. a doula, obstetrician, other family members.

Maria (28 years old) is having her first baby and is 41 weeks' pregnant. Her Birth Plan states that she wants to avoid 'unnecessary intervention' including Pethidine and an epidural. After 12 hours of labouring at home, she came into hospital two hours ago. Her cervix was then 6 cm dilated and her baby's head is well down in her pelvis. She has been coping well, tried Entonox but didn't like it and is now having very strong contractions every two minutes lasting a minute.

Leon is Maria's husband. His first wife had a baby at another hospital five years ago. She had an epidural and ventouse birth and the experience was very distressing for all concerned. He thinks Maria is unprepared for the reality of labour pain and doesn't want her to suffer. He sees his role as advocating for her to make sure she gets an epidural if she needs one.

Teresa is Maria's Mum. She had three babies in the 1970s; all were induced for 'post-maturity'. She had Pethidine for all three labours and chose an epidural when having her last baby. She admires and respects her daughter's wishes but is struggling with seeing her in pain.

Alex is Maria's friend. She had her first baby a year ago in the same hospital. She had a long labour and gave birth in a pool. She felt very proud of herself and is very supportive of Maria, her labour supporters and the midwives.

Grace is an experienced midwife who has been working at this hospital for three years. She is very supportive of women who want to labour without pharmacological pain relief.

Celia is a third-year student midwife who is passionate about promoting normal birth. She is very clear about the evidence for continuous support in labour.

Reassurance in the 'rest and be thankful stage'

Like transition, the 'rest and be thankful' phase of labour – the lull that sometimes occurs before second stage while the baby's head rotates (Long, 2006) – can also bring surprises. Some women switch from frenetic behaviour to a sudden calming, or sleepiness, that can be disconcerting for everyone in the room. Reassurance is required here, explaining to the woman and her supporters that this lull is normal and can be useful. Nicky remembers a somewhat bizarre example of this during a woman's first labour at home:

> She changed from roaring like a demon in a cave to modestly asking us to bring her a mango. During the silence of the next ten minutes she calmly peeled and ate the mango and then said, 'Right I'm ready to push now.'

When women give birth at home, they will often decide at the last moment where the 'best place' is for them to go when they are ready to give birth, a habit we see in animals. Home birth midwives therefore often have their essential birth equipment ready on a tray so that they can follow the woman to wherever she decides to give birth, rather than setting up a birthing area.

Supporting women when contractions are expulsive

Women tend to talk about 'When I was pushing the baby out', rather than 'second stage'. Whilst some women will breathe through contractions while their baby descends, for many women, particularly if it is their first baby, the overwhelming nature of expulsive contractions can be quite shocking. Gentle reassurance to 'go with it' can help:

> When I gave birth the first time, those pushing contractions were such a shock – the strangest bodily sensation, nothing I could do to control it using my will – a complete takeover of my body pushing this baby out, and quite scary when you're not ready for it. So overpowering, nothing you can do to resist it, you have to join in and that's all you can think about. I can imagine that if anyone had told me to do anything else it would have felt very strange.
>
> (Mother, Leap, 2015, unpublished data)

The ways in which midwives facilitate women to give birth during physiological second stage were identified in a systematic review that included 17 studies (Healy *et al.*, 2020). The main conclusions were that women should be supported to adopt positions they choose and to respond to expulsive contractions spontaneously in whatever way feels right for them.

In our experience, when women are given a free rein to get into any position they like in second stage, the majority will respond to the sensations they are feeling by kneeling forward over furniture or dropping onto hands and knees. Occasionally, a supported squat, birth stool or upright kneeling position can be useful when the woman needs help in what is often referred to as 'bringing the baby down'. We have also seen women stand and lunge during contractions with one leg on a chair where their baby's head is descending in a tilted (asynclitic) fashion. It seems that women instinctively choose positions or movements that enable them to ease or wriggle their baby through the largest possible diameter they can make with their pelvis.

Figure 7.9 Supporting women to 'bring the baby down'

Questioning the traditional rituals of second stage

There are a series of traditional rituals associated with second stage that may or may not be useful or appropriate for individual women. We list these here with some examples to promote discussion:

Avoiding 'cheerleading'

In spite of all the evidence that reminds us *not* to tell women to take a deep breath, hold it and push as hard as they can, it seems that, in many maternity units, cheerleading in second stage persists, often with instructions that can feel very counter-productive:

> The midwife kept telling me to push into my bottom as if I was doing a poo. It frightened me – the whole idea of doing a poo in public – and I think I tightened up because of it.
>
> (Mother, Leap, 2015, unpublished data)

Occasionally, directed pushing is a useful intervention, but there are good reasons to encourage women to follow their urges and to respond spontaneously when contractions are expulsive (Healy *et al.*, 2020; Osborne and Hanson, 2012):

> Sometimes the partners start doing that cheer leading, 'Push Push Push' because they've seen it on 'One Born Every Minute' and I gently try to suggest we encourage her to bring the baby down in the way her body is telling her. Sometimes it's appropriate though. There have been times when I've transferred in when a woman isn't progressing in second stage and after a bumpy ride the midwives in the hospital do all that loud, almost bullying, cheer leading and the baby comes out and I think, 'Hmmm . . . I should have done that in the first place'.
>
> (Community midwife, Leap, 2015, unpublished data)

Preventing perineal trauma

The systematic review of midwives' practice during second stage that we highlighted earlier (Healy *et al.*, 2020) found insufficient evidence to make recommendations around the prevention of perineal tears through 'hands on' or 'hands off' techniques but identified strong evidence to promote the use of warm perineal compresses (Aasheim *et al.*, 2017; Magoga *et al.*, 2019). This low-cost practice has been shown to be highly acceptable to both women and midwives and we need to question why it is rarely implemented in maternity care settings and consider challenging this on the basis of evidence informed practice (Dahlen *et al.*, 2007; Dahlen *et al.*, 2009; Dahlen, 2012).

Whether or not warm perineal compresses are being used, no one would dispute the age-old midwifery skill of encouraging the woman to breath slowly as her baby's head is crowning in order to slow down birth and prevent serious tears. We can explain the value of this to women during conversations in pregnancy and invite them to practise sighing their baby out: 'If your mouth is loose and open, your vagina is loose and open'. In relation to this concept we do have to question what happens to our pelvic floors if we are told to 'pant like a little dog' (try it!). A midwife describes the words she uses to encourage a woman to breathe her baby out slowly:

> As the head is coming I'm very directive and say, 'Breathe slowly now, breathe, breathe . . .'. Other midwives tell women to 'Pant', or 'Blow' – one I know tells women to sigh the baby out and shows them how to do that, saying, 'Haarr'. . . . Whatever you're saying needs to help them breathe the baby's head out 'gently' and 'slowly'. It makes such a difference to the care of the woman's perineum. And with the 'hands off the perineum' approach, it's so important that you use your voice to help the woman give birth slowly. Sometimes people forget this when the woman is in the pool and the midwife feels one step removed. 'Hands off' doesn't mean 'voice off'. It doesn't mean do nothing.
>
> (Midwife, Leap, 2015, unpublished data)

This midwife's description of how important it is to slow down the birth of the baby's head and body is, perhaps, more pertinent than ever. As we go to press, debates continue to rage about how to prevent serious perineal trauma. The articles in Box 7.19 highlight some of those debates and the contested ways in which evidence is being translated into practice. You may be interested in looking for follow-on commentaries and discussions about the OASI Care Bundle; meanwhile we recommend these articles as a resource to promote discussion about measures to prevent severe perineal trauma.

Box 7.19   Recommended Resources: Preventing serious perineal injury – contested evidence and practice

Allen, J., Small, K. and Lee, N. (2021). How a perineal care bundle impacts midwifery practice in Australian maternity hospitals: a critical, reflexive thematic analysis. *Women and Birth.* https://doi.org/10.1016/j.wombi.2021.01.012.

Moncrieff, G. and Dahlen, H. (2020). The UK OASI Care Bundle: the results are out but so is the jury. https://www.all4maternity.com/the-uk-oasi-care-bundle-the-results-are-out-but-so-is-the-jury/.

Thornton, J.G. and Dahlen, H.G. (2020). The UK Obstetric Anal Sphincter Injury (OASI) Bundle: a critical review. *Midwifery*, *90*, 102801.

Thakar, R., Gurol-Urganci, I., Bidwiell, P., Sevdalis, N., Silverton, L., Freeman, L. and van der Muelen, J. (2020). Obstetric Anal Sphincter Injury (OASI) Care Bundle: response to a critical review. *Midwifery*, *90*, 102802.

Webb, S. (2020). The OASI Care Bundle – a lively topic for discussion. *MIDIRS Midwifery Digest*, *30*(*4*), 414–417.

Questioning: 'Touch your baby's head'

It has become quite common for midwives to encourage the woman to touch her baby's head as it starts to emerge. However, doing this may not be appropriate for all women and runs the risk of taking women out of the 'zone', as this midwife cautions:

> I've seen people adopt little rituals like saying to the woman, 'Put your fingers inside and feel your baby's head coming down' and they start thinking that all women want to do that. In my experience very few women really want to touch the baby's head – some do it to please the midwife. Occasionally it's exactly the encouragement they need but more often it's taking them away from their inner intensity. It can sort of un-nerve them. Touching the baby's head can completely skew her – she's there to bring the baby down and it's a huge thing. . . . Maybe it's different when women have epidurals. They're not feeling anything so maybe feeling the baby's head is an important connection for them sometimes.
>
> (Midwife, Leap, 2015, unpublished data)

Supporting 'the first embrace'

The World Health Organization's 'First Embrace' initiative identifies the importance of the period immediately after the baby is born and the significant benefits for mothers and babies of immediate, uninterrupted skin-to-skin contact, delayed cord clamping and early breastfeeding:

> The First Embrace refers to immediate skin-to-skin contact shortly after the baby is born. This simple act of love transfers life saving warmth, placental blood and protective bacteria from the mother to the newborn. It also has the added benefit of promoting a natural bond between mother and child that improves the condition of all babies including those who are premature, sick or born by caesarean section.
>
> (WHO Regional Office for the Western Pacific, 2014, p.3)

For most women, greeting their baby is a moment so extraordinary and precious that it cannot and should not be disturbed or hurried. If we believe that the act of giving birth is powerful and belongs to the woman, then, arguably, we might also see the act of picking the baby up following birth as belonging to the woman. Unless the baby is born into water (in which case the woman may need help to reach down and scoop her baby up), we can step back and wait and watch in awe.

Figure 7.10 Greeting the baby

This act of the new mother picking up her baby and taking it to her body for the first embrace can have profound significance for women. At birth, 'seeing is believing'. The first contact with the baby often resonates with shock and stunned amazement. Suddenly the waves of physical intensity are gone; the contrast is extraordinary as the realisation of the baby penetrates the woman's consciousness. It often takes a while for her to come out of the intensity of her labour ('own world') and back into the 'external world' (Reed *et al.*, 2015). She looks at her baby and remembers what it is all about. Sometimes this moment is tinged with echoes of recognition, a feeling of a timeless continuum, characterised by words such as 'I looked at you and it was as if we knew each other'.

We have all seen situations where women in a recumbent position initially recoil when the attendant scoops the baby up and ceremoniously places her/him on their chest (often announcing the baby's gender with a triumphant flourish):

> Often women shrink back because they're not ready. It's like they're in their body and not yet ready to come out of their body and into the baby. You know how sometimes it takes women a while to do that after the baby is born. You see it in birth films: they look around at everyone before concentrating on the baby.
>
> (Midwife, Leap, 2015, unpublished data)

Where the midwife gently dries the baby and lays her/him on a warm surface in front of the woman, it may take several minutes of tentative stroking and exclaiming before the mother is ready to gather up her baby to her body. Once in her arms, the new mother can find out whether her baby is a boy or girl when she is ready. She begins the primeval process of curiosity, searching her baby's body, counting fingers and toes, pointing out familial similarities, checking for uniqueness and difference. For some women it is 'love at first sight'; others need reassurance that many women find their love unfolds gently over the first hours or days.

In the postscript to this chapter Nicky tells a story that illustrates the potential significance of the woman picking up her baby. In some cultures, however, there are taboos around women touching the baby until it has been bathed and wrapped. Ideally, this needs to be explored with the woman during pregnancy. It might mean wrapping the baby in warm towels before she picks up her baby and begins the process of skin-to-skin contact. As we discussed in Chapter 6, though, we should be wary of assumptions that 'cultural traditions' lead to inevitable choices around birth.

Reassuring supporters about the new baby's appearance

It can sometimes be important to reassure the woman's supporters about the range of normal in babies' appearances at birth, in particular, head moulding and colour. We have heard of fathers saying they fretted in silence, thinking that there was something very wrong with the baby. The midwife's reassurance made a big difference for this new father:

> He was beautiful in his own way when he first came out. My partner grabbed him, she was in tears, we were both in tears, big gushes of love, big hugs, and she said, 'Isn't he beautiful, isn't he beautiful?' And I . . . he had his head like a Smurf's hat and he had a huge hand, and he was this sort of greyish pale blue, and he had blood coming out of his nose and he had one eye open, and I said, 'Well, he's gonna be, he's not the most beautiful thing at the moment but he's going to be.' But, you know, I loved him dearly as soon as I saw him. That was incredible.
>
> (Father, Sandall *et al.*, 2010, unpublished data)

Support for women who choose physiological third stage

Women have described to us the important role that the midwife played in supporting their choice to have a physiological third stage when labour is straightforward. This sometimes extends to guidance and encouragement when expelling their placenta:

> So my midwife asked me to push, she said, 'Just push the way you have been pushing to have the baby.' I said, 'I don't want to push again.' She said, 'This one is not a painful one, your placenta is soft and squishy, it will slide out.' And really it was not a painful one, I just pushed and the placenta just came out. It was lovely.
>
> (Midwife, Leap, 2015, unpublished data)

Support in the early hours after birth

In the critical hours following birth, support of the woman and her family continues. Variations of support measures that we have discussed previously – watchful anticipation, reassurance, responding to cues, suggesting comfort measures, respecting privacy – can make a huge difference for the woman and her family as they embark on life with their new baby:

> The long-term effects of the environment in that first hour of birth are so important. It must have an effect on the baby, on its wiring, and the long-term effects of how it grows and develops and its relationships with its parents.
>
> (Midwife, Leap, 2015, unpublished data)

We finish this chapter with an activity that leads us into the next chapter, where we explore how we can best support women who are having complicated labours and births.

Box 7.20   Reflective Activity: Supporting women for 'the first embrace'

In *The Art and Soul of Midwifery: Creativity in Practice* (Davies, 2007), various authors explore how music, art, craft, dance, drama, poetry and other forms of creative expression may be used to enhance learning and practice.

Individual, pair or small group activity:
- Choose a creative art medium to explore 'the first embrace' from different perspectives and experiences. We encourage you to choose circumstances where support promotes the best possible circumstances for a positive experience, including perhaps for a woman who has an instrumental or caesarean birth or where her baby needs resuscitation.
- Present your work to colleagues and facilitate a discussion on the potential learning from this activity.

Postscript: to have and to hold

The woman in this story had made it clear throughout pregnancy that she was somewhat ambivalent about the whole business of growing a baby and becoming a mother.

'To have and to hold'

> After a roaring, intense labour, she gives birth at home in front of a gas fire in a small London flat. We dry the baby and place her on a small, towel-covered electric heat pad (no need to wrap the baby in these warm circumstances). The baby girl wriggles and squints, unfolds slowly before her mother, is alert and peaceful. 'Take it away, take it away', her mother yells, head rolling, eyes everywhere but on her baby.
>
> We had told her during her pregnancy that we would wait for her to pick up her baby when she was ready, that the act of giving birth includes picking up the baby. We sit tight, deal with our discomfort and hope that we've got it right. Minutes pass, the cord is no longer pumping. She is sitting on a soft plastic bedpan; we can see that she is not bleeding.
>
> She writhes a torrent of exclamations and shudders, still reeling from the intensity of it all. It takes a full ten minutes before she calms down, leans forward, starts to touch – slowly, tentatively, with caution; she looks at her baby, begins talking to her, 'Poor little one, are you all right, are you a girl or a boy, oh my goodness, you're so beautiful!' She lifts her baby to her, all that passionate intensity redirected to the tiny girl who blinks back at her mother's all-consuming gaze. She suckles; the placenta plops into the bedpan; we midwives heave a sigh of relief.
>
> Afterwards she tells us that it was really important that we did not pick the baby up, that she needed time to come to terms with this tiny dependent creature, that picking her up was an act of profound acceptance and love.
>
> To have and to hold . . .

(Nicky Leap, personal reflection)

References

Aasheim, V., Nilsen, A.B.V., Lukasse, M. and Reinar, L.M. (2017). Perineal techniques during the second stage of labour for reducing perineal trauma. *Cochrane Database of Systematic Reviews.* doi:10.1002/14651858.CD14006672.pub3.

Abalos, E., Oladapo, O.T., Chamillard, M., Díaz, V., Pasquale, J., Bonet, M., . . . Gülmezoglu, A.M. (2018). Duration of spontaneous labour in 'low-risk' women with 'normal' perinatal outcomes: a systematic review. *European Journal of Obstetrics & Gynecology and Reproductive Biology, 223,* 123–132

Albers, L. (1999). The duration of labour in healthy women. *Journal of Perinatology, 19,* 114–119.

Allen, J., Small, K. and Lee, N. (2021). How a perineal care bundle impacts midwifery practice in Australian maternity hospitals: a critical, reflexive thematic analysis. *Women and Birth.* https://doi.org/10.1016/j.wombi.2021.1001.1012.

Baxter, J. (2007). Care during the latent phase of labour: supporting normal birth. *British Journal of Midwifery, 15*(12), 765–767.

Beake, S., Chang, Y-S., Cheyne, H., Spiby, H., Sandall J. and Bick, D. (2017). Experiences of early labour management from perspectives of women, labour companions and health professionals: a systematic review of qualitative evidence *Midwifery, 57,* 69–84.

Bergstrom, L., Roberts, J., Skillman, L. and Seidel, J. (1992). 'You'll feel me touching you, sweetie': vaginal examinations during the second stage of labor. *Birth, 19*(1), 10–18.

Borrelli, S.E., Walsh, D. and Spiby, H. (2018). 'You are only in early labour, you are not in active labour yet'. Midwives' language and behaviour and the meaning women make of it. *The Practising Midwife, 21(7)*, 25–29.

Buckley, S.J. (2008). *Gentle Birth, Gentle Mothering: A Doctor's Guide to Natural Childbirth and Early Parenting Choices*. New York: Crown Publishing Group.

Buckley, S.J. (2015). *Hormonal Physiology of Childbearing: Evidence and Implications for Women, Babies, and Maternity Care*. Retrieved from Washington, D.C: www.ChildbirthConnection.org/HormonalPhysiology.

Burns, E., Boulton, M.G, Cluett, E.R., Cornelius, V.R. and Smith, L.A. (2012). Characteristics, interventions, and outcomes of women who used a birthing pool: a prospective observational study. *Birth, 39(3)*, 192–201.

Byrne, J., Hauck, Y., Fisher, C., Bayes, S. and Schutze, R. (2014). Effectiveness of a mindfulness-based childbirth education pilot study on maternal self-efficacy and fear of childbirth. *Journal of Midwifery and Women's Health, 59*, 192–197.

Cheyne, H. and Duff, M. (2019). Anatomy and physiology of labour and associated behavioural clues. Chapter 3 in S. Downe and S. Byrom (eds), *Squaring the Circle: Normal Birth Research, Theory and Practice in a Technological Age* (pp.32–46). London: Pinter & Martin.

Clews, C., Church, S. and Ekberg, M. (2020). Women and waterbirth: a systematic metasynthesis of qualitative studies. *Women and Birth, 33*, 566–573.

Cluett, E.R., Burns, E. and Cuthburt, A. (2018). Immersion in water during labour and birth. *Cochrane Database of Systematic Reviews*, Issue 5. Art. No.: CD000111. doi:000110.001002/14651858. CD14000111.pub4.

Dahlberg, U. and Aune, I. (2013). The woman's birth experience – the effect of interpersonal relationships and continuity of care. *Midwifery, 29*, 507–415.

Dahlen, H.G. (2012). Perineal warm compress reduces risk of third- and fourth- degree tears and should be part of second stage care. *Evidence Based Nursing, 15(4)*.

Dahlen, H.G., Dowling, H., Tracy, M., Schmied, V. and Tracy, S. (2013). Maternal and perinatal outcomes amongst low risk women giving birth in water compared to six birth positions on land. A descriptive cross sectional study in a birth centre over 12 years. *Midwifery, 29*, 759–764.

Dahlen, H., Homer, C.S.E., Cooke, M., Upton, A., Nunn, R.A. and Brodrick, B.S. (2007). Perineal outcomes and maternal comfort related to the application of perineal warm packs in the second stage of labor. A randomized control. *Birth, 34(4)*, 282–290.

Dahlen, H.G., Homer, C.S.E., Cooke, M., Upton, A., Nunn, R.A. and Brodrick, B.S. (2009). 'Soothing the ring of fire'. Australian women and midwives experience of using perineal warm packs in the second stage of labour. *Midwifery, 25*, 39–48.

Davey, M-A., McLachlan, H.L., Forster, D. and Flood, M. (2013). Influence of timing of admission in labour and management of labour on method of birth: results from a randomised controlled trial of caseload midwifery (COSMOS trial). *Midwifery, 29*, 1297–1302.

Davies, L. (ed.). (2007). *The Art and Soul of Midwifery: Creativity in Practice, Education and Research*. Edinburgh: Churchill Livingstone/Elsevier.

Davies, L. (2011). Supporting women through a prolonged latent phase of labour. *Essentially MIDIRS, 2(2)*, 38–42.

Davis, J. (2014). Rebozo in an NHS setting. *AIMS Journal, 26(4)*, 6–8.

Dempsey, R. (2013). *Birth with Confidence. Savvy Choices for Normal Birth*. Fairfield, Australia: Boathouse Press.

Dixon, L., Skinner, J. and Foureur, M. (2013a). Women's perspectives of the stages and phases of labour. *Midwifery, 29*, 10–17.

Dixon, L., Skinner, J. and Foureur, M. (2013b). The emotional and hormonal pathways of labour and birth: integrating mind, body and behaviour. *Journal of the New Zealand College of Midwives, 48(1)*, 15–23.

Dixon, L., Skinner, J. and Foureur, M. (2014). The emotional journey of labour – women's perspectives of the experience of labour moving towards birth. *Midwifery, 30*, 371–377.

Downe, S., Gyte, G.M.L., Dahlen, H.G. and Singata, M. (2013). Routine vaginal examinations for assessing progress of labour to improve outcomes for women and babies at term (Review). *Cochrane Database of Systematic Reviews*, Issue 7. Art. No.: CD010088. doi:10.1002/14651858.CD010088. pub2.

Eri, T.S., Blystad, A., Gjengedal, E. and Blaaka, G. (2011). 'Stay home for as long as possible': midwives' priorities and strategies in communicating with first-time mothers in early labour. *Midwifery*, e286–e292.

Feeley, C., Cooper, M., and Burns, E. (2021). A systematic meta-thematic synthesis to examine the views and experiences of women following water immersion during labour and waterbirth. *Journal of Advanced Nursing*. doi:10.1111/jan.14720.

Finlayson, K., Downe, S. and Hinder, S. (2015). Unexpected consequences: women's experiences of a self-hypnosis intervention to help with pain in labour. *BMC Pregnancy and Childbirth*, *15*, 229.

Fumagalli, S., Nespoli, A., Oliva, A., Zobbi, V.F. and Colciago, E. (2020). Maternal postures to promote the rotation of occiput posterior foetal position during labour. *The Practising Midwife*, *23(4)*, 26–30.

Gilkison, A., McAra-Couper, J., Fielder, A., Hunter, M. and Austin, D. (2017). The core of the core: what is at the heart of hospital core midwifery practice in New Zealand? *NZCOM Journal*, *53*, 30–37.

Gould, D. (2000). Normal labour: a concept analysis. *Journal of Advanced Nursing*, *31(2)*, 418–427.

Gupta J.K., Sood, A., Hofmeyr, G., Vogel, J.P. (2017) Position in the second stage of labour for women without epidural anaesthesia. *Cochrane Database of Systematic Reviews*, Issue 5. Art. No.: CD002006. doi:10.1002/14651858.CD002006.pub4.

Healy, M., Nyman, V., Spence, D., Otten, R.H.J., Verhoeven, C.J.. (2020). How do midwives facilitate women to give birth during physiological second stage of labour? A systematic review. *PLoS ONE*, *15(7)*, e0226502.

Hunter, B., Berg, M., Lundgren, I., Ólafsdóttir, Á. and Kirkham, M. (2008). Relationships: the hidden threads in the tapestry of maternity care. *Midwifery*, *24*, 132–137.

Iversen, M.L., Midtgaard, J., Ekelin, M. and Hegaard, H.K. (2016). Danish women's experiences of the rebozo technique during labour: a qualitative explorative study. *Sexual and Reproductive Healthcare*, *11(1)*, 79–85.

Jenkinson, B., Josey, N. and Kruske, S. (2013). *BirthSpace: An Evidence-based Guide to Birth Environment Design*. Queensland Centre for Mothers & Babies. The University of Queensland.

Jones, L., Othman, M., Dowswell, T., Alfirevic, Z., Gates S., Newburn, M., Jordan, S., Lavender, T. and Neilson, J.P. (2012). Pain management for women in labour: an overview of systematic reviews. *Cochrane Database of Systematic Reviews 2012*, Issue 3. Art. No.: CD009234. doi:10.1002/14651858.CD009234.pub2.

Kitzinger, J.V. (1992). Counteracting, not reenacting, the violation women's bodies: the challenge for perinatal caregivers. *Birth*, *19(4)*, 219–220.

Lawrence, A., Lewis, L., Hofmeyr, G.J. and Styles, C. (2013). Maternal positions and mobility during first stage labour (Review). *Cochrane Database of Systematic Reviews*, Issue 10. Art. No.: CD003934. doi:003910.001002/14651858.CD14003934.pub4.

Leap, N. (1996). A midwifery perspective on pain in labour. Unpublished MSc dissertation, South Bank University, London. Available on request from nickyleap@me.com.

Leap, N. (2010). The less we do the more we give. Chapter 2 in M. Kirkham (ed.), *The Midwife–Mother Relationship*, 2nd edn (pp.17–35). London: Palgrave Macmillan.

Leap, N. (2015, unpublished data). Identifying the experiences of receiving and providing support in labour.

Leap, N., Sandall, J., Buckland, S. and Huber, U. (2010). Journey to confidence: women's experiences of pain in labour and relational continuity of care. *Journal of Midwifery and Women's Health*, *55(3)*, 235–242.

Levett, K.M., Smith, C.A., Bensoussan, A. and Dahlen, H.G. (2016). Complementary therapies for labour and birth study: a randomised controlled trial of antenatal integrative medicine for pain management in labour. *BMJ Open Access*, *6*. doi:10.1136/ bmjopen-2015-010691.

Levett, K.M., Smith, C.A., Dahlen, H.G. and Bensoussan, A. (2014). Acupuncture and acupressure for pain management in labour and birth: a critical narrative review of current systematic review evidence. *Complementary Therapies in Medicine, 22*, 523–540.

Long, L. (2006). Redefining the second stage of labour could help to promote normal birth. *British Journal of Midwifery, 14(2)*, 104–106.

Lowe, N.K. (2002). The nature of labor pain. *American Journal of Obstetrics and Gynecology, 186(5)*, S16–S24.

Magoga, G., Saccone, G., Al-Kouatly, H.B., Dahlen, H.G., Thornton, C., Akbarzadeh, M., . . . Berghella, V. (2019). Warm perineal compresses during the second stage of labor for reducing perineal trauma: a meta-analysis. *European Journal of Obstetrics & Gynecology and Reproductive Biology, 240*, 93–98.

Meddings, N. (2017). *How to Have a Baby: Mother-gathered Guidance on Birth and New Babies.* Chipping Norton, Oxfordshire: Eynham Press.

Menakaya, U., Albayati, S., Vella, E., Fenwick, J. and Angstetra, D. (2013). A retrospective comparison of water birth and conventional vaginal birth among women deemed to be low risk in a secondary level hospital in Australia. 114–118.

Milosevic, S., Channon, S., Hunter, B., Nolan, M., Hughes, A., Barlow, C., . . . Sanders, J. (2019). Factors influencing the use of birth pools in the United Kingdom: perspectives of women, midwives and medical staff. *Midwifery, 79*, 102554.

Milosevic, S., Channon, S., Hughes, J., Hunter, B., Nolan, M., Milton, R. and Sanders, J. (2020). Factors influencing water immersion during labour: qualitative case studies of six maternity units in the United Kingdom. *BMC Pregnancy and Childbirth, 20*, 719.

Moncrieff, G. and Dahlen, H. (2020). The UK OASI Care Bundle: the results are out but so is the jury. https://www.all4maternity.com/the-uk-oasi-care-bundle-the-results-are-out-but-so-is-the-jury/.

Neal, J.L., Lowe, N.K., Ahijevych, K.L., Patrick, T.E., Cabbage, L.A. and Corwin, E.J. (2010). 'Active labor' duration and dilation rates among low-risk, nulliparous women with spontaneous labor onset: a systematic review. *Journal of Midwifery and Women's Health, 55*, 308–318.

NICE (2014). Intrapartum care: care of healthy women and their babies during childbirth. Clinical guideline 190. National Collaborating Centre for Women's and Children's Health UK. Commissioned by the National Institute for Health and Care Excellence (NICE): www.nice.org.uk/guidance/cg190.

Nolan, M. (2010). Childbirth education: politics, equality and relevance. Chapter 3 in D. Walsh and S. Downe (eds), *Essential Midwifery Practice: Intrapartum Care* (pp.31–44). Chichester: Wiley-Blackwell.

Osborne, K. and Hanson, L. (2012). Directive versus supportive approaches used by midwives when providing care during the second stage of labor. *Journal of Midwifery Women's Health, 57(1)*, 3–11.

Priddis, H., Dahlen, H.G. and Schmied, V. (2012). What are the facilitators, inhibitors, and implications of birth positioning? A review of the literature. *Women and Birth, 25*, 100–106.

RCM. (2018) *Midwifery Care in Labour Guidance for All Women in All Settings. RCM Midwifery Blue Top Guidance. No. 1.* London: Royal College of Midwives. https://www.rcm.org.uk/media/2539/professionals-blue-top-guidance.pdf.

Reed, R., Barnes, M. and Rowe, J. (2015). Women's experience of birth: childbirth as a rite of passage. *International Journal of Childbirth, 5*, 46–56.

Roberts, L., Gulliver, B., Fisher, J. and Cloyes, K.G. (2010). The coping with labor algorithm: an alternate pain assessment tool for the laboring woman *Journal of Midwifery & Women's Health, 55(2)*, 107–116.

Sandall, J., Leap, N., Grant, J. and Bastos, M.H. (2010). Supporting women to have a normal birth: development and field testing of a learning package for maternity staff. London: Health and Social Care Research Division, King's College London.

Sandall, J., Soltani, H., Gates, S., Shennan, A. and Devane, D. (2016). Midwife-led continuity models versus other models of care for childbearing women. *Cochrane Database of Systematic Reviews,* Issue 4. Art. No.: CD004667. doi:10.1002/14651858.CD004667.pub5.

Simkin, P. (2002). Supportive care during labor: a guide for busy nurses. *JOGNN, 31(6)*, 721–732. doi:10.1177/0884217502239208.

Simkin, P. (2007). *Comfort in Labour: How You Can Help Yourself to a Normal Satisfying Child-birth*. Childbirth Connection. https://www.nationalpartnership.org/our-work/resources/health-care/maternity/comfort-in-labor-simkin.pdf.

Simkin, P., Ancheta, R. and Hanson, L. (2017). *The Labor Progress Handbook: Early Interventions to Prevent and Treat Dystocia*, 4th edn. Chichester, West Sussex: Wiley-Blackwell.

Simkin, P. and Bolding, A. (2004). Update on nonpharmacologic approaches to relieve labor pain and prevent suffering. *Journal of Midwifery and Women's Health*, *49*(6), 489–504.

Simkin, P. with Rohs, K. (2018). *The Birth Partner: A Complete Guide to Childbirth for Dads, Doulas, and All Other Labor Companions*, 5th edn. Boston, MA: Harvard Common Press.

Smith, C.A., Levett, K.M., Collins, C.T. and Crowther, C.A. (2018). Relaxation techniques for pain management in labour. *Cochrane Database of Systematic Reviews*, Issue 3. Art. No.: CD009514. doi:10.1002/14651858.CD009514.pub2.

Smith, C.A., Levett, K.M., Collins, C.T. and Jones, L. (2012). Massage, reflexology and other manual methods for pain management in labour. *Cochrane Database of Systematic Reviews 2012*, Issue 2. Art. No.: CD009290. doi:10.1002/14651858.CD009290.pub2.

Spiby, H., Walsh, D., Green, J.M., Crompton, A. and Bugg, G. (2014). Midwives' beliefs and concerns about telephone conversations with women in early labour. *Midwifery*, *30*, 1036–1042.

Spillane, E. (2018). Small things make a big difference; birth environments matter. *The Practising Midwife*, *21*(*10*), 36–39.

Swahnberg, K., Wijma, B. and Siwe, K. (2011). Strong discomfort during vaginal examination: why consider a history of abuse? *European Journal of Obstetrics & Gynecology and Reproductive Biology*, 200–205.

Thakar, R., Gurol-Urganci, I., Bidwiell, P., Sevdalis, N., Silverton, L., Freeman, L. and van der Muelen, J. (2020). Obstetric Anal Sphincter Injury (OASI) Care Bundle: response to a critical review. *Midwifery*, *90*, 102802.

Thornton, J.G. and Dahlen, H.G. (2020). The UK Obstetric Anal Sphincter Injury (OASI) Bundle: a critical review. *Midwifery*, *90*, 102801.

Walker, D.S, Visger, J.M. and Rossie, D. (2009). Contemporary childbirth education models. *Journal of Midwifery & Women's Health*, *54*(6), 469–476.

Walsh, D. (2001). Are midwives losing the art of keeping birth normal? *British Journal of Midwifery*, *9*(3), 146.

Walsh, D. (2010). Labour rhythms. Chapter 5 in D. Walsh and S. Downe (eds), *Essential Midwifery Practice: Intrapartum Care* (pp.63–80). Chichester: Wiley-Blackwell.

Walsh, D. (2012). Pain in labour. Chapter 7 in D. Walsh (ed.), *Evidence and Skills for Normal Labour and Birth*, 2nd edn (pp.82–100). London: Routledge.

Webb, S. (2020). The OASI Care Bundle – a lively topic for discussion. *MIDIRS Midwifery Digest*, *30*(*4*), 414–417.

Whitburn, L.Y., Jones, L.E., Davy, M-A. and Small, R. (2014). Women's experiences of labour pain and the role of the mind: an exploratory study. *Midwifery*, 1029–1035.

WHO. (2018). *WHO Recommendations: Intrapartum Care for a Positive Childbirth Experience*. Geneva: World Health Organization.

WHO Regional Office for the Western Pacific. (2014). *First Embrace: A Mother's First Embrace, Her Baby's First Breath*. Manila: World Health Organization. Regional Office for the Western Pacific. https://apps.who.int/iris/handle/10665/208239.

8 Supporting women with complex needs in labour

Introduction

In this chapter we'll consider the kind of support that a woman and her birth companions may need in various situations that could be described as 'complex'. This might be due to complications identified during pregnancy or labour; interventions, such as induction of labour; or the use of various forms of technology. It is not possible within the scope of this book to consider all possible situations that could be described in this way, so we have concentrated on the ones that you are most likely to encounter, for example, where women have epidurals, induction of labour, caesarean birth or continuous CTG monitoring.

In any situation, women need authentic support from their attendants. They need to feel that their concerns are really heard, that they are seen as an individual, not a 'case' or a 'high risk woman', and that the professionals are working in partnership with them all the way:

> My birth wasn't the birth that I planned because I ended up having him four weeks early but the overall outcome I suppose was very positive . . . it wasn't what I wanted initially but I was able to work with them to achieve what I wanted out of that situation, if you like. And I remain really positive about it, it wasn't really traumatic but it wasn't at all sort of planned, obviously, at that time, so yeah. . . .
>
> (Mother, Sandall *et al.*, 2010, p.39)

They also need to know that their emotional needs will be attended to with as much attention as their physical needs and that every opportunity will be taken to optimise normal physiology where possible, for example, by ensuring skin-to-skin contact following caesarean birth (Walker and Bewley, 2019). In other words, they need the same quality of attention, care and empathy that women need when labour is normal – as described in the previous chapter.

Throughout this chapter, we refer to 'supporting a woman who . . .'. We would like to make it clear that it is a given that this also means supporting a woman's partner and close family and friends, and trust that you will bear this in mind in all your discussions.

When women are identified as having 'risk'-associated labours

Thinking about the language of 'risk'

Before we start to discuss how best to support women whose labours are viewed as complicated, we shall step back and consider the effect the language and practices associated with 'risk' may have on women, the type of care they receive and the culture of institutionalised care. Most of us are practising in services where even women who do not have complications

DOI: 10.4324/9781003092520-9

hear that risk may be lurking in their 'low risk' status. Sara Wickham (2005, 2018) suggests that we should think about the messages women are getting when they hear the abundance of terms centred on the word 'risk': low risk, high risk, increased risk, relative risk, risk analysis, risk management, risk factors and risk assessment. The research articles profiled in Box 8.1 explore the challenges faced by midwives working in a predominant culture of risk management.

Box 8.1 Research Briefing: The culture of 'risk management' in hospital maternity units

Newnham, E., McKellar, L. and Pincombe, J. (2015). Documenting risk: a comparison of policy and information pamphlets for using epidural or water in labour. *Women and Birth, 28*, 221–227.

This ethnographic study showed how the information given to women in the two hospital leaflets identified epidural analgesia as an acceptable, accessible and relatively safe option while insisting on caution if contemplating the use of water. This presented midwives with the challenge of translating the subtleties of the risk discourse for women in their care.

Seibold, C., Licqurish, S., Rolls, C. and Hopkins, F. (2010). 'Lending the space': midwives perceptions of birth space and clinical risk management. *Midwifery, 26*, 526–531.

In this qualitative study midwives described how clinical risk management, underpinned by a risk discourse, impacted on their practice and efforts to create an ideal birth space for women. The hierarchical culture and rigid practices of risk management prevailed after the move to a new hospital with more comfortable, spacious and private birth spaces. Midwives working in a caseload model thought they had the best opportunity to make a difference to women's experiences during labour and birth as they were able to develop trusting relationships with them during the antenatal period.

Verena Schmid and Soo Downe (2010) make an important contribution to debates about risk and how we define whether a woman's labour is 'normal' or 'abnormal', noting that abnormality has come to mean 'deviation from the average, with the *potential* for pathology' [our emphasis] rather than actual pathology (p.159). They challenge us to move away from seeing all labours as potentially abnormal, to thinking: 'Are this woman and baby actually at imminent risk in this specific situation – or, although what is happening is unusual, could it be normal for them?' (p.159). They advocate the use of the term 'unusual labour' to highlight that a birth may be physiological but unusual in some way, rather than pathological.

Box 8.2 Recommended Resource: Midwifery skills for normalising unusual labours

Schmid, V. and Downe, S. (2010). Midwifery skills for normalising unusual labours. Chapter 10 in D. Walsh and S. Downe (eds), *Essential Midwifery Practice: Intrapartum Care* (pp.159–190). Chichester: Wiley-Blackwell.

This thought-provoking chapter is an excellent resource that provides an overview of the physiology of labour and birth, before considering a broad range of evidence that describes how midwives and other labour attendants can differentiate between unusual physiological births and unusual pathological births.

How risk categorisation impacts on the care women receive

There is a danger that, once women are categorised as not being 'low risk', the approach to their care fundamentally changes. Formal criteria delineating the boundaries between 'low risk' and its deviations into variations or complications are often used to identify which women are 'suitable' for midwife-led care or birth centre care (Hunter and Segrott, 2014). Yet, as midwives and obstetricians know only too well, such boundaries are hazy and movable. For example, in some maternity units a woman may be classified as unsuitable for birth centre care if she has a body mass index (BMI) over 35, whereas in others the cut-off may be a BMI of 40. A 'grey area' is thus created, of women who are not high risk but – it is feared – may become so.

Similarly, although vaginal birth after caesarean (VBAC) is a safe option for the majority of women, in some maternity units, they may be denied access to a midwife-led birth centre or use of a pool for comfort during labour (McKenna and Symon, 2014). They may also not be eligible for midwifery continuity of care, despite the evidence that this can promote positive experiences for women wanting a VBAC, increasing their sense of control and confidence. Indeed, when women wanting a VBAC receive continuity of care, there is an increased likelihood of spontaneous vaginal birth, an active labour, water immersion and giving birth in an upright position (Keedle *et al.,* 2019, 2020).

When women have complicated labours, a standardised approach to care may dominate, one that pays little heed to their individual wishes and concerns. For these women, the homely environment of a birth centre is replaced by the high-tech environment of the labour ward, as this midwife describes:

> I work on the labour ward in a busy maternity unit and I am often concerned about the environment we provide for the women who don't meet the criteria to give birth in the midwife-led unit (MLU). It may be that their blood pressure has gone up towards the end of pregnancy or they have been labouring in the MLU but now they want more pain relief or their labour is getting prolonged. Whatever the situation, they can't stay in that lovely environment with the soft colours and cushions and fairy lights. And no one thinks of making it more homely here, suddenly it's straight up on the bed, monitor on, IV in. We have lovely birth pools on labour ward, but they are hardly ever used. It's like imagination and creativity go out of the window when women come here. People give up on trying to support as normal a birth as possible, but that's just what we should be doing – for everyone we care for on labour ward. Normalise all the bits you can.
>
> (Midwife, Hunter, 2015, unpublished data)

A midwifery model for supporting women with obstetric complications in labour

When there are obstetric complications, pregnant women will still want to be affirmed as an individual mother-to-be, rather than a 'high risk case' (Berg, 2005; Berg and Dahlberg (1998). The practice of caring for each woman as a unique individual and promoting her 'inborn' capacity to give birth and be a mother was identified in Marie Berg's (2005) research, which enabled her to develop an important theory about a midwifery model of care for women at high risk. In Box 8.3 we have profiled the research and use it in a Reflective Activity to facilitate discussion about the essence of woman centred care for women whose labours involve complications.

Box 8.3   Reflective Activity: A midwifery model of care for women at high risk of complications

Berg, M. (2005). A midwifery model of care for childbearing women at high risk: genuine caring in caring for the genuine. *Journal of Perinatal Education,14(1)*, 9–21.

Summary

The ideal midwifery care for women at high risk has three constituents:

1   A dignity protective relationship that includes: mutuality, trust, ongoing dialogue, shared responsibility and enduring presence.
2   The midwife's embodied knowledge: theoretical, practical, intuitive and reflective.
3   A responsibility to balance physiological and medical perspectives by supporting normalcy and exhibiting sensitivity for the genuineness of each woman.

Individually or in pairs
*   Write a story (not more than 2,000 words) about an imaginary woman (give ficti-tious names to all characters) who is having her second baby. She had an emer-gency caesarean birth for her first baby, following a 'routine' induction of labour at 41 weeks. In this pregnancy, she has had midwifery continuity of care and is very keen to have a normal birth this time. The story starts when she is 36 weeks into a healthy pregnancy and includes the way her midwife negotiates with an obstetrician and midwifery manager in order for her to use the birth centre and pool if all is progressing well in labour. The story ends with a discussion between the midwife and mother at a postnatal visit where the woman describes the empowering and healing experience of her labour.
*   In a separate document, list the examples in your story of how the three overarching constituents of Marie Berg's midwifery model of care for childbearing women at risk were enacted and provide a bibliography of other research articles that informed the way you described the midwife's practice and the woman's experiences.

We suggest that this Reflective Activity can be adapted as an assignment.

Normalising the environment for birth

There are other important ways that a midwife can support a woman where technology is being used. It is certainly possible to make a labour ward environment more woman and family friendly, in spite of the technology, and thus more conducive to optimising normal physiologi-cal processes (Brodie and Leap, 2008). This takes empathy and imagination, characteristics that can be enhanced by learning from positive role models, as these student midwives describe:

> It was really good to see that midwife creating the same environment as the birth centre, up on the labour ward. And her approach with women and their partners was lovely . . . they were so thankful towards her; even though they'd only known her for a short period of time they remembered it as being really nice.
>
> (Student midwife, Hunter, 2015, unpublished data)

A midwife working in the community told me that although she loves caseloading, she feels that she made a bigger difference on the labour ward because she knows that she has a particular ability to make that rapport, and to see the women through who may not have a normal birth otherwise.

(Student midwife, Leap, 2015, unpublished data)

Supporting women who are having continuous CTG monitoring

Women having any kind of continuous cardiotocographic (CTG) monitoring will continue to need midwifery support; for example, to remain upright and to find comfortable positions in response to what feels right. They may well need lots of reassurance and explanations about what is happening, particularly if conversations have been taking place between staff outside of the room. Anxiety about how to interpret the CTG trace can run high if the machine is in the room but when central monitoring systems are in place, women and their birth companions are likely to need reassurance that someone is keeping an eye on what is happening.

Enabling movement and upright positions with CTG monitoring

Whilst most guidelines recommend intermittent fetal monitoring in labour for women with healthy pregnancies, continuous CTG monitoring is universally recommended for women most at risk of poor outcomes. This is regarded by some as contentious, however, as highlighted in the literature review in Box 8.4.

Box 8.4   Research Briefing: Intrapartum CTG monitoring for women at risk of poor outcomes

Small, K.A., Sidebotham, M., Fenwick, J. and Gamble, J. (2020). Intrapartum cardiotocograph monitoring and perinatal outcomes for women at risk: literature review. *Women and Birth*, *33*, 411–418.

This systematic review of the research evidence did not demonstrate improvements in perinatal outcome for infants born to women at risk of poor perinatal outcome when intrapartum CTG monitoring is used. The authors conclude that there is an urgent need to verify whether continuous CTG monitoring during pre-term labour contributes to cerebral palsy rates and to identify which women, if any, benefit from intrapartum CTG monitoring.

Wireless and beltless technologies to facilitate freedom of movement

The advantages of using wireless CTG technology – or 'telemetry' – to facilitate freedom of movement and a sense of control for women are widely acknowledged and outlined in the studies in Box 8.5. However, the majority of women with complex pregnancies do not access this form of technology, even when it is available. It is interesting to ponder why this might be the case.

Box 8.5   Research Briefing: CTG technologies to enable mobility for women

Fox, D., Maude, R., Coddington, R., Woodworth, R., Scarf, V., Watson, K. and Foureur, M. (2021). The use of continuous foetal monitoring technologies that enable mobility in labour for women with complex pregnancies: a survey of Australian and New Zealand hospitals. *Midwifery*, *93*, 102887 (in press).

Watson, K., Mills, T.A. and Lavender, T. (2018). The use of telemetry in labour: results of a national online survey of UK maternity units. *British Journal of Midwifery*, *26*, 14–19.

Box 8.6   Reflective Activity: Promoting normal birth around technology

In small groups:
* Discuss the pictures in Figure 8.1 below, which illustrate ways of adapting a labour ward setting to optimise normal labour and birth for women experiencing technology.
* Consider the following questions:

  * Describe how you have seen these or similar positions/approaches being used in a 'high-tech' setting such as a labour ward. If you have not seen this, why might that be?
  * How would you discuss the advantages of trying out these positions with the woman (and her partner)? Write a script for the words you would use and share these with the larger group.
  * How would you advocate enabling women to try these positions with colleagues who are sceptical? Write a script for the words you would use and share these, saying them out loud within the larger group.
  * Identify the high quality research to back up your arguments

---

Figure 8.1 Optimising normal birth around technology

Creating a sense of calm in the birth room

It can be hard to create a positive environment for women in labour when the room is dominated and cramped by the features of technology. Consider the following story of a frightened woman experiencing a complicated labour and how the midwife responded to this, as told to Nicky by an experienced Australian midwife.

Box 8.7   Reflective Activity: Creating a sense of calm in the birth room

I was called into the birth room, and there was an Indigenous woman, curled up in the corner of the room, trying to hide behind the bed, screaming. She had diabetes and cardiac disease and she didn't understand much English. I thought 'Where's the midwife? You can make a difference.' I sat down beside her. The midwife came in wanting to get things done urgently and I thought, 'We've just got to sit down with this woman and help her gain some control before we do anything'. She's in a room with four or five IVs running, strapped to monitors, not able to walk any more. So you get eye contact and you start working as a midwife. Trusting the woman, believing in the woman, helping her to believe in herself, being there for her, being kind, talking so she understands, talking slowly, gently, engaging any support people if she has any, and slowly you try to gain some sort of calm.

(Midwife, Leap, 2015, unpublished data)

In pairs:
- Tell each other a story about a similar situation you have been in and explain what you did to try to help. Remember that this help can often be the 'small things' you did, as the midwife above describes.
- What assisted you in improving the situation, or what might have assisted you?
- Imagine you find yourself in a similar situation next week. How might you handle the situation now?

Supporting a woman who chooses to have an epidural

When a woman has an epidural in labour she will require a particular type of support. First, she will need to know what the epidural insertion process entails and how she might experience having epidural analgesia. It is important to encourage her to ask questions, to listen carefully to these and to allow enough time to answer them fully. Second, she will need support and reassurance during the process of epidural insertion, which can sometimes be tricky and uncomfortable, especially if she's having strong contractions and is finding it difficult to remain still. Eye contact, breathing together and comforting touch by the midwife or the woman's partner can help in such situations, as can using Entonox (nitrous oxide). Third, once the epidural is in place, the woman will need support with trying different positions, or encouragement to keep as mobile as possible.

During labour, when a woman chooses to have an epidural, the type of support that she needs shifts and this can sometimes feel challenging for us, as this midwife suggests:

Sometimes I find it quite difficult to know how best to support her. You go from full on support to her not needing you in the same way. I'm quite busy filling in charts and attending to drips and monitors, blood pressures and the like while she's often eyes shut resting until 'the big push' sort of thing.

You try everything you know to avoid an instrumental birth: different positions, using a mirror to encourage her if the baby's head is visible, and eventually getting her into lithotomy because that's always the last thing you try. But it feels like such hard work, all of that, when she's got an epidural. And all the monitoring and filling in bits of paper get between you and the woman.

(Midwife, Leap, 2015, unpublished data)

What is possible for women in terms of mobility depends, to some extent, on the type of epidural used. It will also depend on how the woman and her baby are responding to the stress of labour. But it is important not to see the woman as inevitably passive just because she has an epidural. There are many aspects of care that are negotiable, as this story of a standing epidural birth vividly illustrates:

Midwife 1:   So she'd been fully (dilated) for an hour and then I got her to start to push. And nothing much was happening. And then she just had this urge and at the same time I thought it would be a really good idea if she'd just get up. I said, 'Well how do your legs feel?. . . . Well if we support you, what about . . .?' And she said, 'Well I'd really like to stand!' and she got up and she started to push and the head was just coming down nicely and she just delivered this – I mean just literally, his face came out and I thought, 'Oh! He's huge!' For one second I thought, 'Oh goodness me! How are his shoulders going to come out?' And he just slid down my arm. [Appreciative noises and laughter from group.] And when we weighed him he was eleven pounds ten ounces!

Midwife 2:   Oh my god!

Midwife 1:   Massive! And he was gorgeous and it was perfect. It was like – so perfect I could cry even now . . . I really could . . . [Voices: Aw!].

(Hunter, 2002, p.178)

This story is particularly interesting as it shows how a 'low-tech' approach to supporting the normal physiology of labour (standing) can be used in conjunction with high-tech childbirth (the epidural) in a way that can be beneficial. Given the size of the baby, there was an increased likelihood of shoulder dystocia, especially if the woman had remained on her back. By standing up, the diameters of the woman's pelvic outlet were increased and the possibility of an obstetric emergency was reduced. Trust is a central theme in this story: both the woman's trust in the midwife's skills and assessment of the situation, and the midwife's trust in normal physiology and the woman's potential ability to give birth normally.

Births involving epidurals are not always straightforward, however, and women's requests for an epidural may present dilemmas for the midwife, particularly if a woman has previously said that she does not want an epidural under any circumstances. As we discussed in Chapter 2, assessing the best response is much easier when the midwife and woman know each other or when the woman's birth support team are confident that she is likely to be glad afterwards that she was encouraged in this way. However, midwives may be wary of being accused of violating the woman's wishes in their efforts to promote normal birth if they do not call for the anaesthetist straight away when a woman is asking for an epidural. We explore this dilemma, using the following student midwife's story as a Reflective Activity.

Box 8.8   Reflective Activity: Epidural dilemmas – a student midwife's story

When a woman is asking for an epidural, it's very difficult to know what to do sometimes. If I had called an anaesthetist for every woman who asked for an epidural then I would have called the anaesthetist for almost everybody.

I remember a woman, a multip who had a really, really quick labour. When she came in the baby's head was visible and she was asking for an epidural. And I said, 'I can see the head, a few more pushes and your baby will be out.' 'I don't care! I want an epidural! I want an epidural now!' And the midwife I was working with said, 'You have to call, you know, if a woman asks for an epidural you have to show that you've acted, you've done something.' And I was like, 'Well the vertex is visible, the baby's going to be out', but she said, 'You have to call the anaesthetist because she's asked. You have to show that you have actually acted on behalf of the woman because she has asked for it.'

(Student midwife, Leap, 2015, unpublished data)

In threes:
- Take it in turns to be the student midwife, the mentor and the woman in three short renditions of this scenario, in order to 'get into the shoes' of each person. Each time, after you have played the situation, engage in a short discussion about how your character was feeling.
- What was motivating their behaviour and attitudes?
- How might the situation have played out differently?
- Try changing one person's words or responses and see how the situation might have changed.

Supporting women faced with induction of labour

In recent years, in many Western countries, induction rates have soared, with more than a third of women having their labours induced. As can be seen in the articles profiled in Box 8.9, there is ongoing debate about the evidence for clinical indications for induction and the practice of offering induction to all women at term. This professional debate contributes to the complexity of decision making for pregnant women when they are offered 'informed choice' about whether or not to have their labours induced. Although there are circumstances where it is clear that an induction is necessary for the wellbeing of a mother or baby, this decision is not so clear-cut for the majority of women who have healthy pregnancies at term.

Box 8.9   Research Briefing: Indications for induction

Coates, D., Makris, A., Catling, C., Henry, A., Scarf, V., Watts, N., . . . Homer, C. (2020). A systematic scoping review of clinical indications for induction of labour. *PLoS ONE, 15(1)*, e0228196.
Seijmonsbergen-Schermers, A.E., Scherjon, S. and de Jonge, A. (2019). *BJOG* debate. Induction of labour should be offered to all women at term. AGAINST: induction should not be offered to all women at term: first, do no harm. *BJOG, 126(13)*, 1599–1599.

Supporting women making decisions about induction

Local and national guidelines inform our discussions with women and their birth supporters, for example the NICE (2008) guidelines *Inducing labour*. It is not as simple as just following guidelines, though. Midwives need to have time to sit with a woman and her birth supporters and discuss all aspects of her individual situation, including: the relative risks of induction versus continued pregnancy; alternative options; what to expect during an induction; and the woman's feelings, thoughts and fears (Jay and Thomas, 2018), As we discussed in Chapter 1, setting aside enough time for such conversations is particularly important when working with women through interpreters, or when women have a limited understanding of the language in which we are communicating.

Supporting women to make decisions about induction requires midwives to have good listening skills, employing the LAURS of communication that we discussed in Chapter 5 (Cyna, 2019) and the ability to share information in a way that is sensitive to what induction might mean for the individual woman. This involves understanding that the notion of 'informed decision making' is complex and fraught with difficulty, particularly in terms of the influence of the person providing the information if they are seen as an authority figure (Leap and Edwards, 2006).

Socioeconomic factors may also influence how confident women feel about engaging in such conversations. A UK study showed that women with fewer educational qualifications and those living in disadvantaged areas were more likely to end up with labour induction and subsequent interventions than women with higher qualifications and those living in advantaged electoral wards (Carter *et al.*, 2020).

Women's experiences of induction

The studies in Box 8.10 identify the shift in expectations and the emotions that women may experience when their labours are induced. For some, the decision can represent relief and a sense of certainty about when their labour will begin; for many women, though, there is a sense of resignation involving disappointment, helplessness and, in some cases, distress about a lack of discussion or consideration of their preferences. When convinced that there are concerns for their baby's wellbeing though, women are often keen to have the best birth possible in spite of any interventions that will be required.

During the induction and subsequent labour, women often describe feeling neglected and powerless as they are processed through a system with set time frames. A lack of information about delays in the induction process and what to expect at each stage is a major contributory feature to the stressful experiences women describe. Midwives not taking seriously their requests for pain relief when contractions are artificially stimulated are also part of the harrowing tales that women tell. It is, perhaps, not surprising that many women state they would not opt for induction of labour in another pregnancy if they had a choice (Schwarz *et al.*, 2016).

Box 8.10   Research Briefing: Women's experiences of induction of labour

Coates, R., Cupples, G., Scamell, A. and McCourt, C. (2019). Women's experiences of induction of labour: qualitative systematic review and thematic synthesis. *Midwifery, 69*, 17–28.

Lou, S., Hvidman, L., Uldbjerg, N., Lone Neumann, L., Jensen, T.F., Haben, J-K. and Carstensen, K. (2019). Women's experiences of post term induction of labour: a systematic review of qualitative studies. *Birth, 46*, 400–410.

Akuamoah-Boateng, J. and Spencer, R. (2018). Woman-centered care: women's experiences and perceptions of induction of labor for uncomplicated post-term pregnancy: a systematic review of qualitative evidence. *Midwifery, 67*, 46–56.

Supporting women whose labours are being induced

It seems that the features of support which we have discussed in previous chapters are often missing for women who have their labours induced, in particular: reassurance, privacy, presence, caring behaviours and the facilitation of a sense of security. The Royal College of Midwives publication *Midwifery Care for Induction of Labour* (RCM, 2019) draws on the evidence highlighted in Box 8.11 in making recommendations for practice to improve women's experiences of induction of labour.

Box 8.11   Recommended Resource: Midwifery care for induction of labour

RCM. (2019). *RCM Blue Top Midwifery Guidance (No 2). Midwifery Care for Induction of Labour*. London: Royal College of Midwives. https://www.rcm.org.uk/media/3552 /midwifery-care-for-induction-of-labour-a4-2019-16pp_2.pdf.

A summary of systematically produced research evidence for women facing induction of labour. Recommendations of midwifery care are provided under the following headings:

- Supporting women to make decisions about induction of labour
- Improving women's experiences of induction of labour
- Membrane sweeps
- Returning home following cervical priming
- Supporting women who wish to use complementary therapies to induce labour

---

Box 8.12   Reflective Activity: Supporting women faced with induction

In preparation for this activity, study the research papers outlined in Box 8.9 and Box 8.10 and the recommendations in the Royal College of Midwives publication *Midwifery Care for Induction of Labour* (RCM, 2019) profiled in Box 8.11.

Scenario:

Faith is a 35-year-old woman having her first baby. You are her primary midwife and have shared all her antenatal care with your midwife partner, Dianne. Either you or Dianne will be her midwife when she is in labour and will be sharing her postnatal care. Faith has had a healthy pregnancy and is now 40 weeks' pregnant. You have set aside time to meet with Faith and her partner Joseph to discuss booking her in for induction at 41 weeks, which is the policy in the maternity unit where you work. Faith tells you that she wants to avoid having an induction unless it's really necessary for her baby's wellbeing. She tells you that she wants to give birth in the birth centre and be able to move around, use the pool and birth ball and do all the things that you have previously discussed to help her body work well. She says her mum always went 'overdue' with her babies and asks you to explain the policy of induction at 41 weeks and what the alternative options are for bringing her labour on.

In pairs or small groups:

- Make a dot-point list of the things you might cover in your conversation with Faith and Joseph, including options to address her wishes for labour if she decides later to have an induction.
- Share this list with the wider group.
- Engage in a facilitated discussion about the changes that might be needed in the environment/s in which you work in order to meet the following 'Good Practice Points' to improve women's experience of induction:

  - Midwives should ask women about their needs during the induction process and wherever possible, provide women with supportive aids, spaces and privacy.
  - Midwives and maternity services should enable women to have access to spaces to mobilise, birthing balls, water immersion, peaceful settings to rest and sleep and access to food and drink.

(RCM, 2019, p.9)

Box 8.13   Recommended Resource: Making decisions about induction

Reed, R. (2018). *Why Induction Matters.* London: Pinter & Martin.

This small book is a mine of information to help women in their decision making around induction; it is also a useful resource for all birth workers who engage in conversations with women faced with making these decisions. Rachel Reed skilfully combines evidence, women's stories about their experiences, and frameworks for thinking about 'risk' and decision making.

Chapter 2 'Complications of pregnancy' discusses the main complications of pregnancy which lead to a recommendation to induce labour: high blood pressure; pre-eclampsia; gestational and existing diabetes; intrahepatic cholestasis of pregnancy; a growth-restricted baby; reduced fetal movements; prolonged pre-term rupture of membranes; and the death of a baby.

Chapter 3 'Variations of pregnancy' explores decision making around the most common reasons for induction of labour: post dates and post term pregnancy. Associated reasons are discussed, including: 'advanced maternal age'; vaginal birth after caesarean; suspected big baby; multiple pregnancy; and pre-labour rupture of membranes after 37 weeks.

Starting with an explanation of the physiology of normal labour, subsequent chapters cover the processes involved in medical induction, alternative methods of induction and creating a birth plan for a medical induction.

Supporting a woman when birth is by caesarean

The support needed when a woman has a caesarean birth will be affected by whether this is planned (elective) or emergency surgery and, if it is elective surgery, whether this was in response to medical or obstetric concerns or maternal request. Whatever the reason for a woman having a caesarean birth, however, it is important to consider the support that *each individual* woman will need and how this support can be provided by *all* members of the maternity team, using woman centred approaches. Attending to a woman's probable anxiety and fear is vital, especially when we acknowledge the complex neuro-hormonal processes that are at play (Schmid and Downe, 2010). Ultimately, all members of the team need to remember the essence and significance of what is happening: this is a woman having a baby.

Supporting a woman when planning a caesarean birth

We discussed the debate about the implications of caesarean birth by maternal request in Chapter 3. In our experience, whether or not women have requested to give birth this way, they often have a lot of anxiety in the time immediately before having a planned caesarean:

> Suddenly they're confronted with the reality and inevitability of it all. Often they are having an elective because they've had a previous emergency caesarean, which was the saving grace at the end of a horrible labour and memories start crowding in. So I do talk about how many people will be in the theatre and suggest that they focus on the midwife and the anaesthetist because they are their link people.
>
> (Midwife, Leap, 2015, unpublished data)

For women, the number of people in theatre can feel overpowering and it may be useful when midwives describe in advance who will be in theatre, particularly if this is a couple's first experience of caesarean birth:

> I have a little 'operating theatre' set of Playmobil toy figures in scrubs complete with theatre equipment and I often use them with parents approaching caesarean section to explain who will be there in theatre and what their roles will be. You could also draw this on a piece of paper.
>
> (Midwife, Leap, 2015, unpublished data)

If you have the privilege of having continuity of care experiences with individual women as a student midwife, there is a lot you can do to support women who are planning to have a caesarean section, as this midwife reflects:

> I was a third-year year student midwife with a mini caseload and was assigned to a woman who was having a repeat caesarean – her first baby had died in utero. I was unhappy about the assumption that she would have another caesarean so I talked this through with my mentor. She encouraged me to help them prepare for the caesarean they were choosing. So I went with them to look around the unit, including theatre and recovery rooms. They said after they'd had their baby that it made a profound difference that I'd been with them all the way through to ease their anxiety – someone who was absolutely their named person. I could be emotionally there for them, even though I was at the bottom of the chain.
>
> (Midwife, Leap, 2015, unpublished data)

Box 8.14   Reflective Activity: Talking through what to expect in theatre

In threes:

- Using creative art forms – for example, toy models, buttons, sketching a picture or diagram – take it in turns to be the midwife (or other health practitioner) explaining to a woman and her partner who will be in theatre and what their roles will be, also what the major pieces of equipment will be for and where these will be placed.
- Alternatively, you might like to stage an imaginary visit to the labour ward and theatre, giving the same explanations.
- When everyone has had a turn at providing this information, discuss the phrases that worked well in terms of their potential to allay fear and anxiety.

Enabling choice and control around caesarean birth

In Chapter 5, we raised a note of caution about the concept of the 'natural caesarean section' (Newman and Hancock, 2009; Smith *et al.*, 2008) and the framing of it as woman centred. Leaving such philosophical concerns to one side, we think it is worth considering the techniques that are suggested in the article when planning a caesarean in all situations where the woman and her baby are healthy. There appears to be increasing awareness about the importance of enabling women and their partners to be actively involved in making choices about the sort of support they would like during and after a caesarean in order to greet their baby; for example: ambience (lighting, music, clothing); slow, gentle birthing with late cord-clamping allowing the baby to establish breathing physiologically; immediate skin-to-skin contact; minimal separation of mother and baby; and early breastfeeding (Walker and Bewley, 2019). For some parents this also includes: dropping the drape (or having a see-through drape) and tilting the bed so that they can watch the baby emerge and identify whether it is a boy or girl.

You may also come across parents who have watched the documentary *Microbirth* and who are concerned about the microbiological effects of caesarean birth on the immune system and potential epigenetic changes to the microbiome (Dahlen *et al.*, 2014; Jenkins *et al.*, 2019). In some cases this leads them to request 'vaginal seeding': transferring a swab from the mother's vagina and smearing the mucous around their baby's nose, mouth and skin, in order to stimulate microbiome development. Paediatricians and infection control experts have expressed concerns about this practice in terms of babies being exposed to severe infections and pathogens that the mother might carry asymptomatically. They recommend that the practice should not be performed; however, they note that, having been fully informed of the risks, if mothers choose to do vaginal seeding themselves, their autonomy should be respected. Promoting breastfeeding and the avoidance of unnecessary antibiotics are suggested as more important strategies to protect babies' developing microbiota (Cunnington *et al.*, 2016).

At the more unusual end of responding to women's requests, we know of situations where obstetricians have enabled a 'lotus birth' after a caesarean birth (leaving the cord uncut until it falls off, still attached to the placenta, a few days after birth); women request 'lotus birth' for a number of reasons, including seeing it as the ultimate way to conclude a physiological birth; to promote uninterrupted bonding and attachment; and as part of spiritual beliefs, allowing the baby to release the placenta when ready (Monroe *et al.*, 2019; Zinsser, 2016).

**Box 8.15   Reflective Activity: Planned caesarean birth –
exploring choices**

In pairs or small groups:

*   Brainstorm a list of choices that (in an ideal world) parents might make in plan-
    ning a caesarean birth – with individualised features for a safe and positive experi-
    ence for both their baby and themselves.
*   Individually, identify which items on this list you might like to plan for if you
    were having a caesarean birth yourself.
*   Discuss your choices in your pair/group and identify how you might overcome
    any potential barriers to enabling these choices. How many of these approaches
    could also be applied where an unplanned caesarean is needed?

Supporting a woman during a planned caesarean birth

However much a woman has prepared for a planned caesarean, she is likely to have many concerns. When she has chosen this way to have her baby she may have unspoken anxieties that she feels she should not express:

> It depends on the reason for the caesarean, but explanations are really important about what is happening. It's not just about asking questions. It's about really attentive lis-tening to what she's saying and picking up on what her angle is – because sometimes they'll say things that they think you want to hear, or things that they think they should say, but somewhere in there is the clue to what she's really thinking and how she feels about what is happening. As with all caesareans, it's about trying to work out what is absolutely quintessentially important to her.
>
> (Midwife, Leap, 2015, unpublished data)

This story describes beautifully how an elective caesarean birth can be an intimate event if women and their partners are supported to create the experience they want:

> This was their eighth baby; their last one had been an emergency caesarean and they decided to have another caesarean this time. You could see that the couple were really intimate, really close. He talked about the other children and how much they loved their kids and that's what their whole life is about, having the children. It was just beautiful, lots of skin-to-skin and he knew all about how important that was. They managed to create a feeling of intimacy, that this was a really extraordinary event, even though they were in an operating theatre with strangers.
>
> (Midwife, Leap, 2015, unpublished data)

Supporting a woman when an emergency caesarean birth is needed

When supporting women during labour, we are often aware that a caesarean is looking likely. This can pose dilemmas for us in terms of when to introduce the possibility and how to sup-port women who are scared about having a caesarean:

> Sometimes when it's looking inevitable, I mention the caesarean word – maybe earlier than other midwives might because I want almost to prepare them for when the doctor

mentions it because that will be the next thing. I think it can be so shocking for some people when they hadn't considered it.

I often say, 'They're really good at doing caesareans' because women usually find it really scary and say, 'I really don't want a caesarean.' I say that it will be quite quick and it will be the end point of having tried everything possible to birth the baby without having a caesarean. I tell her that she's done everything she could and that she will be having her baby in her arms quite soon.

Some women are really scared because they've had an epidural and it hasn't been working well and they're worried about the caesarean being done without that working properly. That's when I work closely with the anaesthetist to try and allay some of those fears.

The anaesthetists have a really important role. They're the ones who calm everything down, the main communicator with the woman during the caesarean. They do it very well in my experience. They explain to the woman what she might feel – I think a lot of women are shocked at how much they feel – 'the washing machine' thing. The anaesthetist is often also very lovely around the greeting of the baby.

(Midwife, Leap, 2015, unpublished data)

The importance of 'talking it through' after emergency caesarean birth

When women need to have an emergency caesarean there are particular communication challenges, as this midwife describes. She emphasises the importance of talking through the experience with the woman afterwards; even if, at the time it's not possible to explain the reasons in detail, this should certainly happen retrospectively:

> I think it's about supporting them to understand what is happening and why it's happening as much as you can through that very tense time when you're making the transfer to theatre and thereafter. Then going back afterwards and de-briefing, talking about why it happened and making sure they understand and giving them space to talk about how it was for them. You see if you can find anything that might be a doubt lurking there, something that they didn't really understand. Sometimes you have to push a little to enable women to tell you about those lurking doubts, they don't necessarily come straight out with them. 'Did I do something wrong . . .? Could anything else have been done . . .?' Almost like, 'Was it my fault?' I always try to get hold of the notes so that we can go over what happened.
>
> (Midwife, Leap, 2015, unpublished data)

Supporting a woman when an emergency occurs

Whenever a multi-professional team is providing care for a woman, it is essential that her support needs are foremost in everyone's minds. Particularly when there is an emergency, it is easy (and understandable) for the focus to shift to clinical care and the tasks that need to be completed quickly to ensure safety; all those caring for the woman, however, need to be highly tuned to how she may be feeling. The continuous presence of a supportive midwife can make a huge difference to the woman and her partner in the potentially frightening environment in which they find themselves, mainly through the midwife's reassuring presence but also through her role as interpreter, go-between, advocate and protector:

> I had a haemorrhage at home, and what was so wonderful was that I really felt that I trusted them completely, and we had to go into hospital but the midwives were just, from

standing back and being very empowering and enabling me to do what I needed to do to have my baby, they then went straight into action, and they dealt with the emergency. And I just lay there with my baby on my chest just feeling very relaxed and calm. They came with me to the hospital; one of them was with me all the way and visited me every day when I was there. And so I didn't feel traumatised by it at all. I kind of felt that they just supported me right the way through.

(Mother, Sandall *et al.*, 2010, unpublished data)

This midwife describes what she thinks is most important during an emergency:

The most important thing is to stay in their view – while they're getting their spinal or whether you're rushing along the corridor with them to get to theatre, you make a difference – because you're often the only person they know in the room. On the way there, I always talk about how many people are going to be there and prepare them for what they're going to see. And I try to protect them from any negative energy that we occasionally get from theatre staff. Sometimes they're just wonderful and understand that this is about the birth of a baby and something that a woman will remember vividly for the rest of her life. But some can be quite grumpy and treat it like just another operation. So you take the negativity and try not to let it get through to the woman or her partner.

Sometimes partners get sat down somewhere to wait while they all get ready and that can be hard because you need to be with the woman but you try to duck in and out to reassure the partner. It's about giving them every bit of information that you can because they're in a very alien environment usually and it's about being there for them to be scared or sad or whatever.

Afterwards, if the baby's well it's about doing everything in your power to keep the baby from being separated from them. Keeping the baby with the mother, ensuring skin-to-skin and early breastfeeding – all the Baby Friendly initiatives. Often the anaesthetists are really good at liaising with the theatre staff over those things, because they have more authority.

(Midwife, Leap, 2015, unpublished data)

The midwife can play a critical role in making the experience as positive as possible. Nicky has recently had a personal experience of observing this:

I was meant to be providing labour support for a family friend who was planning a home birth for her second baby – she'd had a home birth for her first baby and her mother had had six babies at home. So she was very confident about giving birth at home. She rang me at about 37 weeks to say she'd had a show. I asked about the blood loss and she said rather vaguely that it had filled a pad. So of course I said that she should go straight to hospital and that I would meet her there.

They were wonderful at the hospital. They gave her every chance before deciding they really had to do a caesarean; they waited to see if labour would progress fast so that she could push the baby out quickly. But that wasn't happening – there was more blood and the baby was getting a tachycardia and I was thinking, 'Oh please do a caesarean.' But the staff were fantastic. What I saw was amazing inter-professional working.

The midwife was young and so skilled, multitasking and maintaining really empathetic communication with the woman, and her partner but also managing to be calm and really clear with the junior doctor and then the consultant – it was phenomenal. The woman feels so lucky, even though it was a big shock. Everyone was great but it was the midwife who was really there for her. It made me think that, whether you're attending a normal birth or rushing along the corridor to theatre, how you are makes a difference to that woman's experience and how she remembers it forever.

Supporting a woman who is disappointed or traumatised by her experiences

It is possible for women to describe their complicated labours as positive and empowering, as suggested by obstetrician Amali Lokugamage in her book *The Heart in the Womb: An Exploration of the Roots of Human Love and Social Cohesion* (which we heartily recommend):

> Birth can be an empowering experience, and although a natural process may not always be possible due to specific circumstances, even to attempt it brings great richness to a woman's life.
>
> (Lokugamage, 2011, p.3)

Unfortunately, however, not all women feel enriched by their experiences. For many women whose birth experience is very different from the one that they hoped for, there is bitter disappointment and a feeling of loss. Sadly, some may also feel traumatised. These feelings are vividly described in the postscript to this chapter.

The research evidence suggests that feelings of trauma can have long-term effects and be experienced as post-traumatic stress disorder (PTSD) (Olde *et al.*, 2006). Women may be particularly at risk of developing PTSD when they feel they have no control over what is happening, when they lack support from their partner and when there have been negative interactions with staff (Olde *et al.*, 2006). While there are many aspects of an emergency or difficult birth that midwives will not be able to influence, there is certainly potential to find ways to ensure that women feel as much in control as possible, for example by consulting them whenever possible and giving every opportunity for them to be included in decision making. And it is *always* possible to ensure that interactions with maternity staff are supportive and positive:

> The care provided by midwives has the potential to shape women's experiences and (at best) buffer against adverse events or (at worst) form part of the trauma.
>
> (Ayers, 2013, p.147)

In an editorial for a special edition of *Midwifery* about fear of childbirth and postnatal PTSD, psychologist Susan Ayers argues that the focus should always be on prevention of PTSD rather than treatment. In other words, it is much better to prevent or minimise fear of childbirth and PTSD through changes to maternity care (Ayers, 2013). In recent years, Ayers (2017) has suggested that these changes should be informed by new understandings of resilience and post-traumatic growth, in order to identify ways to enhance women's capacity to adapt and thrive, as well as identifying risk factors.

There is some debate about how best to support women after a traumatic birth. Australian researchers Jenny Gamble and Debra Creedy have shown the benefits of counselling after traumatic birth (Gamble and Creedy, 2009; Gamble *et al.*, 2005) However, the 'debriefing' approach to support that was popular several years ago has been criticised as lacking a strong evidence base and also for being potentially damaging in unskilled hands (Ayers, 2013).

Ayers (2013) points to studies that show how women value the opportunity to discuss their experiences after the birth. The value of 'talking it through' is also evident in many of the stories we collected for this book. In particular, women who had experienced a complicated labour and birth described to us the critical role played by the midwife in helping them to understand what was happening and why, both at the time and after the event, as is shown in the next activity.

Box 8.16   Reflective Activity: Support for a breech birth –
**   Tanya's story**

In the following story, Tanya (not her real name) describes how she experienced the complications that resulted when her first baby was in a breech presentation:

> From 28 weeks my baby was breech. Late weeks of pregnancy became a terrain full of conflict and worry, with people I knew supporting me but telling me how brave I was in attempting to have a vaginal birth with a breech baby.
>
> I spent a couple of days experiencing latent labour on and off at home. This was the most challenging time, because we were post-dates and had to negotiate hard to stay at home for as long as possible.
>
> At 42 weeks we arrived at the hospital to be met by the most wonderful midwife. For the first time someone listened to what I wanted: to birth my baby myself rather than 'elect' for an unwanted caesarean. She treated me the same as everyone else. Finally I felt like someone understood why normal birth was so important to me.
>
> My doula was there all the way through, with my husband supporting me to be myself. My waters broke with meconium, but I knew it was OK, normal for breech; my midwife wasn't fazed at all, just kept inspiring me that I could do it, to follow my body.
>
> Pushing was hard work. I was so tired – tired from the long latent stage, tired from the antenatal fighting, tired from the vomiting, tired from the anxiety about whom we would 'get' when we arrived at the hospital.
>
> After 2 hours, I could reach down and touch him; he seemed so close to being here. I hadn't noticed the constant monitoring, but the doctors wanted to know what was going on. My midwife kept them behind the curtains, advocating for my wishes. I trusted her implicitly.
>
> After 3 hours of pushing and what I know now was a less than great trace, she gently broached the subject that things didn't seem to be progressing as would be expected. We discussed a caesarean, and she left us to have some space when I was overcome with disappointment and sadness that I wasn't going to get the birth I had envisaged.
>
> My midwife arranged for me to have my doula and husband in theatre. She had already stayed well beyond the end of her shift and so another midwife cared for us in theatre.

The following days in hospital she came in before her shift, sorting out my breakfast and sitting with me. I will never forget her extra attention after Alex [not his real name] was born; it made such a huge difference. I often wonder what it would have been like to have met her earlier in my pregnancy process.

In pairs:
- Read through the story aloud (take turns to read each paragraph) and then make a list of a) the positive and b) the negative words/phrases that Tanya uses to describe her experience.
- Discuss how you think, overall, Tanya will remember her birth experience.
- How might the support she received from her midwife, partner and doula have affected her experience?
- Read the reviews by Ayers (2013) and Olde *et al.* (2006), described above, and consider the factors that they identify which might contribute to, or prevent, childbirth trauma. You may also wish to read some of the papers that they include in their reviews and the research papers by Gamble and Creedy (2009) and Gamble *et al.* (2005).
- Compare the factors identified in the research reviews with the words you have identified from Tanya's story. Are there any similarities or differences? What can you conclude from this?
- What can you learn from this activity about providing care for women who are potentially distressed or traumatised by their experiences?

Supporting a woman with health concerns

The 2020 UK and Ireland Confidential Enquiries into maternal mortality, *Saving Lives, Improving Mothers' Care* (Knight *et al.*, 2020), found that, in 2016–2018, almost three-quarters of maternal deaths were to women who had pre-existing physical or mental health concerns. It is not surprising then that, for women with existing health concerns, pregnancy and birth may be a particularly anxious time, and there is much that midwives can do to support them as they navigate their way through appointments with obstetric and medical specialties. This is described by a woman whose midwife helped her to steer her way through the system, including going with her to medical appointments:

I was at the hospital nearly every week for an appointment, for outpatients' appointments, and so many scans. I had so much going on, and I think one of the big things that my midwife was able to do was to really sort of advocate for me. So to be able to speak to the consultants at the hospital, speak to the staff there. I'd voice it myself but just to be supportive in that process. And once he was born as well, I think, we were advised to do certain things, to give formula, to do all these things that we didn't really want to do, and then the midwife would come in and say, 'No, actually you don't have to do that, let's look at doing this, or let's look at doing that instead.' So they were able to give us more options, but also to advocate for us, which was really important. *Really* important.
(Mother, Sandall *et al.*, 2010, unpublished data)

Box 8.17   Reflective Activity: 'Pilots through stormy seas' – Carol's story

Carol (not her real name) has Type 1 diabetes. She describes her experiences of midwifery support when pregnant with her first baby:

> I'm diabetic and when I went to the midwives in early pregnancy, they were like, 'Yeah we'll take you on.' They were just like, 'You're a woman, you're pregnant, that's what we do.' And they didn't ever bat an eyelid about my condition, I'd been feeling so negative about it and they made me feel great, instantly, just by that acceptance of me. In fact what she said was, 'Oh we like a challenge.' [Laughs] It was just like, 'Oh great, I'm just a challenge, I'm not a problem, I'm something to be excited about', which was fantastic.
>
> On the Tuesday morning I would go to the hospital clinic and be told I had much more of a chance of having a dead baby being a diabetic mother and I would go to the midwives on the Tuesday afternoon and speak to whoever was on that day. And they would always make me feel so much more positive, they would sort of question with me, sort of deconstruct whatever the doctor had said with me, and so I would always leave there feeling much better.
>
> I just found the midwives incredibly empowering and they completely allowed me to have the birth that I wanted. . . . It could have ended up in a caesarean at 38 weeks, which is what the doctors were kind of moving towards, plus having preeclampsia in the end as well, and Group B strep [laughs]. And I still managed to have a natural birth, but I managed to stay at home for 40 hours of a 48-hour labour and just go in for the last bit, and yeah, had a natural birth, no drugs, and completely doctor-free, which is what I wanted, and it was fantastic.
>
> In labour I wanted to not have an IV drip and all the rest of it; I know how to control my own diabetes with my own insulin what-have-you, which I did, and I kept it at exactly the number that I said I would all the way through. So anyway, when he was born it was really important that he fed straightaway and they were just great in helping me with that. When the staff there wanted to give him formula the midwife was really supporting me in not doing that and she went up and got me some donated breast milk instead.
>
> We were in awe of their tact and diplomacy. They just literally would do this really delicate and subtle dance in advocating for us so no one ever felt bad. They're incredibly skilled at negotiating. I thought I was diplomatic but that's a new level, that. They're highly skilled at dealing with people. They don't just make you feel good they make everyone around them feel good.
>
> What was incredibly useful for me is that the midwives are very well informed. What I needed was someone I could trust but also that had a medical knowledge. It wasn't enough that I had my partner there and another friend of mine was there as well – they were there for me to support me emotionally – but I wanted someone who I could say, 'This doctor, what they're saying, does it make sense to you? Do you understand what he's saying?' You know, so if she said, 'Right, you need to have this intervention now', I could totally just trust her, you know. . . .

And I trusted her to trust me in making the right decisions as well, do you know what I mean? It was like this mutual, we trust each other, which I felt was really important. Yeah, that thing of knowing that they had not only the sort of spiritual and emotional knowledge but the medical oomph as well, they really know their stuff. . . . They're not just all frou-frou; they're hard core, they know their stuff, they've done their work, and they actually researched stuff about my condition when they didn't know about it, they looked into it and they came back with information. And I did research and showed them my stuff, they showed me what they had, and it felt like, OK, this is really great, we're doing this together. They really helped me with my research as well, which was like, that's just wonderful, really wonderful.

I wrote them a card afterwards and said it was like having sort of pilots through stormy seas, literally, I felt like I was being circled by these doctors, not that they're bad but I just felt like they were really pressuring me, because that's their model, it's a medical model, and they didn't see any of the more spiritual or more natural or more beautiful aspects of it, you know? And the midwives kind of kept that alive for me; they sort of allowed me to feel happy and healthy and like a pregnant woman rather than a diabetic freak that didn't deserve a proper birth, which is how I had felt, you know. But they made me feel like I did deserve a good birth and it would all be fine and I was perfectly normal, so yeah it was amazing. Really amazing.

(Mother, Sandall *et al.*, 2010, unpublished data)

In pairs or small groups:
- Discuss why Carol describes her pregnancy so positively.
- Use these points to write some guidance notes for midwives giving care and support for women with existing health concerns.

Supporting women who are considered 'high risk'

Carol's story is an example of how sensitive midwifery support can make a difference for women who are categorised as 'high risk' during their pregnancies. This may be their first experience of being classified as 'unhealthy'; not only will this be worrying for their own well-being and that of their baby, but it may also challenge their personal identity and self-image.

An important contemporary example of this is pregnant women who have a raised body mass index (BMI) and who are likely to be treated as 'high risk'. A systematic review showed that labour complications were more common in heavier women and could lead to more assisted and caesarean births (Heslehurst *et al.*, 2008). However, although there may be physiological reasons for increased complications, we should also not assume that a difficult labour is inevitable:

A large woman came in the other day and the midwives at the desk were all, you know, 'Might as well put your scrubs on now.' But she pushed her baby out so easily. I think it's really important not to have expectations that all large women will need a caesarean.

(Midwife, Leap, 2015, unpublished data)

Christine Furber and Linda McGowan (2011) conducted a qualitative study that explored how pregnant women who were obese felt about their care. Their study provides some important insights: women described how health professionals made value judgements about their size and stereotyped them as unfit, lazy and unable to control their eating. Women felt ignored, stigmatised and humiliated, and few choices were offered to them: a medicalised approach to care was automatic.

As highlighted during recruitment of overweight women to a group antenatal care scheme in Sydney, Australia, midwives are often anxious about how to raise the issue of women's weight without causing offence, particularly if women appear defensive or distressed (Davis *et al.*, 2012). Training in the use of motivational interviewing techniques was shown to increase the midwives' confidence in having enabling conversations in a way that helped women explore their desire for change and find their own solutions (Raymond and Clements, 2013).

Given the current 'obesity epidemic', it is likely that midwives will care for increasing numbers of women who are overweight when pregnant. It is important therefore that we consider the experiences and needs of such women so that we provide sensitive and tailored care. We also need to be self-aware, challenging ourselves and our colleagues when we are in danger of stereotyping or making assumptions.

The importance of interprofessional communication and cooperative working when women are considered 'high risk'

Supporting women who have been identified as being at 'higher risk' can test our skills of adaptability, interprofessional communication and negotiation:

> It's quite a challenge sometimes because you're sandwiched between knowing a normal outcome is less likely and keeping your medical colleagues at arm's length while you give things a little try.
>
> (Midwife, Leap, 2015, unpublished data)

However much experience we have, it can be challenging supporting women in labour who require a lot of technological assistance, particularly when we are working in an unfamiliar environment. The following story is an example of breaking down the hierarchical boundaries that can inhibit us in asking for help and working cooperatively:

> I was in a new role, developing midwifery models of care in an area health service and decided to do a shift on the labour ward of a large hospital. I was assigned to a woman having her first baby, who was in early labour. She had diabetes; she was on insulin; and she was being induced. She also had reduced fetal movements so it was all feeling rather urgent. She'd had no continuity so I'd never met her before.
>
> Her first words when I introduced myself were, 'Do what you like but I don't want any pain.' She was obviously incredibly fearful and she'd heard so much about things that could go wrong that she had no confidence at all. Her husband was very fearful too. He was almost trembling.
>
> The first thing I did was reassure her that there were lots of options open to her if that's what she wanted. And I sat with her for about 15 minutes and just let her talk about what she wanted to talk about – instead of talking about: 'The Induction', 'The Diabetes', 'The Epidural', 'The Risks to the Baby' etcetera [sic]. And while I was doing that I had my hand on her tummy and was able to get a sort of personal closeness through touch – I

did ask her first and she was very comfortable with me touching her. I turned the monitor right down so that we couldn't hear it – it was so distracting and it didn't need to dominate the room. You can so easily get into a situation where men – and midwives – concentrate on looking at the monitor and forget about being focussed on the woman.

I very soon realised that I was out of my depth with all the technology. It was a new hospital for me and I wasn't familiar with some of the machinery. We were about to get a third pump going. So after I'd got to know her a little bit I left the room and the first person to come down the corridor was a student midwife. And I said, 'Ooh, you'll know all about how to work these machines, come here, you're working with me today!' [laughter] She was a final-year student and was very familiar with all of it.

So we worked it out between us – that this is what we needed to think about. We went through all of the notes together so that we were really clear about what needed to happen. And I told her what I wasn't really good at. 'I need some help with the machinery. I understand exactly what it does, but I'm not familiar with it or the dosages.' Of course, we had to check all of that with a third midwife who was familiar with everything as this was a student.

So we were looking after each other a bit, me and the student. It was really good.

The woman had an epidural, predictably very quickly and far earlier than I would normally predict for someone who is in early labour. The student was turning up the Synto – it was, after all, an induction of labour. And the woman was very unhappy and in so much pain. And I said, 'Let's just turn the Synto off – even if it's just for half an hour while we get the epidural working.' The student was very worried about not going by the book. It can be so distracting to have those instructions: 'You will turn up the pump every so many minutes until she's contracting four in ten or whatever . . .'. That was the task and the student was totally taken up with it. She forgot to see that the woman wasn't actually coping with it and her pulse was racing; she was in a sweat and she was miserable.

I said, 'What we do is, we stop. We get the anaesthetist back. That's his skill to get it working well. And we'll get the Synto working when the epidural is working properly.' She was really impressed by that! 'You can really do that?' So I learnt something and the student learnt something and the woman felt heard – which was really important to her. She was listened to and nobody did anything without checking out with her how she was feeling at the time.

The partner was predictably fascinated with all the things that went ping in the room but he actually took his cue from the way we were really focussed on the woman. Sometimes partners get distracted by the things we're distracted by. When we calm everything down, then we can be dealing with all the other stuff, like focussing on the woman and thinking about everything that's going on and what sort of support we should be giving her – and her partner.

She did have a lovely birth. Everything was good about it, especially given her particular circumstances.

(Midwife, Leap, 2015, unpublished data)

Supporting a woman whose baby needs medical care

Women who have complicated labours often give birth to babies needing medical care and admission to the neonatal unit (NNU). In these situations, a woman's existing anxieties and fears will be exacerbated. Her partner, family and close friends may also be very distressed and need a lot of support.

Women still need midwifery support when the baby's care has been transferred to the neonatal team. This support may be particularly crucial if the baby needs to be resuscitated and is taken to the NNU very quickly. The midwife's support can take the form of explaining what is happening, being a 'go-between', interpreting what the neonatologists are saying and ensuring that the parents understand, or simply just 'being there' and listening. This can be a challenging situation for the midwife, particularly if the baby's condition is poor. There is a fine line to tread between being over-reassuring ('I'm sure everything will be just fine') and being realistically supportive, as in the following story:

> It was all so frightening. Suddenly there were lots of people in the room, all doing things to my baby. Everyone was over by the resuscitation machine. There was lots of activity but no one was saying anything to me. And there was that awful silence . . . my baby wasn't crying, not a peep. Except the midwife, she was still right by me, and she just squeezed my hand and said 'He's having a tough time with his breathing, but they're very skilled. Come on little one'. Afterwards – when he was fine but up in the neonatal unit – I thought, 'I'm glad that she didn't just say, "Don't worry, he'll be okay".' I wouldn't have believed her given the worry on the doctors' faces. She just kept squeezing my hand and I felt that we were all willing him to be okay. And the lovely thing was that she came up to see me on the ward a few times, and even came to see the baby with me. I thought that was lovely, it meant a lot that she remembered and cared enough to come and spend time with us.
>
> (Mother, Hunter, 2015, unpublished data)

There is an extensive body of literature relating to the experiences of parents whose babies are ill and admitted to the NNU, and it is not possible to do justice to this evidence in a few sentences. But, to summarise briefly: studies show that mothers may feel frightened, guilty, isolated and confused (Turrill and Crathern, 2010). They also experience a sense of grief and loss that they have not given birth to the perfect baby as they expected and that their 'real' baby needs specialist care from the experts on NNU rather than its parents (Fenwick *et al.*, 2000, 2008; Lupton and Fenwick, 2001). It is known that levels of postnatal depression and PTSD can be relatively high in these mothers (Aagard and Hall, 2008). Clearly, support from midwives and NNU staff is vital to enable parents to talk through these feelings, as well as more specialist psychological support if needed.

Supporting a woman whose baby has died

Supporting a woman who has been told that her baby is not going to live or whose baby has already died is immensely challenging for all concerned (Kenworthy and Kirkham, 2011). The dreadful paradox of death where there should be new life triggers profound emotions, and we can often feel at a complete loss as to how best to provide support for a woman who is deeply shocked and has only just begun to grieve.

The following story challenges us not to make assumptions about what women need at this time, but to listen to what women tell us they need, even if this is uncomfortable for us or challenges what we think is best practice. For example, women may not need to be protected from their emotional and physical pain, but be supported to experience this. What stands out in this story is the importance of support.

Box 8.18   The birth of Ella

When I was 20 weeks' pregnant I realised that my baby was no longer moving. My midwife couldn't hear a heartbeat and I was sent for an ultrasound that confirmed my baby had died. Looking back, I was in a state of shock, quite numb and just focused on what needed to be done practically.

I'd been planning a home birth, having a lovely birth at home with no pain relief as I'd done three years before. But I'd felt very ill during this pregnancy, unlike the earlier one and actually I think I knew deep down that something wasn't right. So even though I was so upset about the baby, on some level perhaps I was prepared. What I wasn't prepared for was that my labour and birth would need to be induced. And I also wasn't prepared for the responses of some of those around me.

What stands out for me now, many years later, was the importance of support and feeling that my wishes were really being listened to. There was an assumption from many midwives and doctors that I would want to have strong pain relief to protect me from the physical – but mostly the emotional – pain. But I didn't want that at all. This was still my birth; even though it would be the birth of a baby who had died half way through my pregnancy, she was still my baby and I wanted to experience the whole event as much as if all had been well. This really troubled the staff. 'This is so hard for you – why put yourself through any more pain?' Luckily there was one wonderful midwife who really listened and got what I was saying. And also my partner and a close friend were with me – really with me – backing me up.

I coped with the pains the same as with my first birth – moving around, rocking, focusing on my breathing. When the baby was born she just slithered out; she was so tiny.

The midwife behaved like she would have done at any birth. What I remember now was how gently she talked to the baby, how she wrapped her up so tenderly and then showed me and my partner all the perfect things about her. In fact she had multiple abnormalities and it must have needed a lot of quick thinking and empathy to do that.

Her approach made such a difference to me afterwards. Not only how she behaved with the baby but also how she respected my wishes and didn't try to protect me or do that 'I'm the expert, I know best' thing. She was really with me, saying, 'Yes you can do this'. She also encouraged us to cuddle the baby, take photos and plan a funeral.

Even though it is sad to remember the birth of Ella, the baby who never really was, I wasn't left with a huge grief. I think being able to really engage with the toughness of the event, and having such sensitive support, helped me to make some sense of it and integrate her birth into who I am.

Supporting a woman whose baby is removed into the care of social services

Women will also experience a sense of huge grief and loss if their baby is removed into the care of social services because of concerns that the baby will be at risk of serious harm in the home of its parent(s) or carer(s). Although there are many differences between these women's experiences and those of a woman whose baby has died, there are also many similarities.

Supporting a woman who has been told that her baby will be removed is also challenging for the staff who are involved. This is not how things should turn out, and we can struggle with knowing how best to provide support.

Box 8.19   Research Briefing: Mothers and midwives' experiences of compulsory removal of babies at birth

Marsh, W., Robinson, A. and Shawe, J. (2015). Mothers' experiences of compulsory removal of babies at birth: a review of the evidence. Part 1. *MIDIRS Midwifery Digest, 25*(3), 341–346.

Everitt, L., Fenwick, J. and Homer, C. (2015). Midwives experiences of removal of a newborn baby in New South Wales, Australia: being in the 'head' and 'heart' space. *Women and Birth, 28*, 95–100.

When there is compulsory removal of a baby, planning can be crucial as this midwifery manager suggests:

> What we try to do antenatally is to have a plan around how it is going to happen. We always try to make a plan for the woman to give the baby up rather than have it taken from her. Giving a baby up is like breaking your arms off, but actually when they decide they are ready, the midwife can make a phone call to the social worker to say, 'She's come to a place where she's ready.' The grief is still as raw, but in a way, the woman has the power to give her baby up, rather than the powerlessness of having it taken from her.

A midwife who works with women in prison describes how hard it is supporting women during labour when they know that their baby is going to be removed:

> There's a lot of grief in the labours. These women cry a lot and there's so much emotion that is nothing to do with pain in labour. Pain in labour is almost nothing; it's nothing to them. They hardly ever have pain relief. It's like the labour has become secondary to the loss of their baby. So you see a very raw grief and emotion. Not just crying, but howling – big cries straight from the heart.
>
> It has felt slightly better recently as we've started expressing breast milk and sending that out into the community for babies placed with foster carers or babies who are in the neonatal unit – the women really latch onto that one because that's a form of parenting that they can do.

In a filmed interview for a learning resource (Australian Centre for Child Protection, 2010), Margaret, a nurse and social worker, acknowledges the ambiguity and distress that staff may experience in these circumstances. She discusses the importance of acknowledging the parents' grief and provides some practical suggestions for supporting them in the same way that we would support any parents facing the loss of a baby.

Box 8.20   Supporting a woman when her baby is taken into care

From my own experience of being on maternity wards when a baby is removed, staff often don't know how to react to this. They've often been the ones that have made the notifications, so there's a sense of fear about how the parent might react to them. There can be a sense of guilt that, 'I've brought this upon this person, even though, professionally and morally I've had to'. But still feeling, 'Could there have been another way?' I suppose one way of handling it is to avoid it and let the social workers deal with it but often the parent has had the relationship with the midwives because they're the ones that are there 24 hours a day.

What we do know is that where grief of a patient is handled well, then nursing staff have a sense that they've achieved something. If we look at palliative care, a good death is a good death for the staff too if they've been able to provide the care that they wanted to provide. And I think the same with these parents. It's about being able to understand, being able to deal with your own feelings in it. So I think that, when a child is removed by child protection, particularly after birth, then staff need to talk about how they feel about that.

My experience is that what parents find hardest is where people are not understanding that they're hurting. And so for someone just to acknowledge and to be empathetic that this is really tough and that this is really painful is all the parent needs to hear.

We've become so much more sensitive to issues around mothers who have a miscarriage, a stillborn child, a child who dies after birth. We've become much better at that but there's a group of parents who have their children removed and their grief is just not even acknowledged. It's as if, because they're a bad parent or a neglectful parent, their grief is not as legitimate as the grief of a parent who loses their child in some other way. And what we see particularly in this group of parents is there's the unresolved ongoing grief that sits with these women and has an effect on their mental health. It's those things we need to acknowledge in this group – they hurt just as much as a parent whose child has died. These parents need to have their grief issues looked at in that context, just as sensitively as we would with other parents.

Do what you would do with another parent who's had a loss. Take some photos of them and their baby before the child is removed. When they are coming to remove the baby from the hospital, have it planned so that it doesn't become a situation where we have to have security guards around. Perhaps discharge the mother before the baby's discharged. Allow the parents and their extended family to be able to say goodbye. Allow the mother to be able to dress the baby in whatever she wants the baby to be dressed in to leave the hospital. Offer things such as the nightie that the baby has been in so that the mother can take that with her. Make sure that the cards from the top of the crib are given to the parents, that they do have photos. Some of those things can be for staff a way of entering in to what's happening and doing that in an empathetic way.

It's all of those things that midwives and nurses have been taught how to do with a parent who loses a child. This is a loss. It's a different kind of loss but it's a loss. So it's respecting the loss, acknowledging the loss, ritualising the loss, which is very important. So rather than avoiding that confrontation, it's important to enter into that grief as we would with any other mother. And to do all of those rituals that are really important.

Box 8.21   **Reflective Activity: Supporting women around the loss of a baby**

In pairs:
- Read aloud the accounts in Box 8.18 and Box 8.20 and then discuss:

  - What can a midwife *do* to best support women at such a difficult time?
  - How should a midwife *be* to best support women at such a difficult time?
  - What have you learnt from this activity that will inform your practice?

This chapter ends with a postscript, which tells a birth story of profound disappointment and sadness. Laura's story is a thought-provoking and fitting end to this chapter, as it vividly illustrates many of the issues that we have discussed and shows how crucial it is to provide support to women who are experiencing complications in their labour. It is also a story of how healing eventually happened with the support of a midwife. In addition, it also helps us to think about what was going on for the midwives, obstetricians and anaesthetists in a highly charged atmosphere, as they were faced with her requests to do things differently. This sets the scene for the next chapter, which is about the emotional work of supporting women for labour and birth.

Postscript: redeeming birth – Laura's* story

When James was 40 days old, I dreamt his birth anew and oh how lovely and light it was. I sat on the golden wooden floor in front of the fire with my legs apart and with one delicious contraction James slid out of me with ease. I picked him up from the floor and all was well. Just as I had always imagined it.

But James wasn't born by fire shine in our warm and lovely living room as we had intended, as I will tell.

Early labour at home

The birth started off so beautifully, the whole Wednesday and half the night was wonderful. In the evening a community midwife came – she was wonderful. She gave us space but also encouraged and praised me.

But then all my fears became true. At midnight she examined me, I was 6cm dilated but I was bleeding. When I saw the red glove I knew that this was the end of my homebirth. Inside me I knew that I was not bleeding dangerously but naturally the midwife could not allow us to stay.

Going to hospital

Going to hospital meant that I had to meet my greatest fears. I am a nurse and fear to be a patient. It was a struggle in hospital because I did not want to be there and the hospital midwife could not acknowledge that. She also could not understand that I did not want any pain relief and repeatedly said: 'I don't know how you manage without pain relief'.

I love the waves. I would breathe out making deep long and loving sounds and as long as I was fully concentrated I could ride the waves beautifully. The bleeding was indeed nothing to worry about and I went into the birthing pool – wonderful.

But the communication was difficult between the midwives and me, I felt so disturbed by them.

The waves became bigger and longer – I loved them and I thought I am safe you can't reach me here. My husband Robert was my blessing in gently supporting me.

In the early morning hours the midwife measured my blood pressure and pulse. My pulse was racing at 130 beats per minute. I didn't feel so well either, and the midwife started blaming me for being so uncooperative. I got out of the bath onto the bed, and the doctor came and re-examined me. The baby was fine but I was still 6cm; after nine hours I hadn't opened further. I was devastated and all my energy left me. I felt so sad, so disappointed with myself.

Agreeing to an epidural

I agreed to an epidural which, since starting my nursing training I feared more than a nightmare. I was hopeful that with some sleep I would have the strength to carry on. The anaesthetist came and I liked her, she was kind and gentle. She was also good because it worked just as it should. The baby was fine, Robert was sad and exhausted, and I fell asleep.

The wonderful obstetrician

I was woken by a new midwife, who told me that the baby's heart was tired. During the sleep I had dilated to 8cm but because of the baby's heart they urged me to have a caesarean. I was defeated and sad; how I had longed to belong to the circle of women who can give birth naturally.

Mr Z., the consultant, came in and examined me. He was wonderful and kind, he smiled and told me that he had been in the same situation with his wife when their first child was born. He told me the different options and he listened to my wishes of how I wanted the caesarean to be done if it had to be. I wanted to be re-examined just before the operation and, if it still was necessary for the caesarean, that I wanted to see what was happening – no screen between me and the surgeon – and then have the baby given to me on my chest straight away with the cord and placenta still attached. He said he had never done it that way, and he was unsure if it was a safe way but he said he would give it a try. I asked him: 'Will you really try or just pretend to try?' He smiled and said 'No I will really try'.

After our conversation Mr Z. examined me and said that I was 8cm dilated and that he would be happy to increase the strength of my contractions with hormones and see if that would help the labour. The hormones worked immediately but the baby showed signs of distress so he stopped it. He told me that his shift ended now and that he couldn't do the operation himself; however, he would tell his colleague about my wishes.

The arrogant obstetrician

Oh and I had to battle so hard with the other surgeon who was as arrogant as the other was kind. I told him my wishes but he didn't listen and told me that this was impossible before even considering it. He turned to one of the anaesthetists and said: 'You wouldn't allow it, would you? It wouldn't be safe for you with all the blood spluttering, would it?' It made me feel like a child that has been lied to.

One anaesthetist said: 'You have come here seeking help. You now can't dictate to the doctors how to help you.' Robert replied: 'In some countries patients might not have any rights, but in England patients do have rights'. The anaesthetist didn't object any more.

I looked the surgeon in his eyes and said: 'I do not trust you'. He said: 'Why don't you trust me!' I replied: 'I do not need to be able to explain my feelings; all I can tell you is that I do not trust you'. He then said: 'But then I can't do the operation – but it won't be easy to find another surgeon'. I asked the surgeon to give me his hand and to tell me his name. He answered: 'Howard, you can call me Howard'. I could sense that the other doctors were surprised.

We found a compromise, which was that he would re-examine me just before the operation and that he would leave the umbilical cord attached as long as possible.

At the end of our conversation I was at peace with the idea that he would be my surgeon. All along I was inwardly saying like a mantra: 'I open myself wide'. It was strange on the one hand praying to relax and release, and on the other hand to demand to be heard and not let my power be taken away, but it was possible!

In the theatre he re-examined me and I was fully dilated. However the baby's head was in the wrong position and he tried with forceps to correct it while the midwife told me when to push. In that moment, by angel hand, the lovely surgeon Mr Z. came back and he tried as well but with no success. I trusted him completely and when he told me that it wasn't safe any longer, it wasn't difficult to consent to the operation. I asked him if he could be the surgeon and he agreed.

A caesarean on my terms

The anaesthetists put up the screen even though I asked them not to. One of them said in a condescending and forceful manner that because of health and safety and infection control it had to be done. But Mr Z. told the anaesthetists in a calm and friendly manner: 'No, no, I have discussed this with her, there is no screen'. Without further argument the screen was put down. I was happy. It seemed to me that a wonderful little miracle had come true that Mr Z. would be my surgeon and the first to touch my baby. I felt safe.

The cut was made and I could see my baby lifted out of my belly and put straight on to my chest. I was flooded by happiness and love. It was wonderful to touch my baby wet and creamy skin with my hands. I couldn't help but love him. The cord was eventually clamped and after I was stitched up the cord was cut by Robert. James cried a little but just a little. He was still on my chest and only given to Robert when I was ready to be transferred to my bed. Back in the labour ward James drank for the first time from my breast. He drank for one sweet hour.

We left the hospital as soon as James and I had been given the all clear. Finally I was back where I most longed to be: Home.

As you can see, James's birth was not easy but it definitely had its blessings. I faced my fears and I grew strong like a lioness, nonetheless I am still sad that my wish of a homebirth was not granted. What was hard was that I felt excluded from the mothers where a natural birth is portrayed as, 'If you only are committed enough, you can do it'.

A year on

A year later I had a dream: I was telling a woman James's birth story and she told me that she could help me heal that great sadness. I woke up with bewilderment – did 'great sadness' truly express my feelings about James's birth? After all he was now a gorgeous, healthy boy and some time had passed. I had to admit to myself: yes indeed I still felt this great sense of sadness. I had tried many things and talked to many people to help me come to terms with the birth but the feelings presided against everyone's advice.

I asked a birth story midwife, Sue, if she could do a session with me about James's birth. Sue had requested my maternity notes and had read them as well as my personal story of events. She asked me how I felt about the birth now. I had mixed feelings: I was proud that I hadn't given away my power to the midwives and doctors but l also felt I had failed; I was ashamed that I had not been able to birth my baby.

Sue and I went through the notes together and I gained another perspective: through the many hours of labour James's head had never descended into my pelvis even though he was in a good position. Reading these facts and seeing an objective account, I was finally at peace. My inner judge changed the verdict from guilty to INNOCENT!

I also could understand the midwife, who had found it so difficult to gain my trust, and how difficult that night had been for her. How she lacked support from the Midwifery Sister who pressured her to follow the protocol, which did not meet my needs of being trusted and left in peace.

Now that I have seen the notes, my questions have been answered, the journey feels complete. It feels like the emotional room of my mind, which is inhabited by James's birth, is no longer a mess. I am free – I am innocent and just a little sad.

Birth memories are powerful but knowing the facts of the birth stories is redeeming. Please give those who try with all their heart's might and fall short of this sweet aim also a place of healing – a star with a scar.

* Note: All names have been changed in this account.

References

Aagard, H. and Hall, E.O.C. (2008). Mothers' experiences of having a preterm infant in the neonatal care unit: a meta-synthesis. *Journal of Paediatric Nursing, 23(3)*, e26–e36.

Akuamoah-Boateng, J. and Spencer, R. (2018). Woman-centered care: women's experiences and perceptions of induction of labor for uncomplicated post-term pregnancy: a systematic review of qualitative evidence. *Midwifery, 67*, 46–56.

Australian Centre for Child Protection. (2010). Nurturing and protecting children: a public health approach. A learning resource for midwives and child and family health nurses. In N. Leap, C. Fowler and C.S.E. Homer (eds). Adelaide: University of South Australia.

Ayers, S. (2013). Fear of childbirth, postnatal post-traumatic stress disorder and midwifery care. *Midwifery, 30*, 145–148.

Ayers, S. (2017). Birth trauma and post-traumatic stress disorder: the importance of risk and resilience. *Journal of Reproductive and Infant Psychology, 35(5)*, 427–430.

Berg, M. (2005). A midwifery model of care for childbearing women at high risk: genuine caring in caring for the genuine. *Journal of Perinatal Education, 14(1)*, 9–21.

Berg, M. and Dahlberg, K. (1998). A phenomenological study of women's experiences of complicated childbirth. *Midwifery, 14*, 23–29.

Brodie, P. and Leap, N. (2008). From ideal to real: the interface between birth territory and the maternity service organisation. Chapter 10 in K. Fahy, M. Foureur and C. Hastie (eds), *Birth Territory and Midwifery Guardianship*. Edinburgh: Butterworth Heinemann/Elsevier.

Carter, S., Channon, A. and Berrington, A. (2020). Socioeconomic risk factors for labour induction in the United Kingdom. *BMC Pregnancy & Childbirth, 20*, 146.

Coates, R., Cupples, G., Scamell, A. and McCourt, C. (2019). Women's experiences of induction of labour: qualitative systematic review and thematic synthesis. *Midwifery, 69*, 17–28.

Coates, D., Makris, A., Catling, C., Henry, A., Scarf, V., Watts, N., . . . Homer, C. (2020). A systematic scoping review of clinical indications for induction of labour. *PLoS ONE, 15(1)*, e0228196.

Cunnington, A.J., Sim, K., Deierl, A., Kroll, J.S., Brannigan, E. and Darby, J. (2016). 'Vaginal seeding' of infants born by caesarean section. How should health professionals engage with this increasingly popular but unproved practice? *BMJ, 352*, i227–i227.

Cyna A.M. (2019). The Laurs of hypnotic communication and the 'lived in imagination' technique in medical practice. *International Journal of Clinical and Experimental Hypnosis, 67(3)*, 247–261.

Dahlen, H.G., Downe, S., Kennedy, H.P. and Foureur, M. (2014). Is society being reshaped on a micro-biological and epigenetic level by the way women give birth? *Midwifery*, 1149–1151.

Davis D.L., Raymond J.E., Clements V., Adams C., Mollart L.J., Teate, A. and Foureur, M.J. (2012). Addressing obesity in pregnancy: the design and feasibility of an innovative intervention in NSW, Australia. *Women and Birth*, 25, 174–180.

Everitt, L., Fenwick, J. and Homer, C. (2015). Midwives experiences of removal of a newborn baby in New South Wales, Australia: being in the 'head' and 'heart' space. *Women and Birth*, 28, 95–100.

Fenwick, J., Barclay, L. and Schmied, V. (2000). Interactions in neonatal nurseries: women's perceptions of nurses and nursing. *Journal of Neonatal Nursing*, 6(6), 197–203.

Fenwick, J., Barclay, L. and Schmied, V. (2008). Craving closeness: a grounded theory analysis of women's experiences of mothering in the special care nursery. *Women and Birth*, 21(2), 71–85.

Fox, D., Maude, R., Coddington, R., Woodworth, R., Scarf, V., Watson, K. and Foureur, M. (2021). The use of continuous foetal monitoring technologies that enable mobility in labour for women with complex pregnancies: a survey of Australian and New Zealand hospitals. *Midwifery*, 93, 102887.

Furber, C.M. and McGowan L. (2011). A qualitative study of the experiences of women who are obese and pregnant in the UK. *Midwifery*, 27, 437–444.

Gamble, J. and Creedy, D.K. (2009). A counselling model for postpartum women after distressing birth experiences. *Midwifery*, 25, e21–e30.

Gamble, J., Creedy, D.K, Moyle, W., Webster, J., McAllister, M. and Dickson, P. (2005). Effectiveness of a counseling intervention after a traumatic childbirth: a randomized controlled trial. *Birth*, 32(1), 11–19.

Heslehurst, N., Simpson, L., Ells, J., Rankin, J., Wilkinson, J., Lang, R. . . . Summerbell, C.D. (2008). The impact of maternal BMI on pregnancy outcomes with immediate short-term obstetric resource implications: a meta-analysis. *Obesity*, 9, 635–683.

Hunter, B. (2002). Emotion work in midwifery: an ethnographic study of the emotional work undertaken by a sample of student and qualified midwives in Wales. Unpublished Ph.D. University of Wales, Swansea.

Hunter, B. (2015, unpublished data). Identifying the experiences of receiving and providing support in labour.

Hunter, B. and Segrott, J. (2014). Renegotiating interprofessional boundaries in maternity care: implementing a clinical pathway for normal labour. *Sociology of Health & Illness*, 36(5), 719–737.

Jay, A. and Thomas, H. (2018). Induction of labour: how do women get information and make decisions? Findings of a qualitative study. *British Journal of Midwifery*, 26(1), 22–29.

Jenkins, H.J. and Hyde, M.J. (2019). The microbiome relating to labour and birth. Chapter 14 in S. Downe and S. Byrom (eds), *Squaring the Circle: Normal Birth Research, Theory and Practice in a Technological Age* (pp. 171–179). London: Pinter & Martin.

Keedle, H., Peters, L., Schmied, V., Burns, E., Keedle, W. and Dahlen, H.G. (2020). Women's experiences of planning a vaginal birth after caesarean in different models of maternity care in Australia. *BMC Pregnancy & Childbirth*, 381.

Keedle, H., Schmied, V., Burns, E. and Dahlen, H.G. (2019). A narrative analysis of women's experiences of planning a vaginal birth after caesarean (VBAC) in Australia using critical feminist theory. *BMC Pregnancy Childbirth*, 19, 142.

Kenworthy, D. and Kirkham, M. (2011). *Midwives Coping with Loss and Grief*. London: Radcliffe Publishing.

Knight, M., Bunch, K., Tuffnell, D., Shakespeare, J., Kotnis, R., Kenyon, S. *et al.* (eds). (2020). *Saving Lives, Improving Mothers' Care – Lessons Learned to Inform Maternity Care from the UK and Ireland Confidential Enquiries into Maternal Deaths and Morbidity 2016–18*. Oxford: National Perinatal Epidemiology Unit, University of Oxford.

Leap, N. (2015, unpublished data). Identifying the experiences of receiving and providing support in labour.

Leap, N. and Edwards, N. (2006). The politics of involving women in decision making. Chapter 5 in L.A. Page and R. Campbell (eds), *The New Midwifery: Science and Sensitivity in Practice*, 2nd edn. London: Churchill Livingstone/Elsevier.

Lokugamage, A. (2011). *The Heart in the Womb: An Exploration of the Roots of Human Love and Social Cohesion*. London: Docamali.

Lou, S., Hvidman, L., Uldbjerg, N., Lone Neumann, L., Jensen, T.F., Haben, J-K. and Carstensen, K. (2019). Women's experiences of post term induction of labour: a systematic review of qualitative studies. *Birth*, *46*, 400–410.

Lupton, D. and Fenwick, J. (2001). 'They've forgotten that I'm the mum': constructing and practising motherhood in special care nurseries. *Social Science and Medicine*, *53(8)*, 1011–1021.

Marsh, W., Robinson, A. and Shawe, J. (2015). Mothers' experiences of compulsory removal of babies at birth: a review of the evidence. Part 1. *MIDIRS Midwifery Digest*, *25(3)*, 341–346.

McKenna, J.A. and Symon, A.G. (2014). Water VBAC: exploring a new frontier for women's autonomy. *Midwifery*, *30*, e20–e25.

Monroe, K.K., Rubin, A., Mychaliska, K.P., Skoczylas, M. and Burrows, H.L. (2019). Lotus Birth: A Case Series Report on Umbilical Nonseverance. *Clinical Pediatrics*, *58(1)*, 88–94.

Newman, L. and Hancock, H. (2009). How natural can major surgery really be? A critique of 'the natural caesarean' technique. *Birth*, *36(2)*, 168–170.

Newnham, E., McKellar, L. and Pincombe, J. (2015). Documenting risk: a comparison of policy and information pamphlets for using epidural or water in labour. *Women and Birth*, *28*, 221–227.

NICE. (2008). *Inducing Labour. Clinical Guideline [CG70]*. www.nice.org.uk/guidance/cg70.

Olde, E., van der Hart, O., Kleber, R. and van Son, M. (2006). Post traumatic stress following childbirth: a review. *Clinical Pschology Review*, *2(1)*, 1–16.

Raymond J., and Clements, V. (2013). Motivational interviewing for midwives: creating 'enabling' conversations with women. *MIDIRS Midwifery Digest*, *23(4)*, 435–440.

RCM. (2019). *RCM Blue Top Midwifery Guidance (No 2). Midwifery Care for Induction of Labour*. London: Royal College of Midwives. https://www.rcm.org.uk/media/3552/midwifery-care-for-induction-of-labour-a4-2019-16pp_2.pdf.

Reed, R. (2018). *Why Induction Matters*. London: Pinter & Martin.

Sandall, J., Leap, N., Grant, J. and Bastos, M.H. (2010). Supporting women to have a normal birth: development and field testing of a learning package for maternity staff. Health and Social Care Research Division, King's College London.

Schmid, V. and Downe, S. (2010). Midwifery skills for normalising unusual labours. Chapter 10 in D. Walsh and S. Downe (eds), *Essential Midwifery Practice: Intrapartum Care* (pp.159–190). Chichester: Wiley-Blackwell.

Schwarz, C., Gross, M.M., Heusser, P. and Berge, B. (2016). Women's perceptions of induction of labour outcomes: results of an online-survey in Germany. *Midwifery*, *35*, 3–10.

Seibold, C., Licqurish, S., Rolls, C. and Hopkins, F. (2010). 'Lending the space': midwives perceptions of birth space and clinical risk management. *Midwifery*, *26*, 526–531.

Seijmonsbergen-Schermers, A.E., Scherjon, S. and de Jonge, A. (2019). BJOG debate. Induction of labour should be offered to all women at term. AGAINST: induction should not be offered to all women at term: first, do no harm. *BJOG*, *126(13)*, 1599–1599.

Small, K.A., Sidebotham, M., Fenwick, J. and Gamble, J. (2020). Intrapartum cardiotocograph monitoring and perinatal outcomes for women at risk: literature review. *Women and Birth*, *33*, 411–418.

Smith, J., Plaat, F. and Fisk, N.M. (2008). The natural caesarean: a woman-centred technique. *British Journal of Obstetrics and Gynaecology*, *115*, 1037–1042.

Turrill, S.C. and Crathern, L. (2010). Families in NICU. In G. Boxwell (ed.), *Neonatal Intensive Care Nursing*. London: Routledge.

Walker, S. and Bewley, S. (2019). Optimising physiological birth for women and babies with complex needs. Chapter 22 in S. Downe and S. Byrom (eds), *Squaring the Circle: Normal Birth Research, Theory and Practice in a Technological Age* (pp. 269–278). London: Pinter & Martin.

Watson, K., Mills, T.A. and Lavender, T. (2018). The use of telemetry in labour: results of a national online survey of UK maternity units. *British Journal of Midwifery*, *26*, 14–19.

Wickham, S. (2005). Language of the complicated. *Practising Midwife*, *8(9)*, 33.

Wickham, S. (2018). The language of the complicated. Retrieved from: https://www.sarawickham.com/articles-2/the-language-of-the-complicated/.

Zinsser, L.A., Stoll, K. and Gross, M.M. (2016). Midwives' attitudes towards supporting normal labour and birth – a cross-sectional study in South Germany. *Midwifery*, *39*, 98–102.

9 Emotions and labour support

Introduction

As we have discussed throughout the preceding chapters, it is essential to recognise and respond to the emotional needs of women and their birth supporters. What is often neglected, though, is the emotional effect of caregiving on the carers. As we shall see, these emotional effects are very important, not only for our personal wellbeing, but also because they may have a knock-on effect on our practice and the quality of care we provide. How well we are able to recognise, interpret, express and manage the emotions of ourselves and others is critical to giving good care. It is also critical to our own experiences of working life.

We begin this chapter by setting the scene in relation to emotions and labour support, before explaining theoretical perspectives about how emotions are experienced and managed in the workplace (known as emotion work or emotional labour). We then briefly describe the research evidence that relates to the emotion work of healthcare practitioners in general, before focusing on the evidence relating to maternity care.

Based on our own experiences and research, and from talking with other midwives, women and their birth supporters, we understand that labour and birth are intense times of huge emotional upheaval and that this emotional turbulence inevitably affects those who are caring for women. To illustrate this, in the second part of the chapter we draw on evidence from midwives, which vividly demonstrates how supporting women through labour and birth can make us *feel*. In the final part of the chapter, we explore some of the strategies and resources that may help us manage the emotional aspects of our work.

The emotional aspects of labour support

The words in Box 9.1 were collected during discussions with a group of UK student midwives who were asked to respond to the question: 'What emotions do you feel when caring for a woman in labour?' Their words suggest that emotions are strongly felt and cover a range of feelings. This raises important questions for all of us:

- What is it like to work in such emotionally charged settings?
- How often do we fully acknowledge our own emotions and the impact that they may have on the care we provide?
- How do we cope with our feelings and how do we manage our emotions when we are at work?

DOI: 10.4324/9781003092520-10

Box 9.1   Student midwives' identified emotions when caring for a woman in labour

Hope   Anxiety   Exhilaration   Impatience   Surprise   Boredom
Frustration   Fear   Amazed   Shocked   Scared   Useless   Stunned
Impotent   Joy   In awe   Out of my depth   Exhausted   Gob-smacked
My mentor is all important

Box 9.2   Reflective Activity: Identifying our emotions when caring for a woman in labour

Individually:
- Start the activity by taking time to look at the list of words given to us by student midwives (in Box 9.1). Circle any emotions that you have also felt when being alongside women in labour.
- Can you add other words to this list based on your own experiences?
- Select the ten words that are most significant to you.

In pairs or small groups:
- Swap your sheet of paper with your colleague/s. Compare your list with their list of words.
- Are there any notable differences or similarities? What might this signify?
- Share stories about situations you have been in where these emotions were significant for you:

    - How did you feel at the time?
    - How might this have affected the support you gave to the woman?
    - How do you feel now as you tell the story?
    - What did you learn from the situation?
    - What would you do in a similar situation in the future?

There are many aspects of labour support that can be seen as contributing to our emotional responses, for example:

'Being there' for women

We know that 'being there' continuously for women in labour is a crucial element of good quality care, yet providing this physical presence and emotional engagement, hour after hour, demands a particular quality of interpersonal connection. This can sometimes feel exhausting.

Managing uncertainty

Labour length is not predictable, so it is difficult for the midwife to pace herself or prepare the woman and her birth partner when they ask, 'How long is it going to take?' Even when labour is straightforward, it is usually coloured by uncertainty, so that providing support can be tinged with anxiety. When labour becomes complicated, these worries may escalate into fear.

Working with intimacy

Labour and birth also require intimate work, for example managing the bodily secretions and excretions of the woman and her baby. This intimate work often also means that midwives have a window into a couple's relationship and sexuality, at a time when it is under great pressure. This intimate 'body work' is rarely discussed (Hunter, 2010), although there is now increased recognition of the potential for intimate care to trigger memories of childhood sexual abuse for women or their caregivers (Dempsey, 2020; Montgomery, 2013).

Working in a culture of contested ideologies

As we have seen throughout the previous chapters, childbirth is not a neutral space; there may be professional politics and rivalries at play, underpinned by differing ideologies and models of what constitutes best care and a 'good birth' (Hunter, 2004, 2005; Mander and Murphy-Lawless, 2013). Raymond de Vries (2004) makes the important point that, compared with other types of healthcare, maternity care is particularly emotionally laden and is 'a highly charged mix of medical science, cultural ideas and structural forces' (p.15).

When there is loss or grief

Midwives experience extreme emotions when there is loss and grief, for example when a mother dies or when there is a stillbirth, neonatal death or personal loss. Research can help us to understand the emotionally charged work of the midwife in such situations and enhance our understanding of the psychological processes in play during challenging times, as well as offering practical suggestions for ways of coping (Halperin *et al.*, 2011; Kenworthy and Kirkham, 2011; Mander, 2006; Sheen *et al.*, 2015; Slade *et al.*, 2018). We will return to a discussion of these particularly stressful experiences later in the chapter.

Given all these factors, it is not surprising that working in maternity care can feel like emotionally hard work. What is surprising, however, is that this hard work tends to be brushed under the carpet or treated as 'just part of the job'.

Box 9.3   Reflective Activity: Acknowledging emotional work in maternity care

In pairs or small groups:
- Discuss the following questions:

  - In your experience of maternity care, how much recognition is given to the emotional hard work that is often needed?
  - Can you give an example of a situation you've experienced where this emotional work was acknowledged? Who by? What was the effect?
  - Can you think of an example where this emotional work was *not* acknowledged? Again, who did not acknowledge it and what was the effect?
  - How did you feel at the time in these situations? How do you feel about them now? What did you learn; and how might you respond in similar situations in the future?

Managing emotions: emotional labour and emotion work

Put simply, emotional labour (often referred to as emotion work) is the work that we do when managing emotions so that they are appropriate for the situation we are in. These may be our own emotions, or those of others. The idea that workers are involved in emotional labour as well as physical labour was developed by the sociologist Arlie Russell Hochschild in her influential book, *The Managed Heart* (Hochschild, 1983). Hochschild defined emotional labour as: 'the induction or suppression of feeling in order to sustain an outward appearance that produces in others a sense of being cared for in a convivial, safe place' (Hochschild, 1983, p.7).

Hochschild (1983) based her theory on her ethnographic observations of North American flight attendants, so her focus is primarily on commercial organisations where workers are required to present a corporate image of hospitality to maximise profit making (for example, the 'switch on smile' of flight attendants). Her ideas have been taken up by researchers investigating many other workplaces, and they have particular resonance for understanding the experiences of healthcare workers.

Hochschild (1983) proposed that workers manage the emotions they feel so that they fit the situation they are in, using what she describes as 'surface and deep acting' (p.3). She argues that sometimes this acting may alienate workers from what they are really feeling. The 'feeling rules' (p.18) of the situation are all important, as they are the social norms that determine what feelings should be felt and displayed. Importantly, Hochschild makes the observation that emotional labour is hard work, which is often invisible, unrecognised and undervalued.

So how can Hochschild's theories be applied to healthcare work? The following section provides an overview of the research evidence relating to managing emotions in healthcare in general. We shall then move on to consider managing emotions in maternity care.

Managing emotions in healthcare work

The emotional aspects of healthcare work, especially nursing, have been studied for over 50 years, beginning with pioneering research by Reginald Revans (1964) and Isabel Menzies (1970). Menzies proposed that nurses 'defended' themselves against the anxieties created in their work by a task-orientated approach to care, de-personalisation and distancing themselves from patients, and denial of feelings.

Although these studies focus on nurses rather than midwives, there is much that may be relevant to midwives and midwifery practice. For example, studies of the emotional labour of nurses by nurse researchers such as Bolton (2000), James (1992), Smith (1992) and Allan (2009) provide insights into how emotion management skills are learned 'on the job' and seen as innate female skills.

Pam Smith (1992) explored how student nurses learnt to 'do' emotional labour. She observed that students used senior nurses as role models and that their emotional responses changed over time. By their final year, most students had developed self-protective coping strategies to cope with the inevitable distress and grief of some nursing work. These strategies included distancing themselves from patients and using a task-orientated approach to care. There is also evidence that midwives may sometimes use similar strategies (Deery, 2009; Hunter, 2005; Hunter *et al.*, 2015).

Sharon Bolton (2000) raises some interesting questions about how emotional labour in healthcare (and other public service work) may differ from emotional labour in profit-making organisations. Based on her study of gynaecology nurses, she proposes that nurses have considerable autonomy in their emotional labour, rather than having their emotional labour controlled by their employer. She sees nurses' emotional labour as a 'gift' that they offer to their patients. Once again, this may have relevance for midwifery.

Managing emotions in maternity care

Maternity care may create particular emotions, especially in relation to intrapartum care. As we noted earlier, maternity care is 'highly charged', both for the individuals concerned and for society more generally (de Vries, 2004). Studies of maternity practitioners' emotions have focused mainly on midwives and have identified a number of key themes that are linked to emotions and emotion work. These relate to emotions arising from the context and politics of maternity care, from differing professional perspectives on safety and risk in childbirth, and from professional and collegial relationships.

Along with Ruth Deery, Billie has studied the emotional aspects of midwifery extensively. Between them they have many publications in this area, including an edited book, *Emotions in Midwifery and Reproduction* (Hunter and Deery, 2009), that brings together other key authors interested in these issues. Recent emotions-related research has tended to focus on negative experiences related to stress and burnout, rather than exploring the emotions inherent in midwifery work more generally (see, for example, Creedy *et al.*, 2017; Hunter *et al.*, 2019; Mollart *et al.*, 2013; Pezaro *et al.*, 2015). Erin Wright and colleagues (Wright *et al.*, 2017) provide a useful scoping review of literature in this area. However, it is important that emotions in midwifery should not be seen as synonymous with stress – there is much more to the emotional aspects of midwifery practice, as we shall see.

The three papers in Box 9.4 are all based on the findings of Billie's ethnographic research. They offer an in-depth exploration of the key sources of emotion for midwives working in different settings in the UK.

Box 9.4   Research Briefing: Managing emotions in maternity care – midwives' experiences

Hunter, B. (2004) Conflicting ideologies as a source of emotion work in midwifery. *Midwifery*, *20*, 261–272.

Billie Hunter's ethnographic research focused on how a range of UK student and qualified midwives experienced and managed their emotions in the workplace. A key emotional concern for midwives was how to manage the tension created by conflicting ideologies of practice: a 'with woman' ideal of good practice, versus the 'with institution' demands of the workplace.

Hunter, B. (2005). Emotion work and boundary maintenance in hospital-based midwifery. *Midwifery*, *21*, 253–266.

This paper explores the emotion work experiences of recently qualified and student midwives and how they negotiate intra-professional boundaries with midwifery colleagues. Their emotional experiences were dominated by the needs of the maternity unit to 'process' women and their babies efficiently through the system, but they learned how to navigate the hierarchical workplace, by 'sussing' out the unwritten rules and using subversive strategies to pretend to comply.

Hunter, B. (2006). The importance of reciprocity in relationships between community-based midwives and mothers. *Midwifery*, *22*, 308–322.

For community midwives, being 'with woman' was much easier than for hospital midwives, especially within continuity of care schemes. Midwives consequently experienced their work as more emotionally rewarding. Emotion work was still needed, but this was focused on their relationships with women. A key ingredient in these midwife–woman relationships was reciprocity.

Box 9.5   Reflective Activity: Discussing emotions in midwifery

In pairs or small groups:
- Select one of the three papers in Box 9.4.
- Make a list of the key points in the paper that might interest your colleagues, and which you could discuss in a journal club or similar.
- Think of a creative way to present these key points that would catch their attention, stimulate discussion and highlight the relevance to everyday practice.
- Discuss how the key points that you have identified are relevant to the context in which you practise and the emotional work that you are familiar with.

If we apply Hochschild's (1983) theory of emotional labour to the work of midwives, as both Billie and Ruth Deery have done (Hunter and Deery, 2009), we can see that there is a natural 'fit': midwives manage their emotions so that they present a caring, professional face in the workplace.

Take a look at Figure 9.1, which gives an illustration of this theory in action. If we take the example of a midwife supporting a woman during a long labour, the midwife may feel anxiety about the length of time that labour is taking and whether there may be delayed progress (this is her 'felt emotion'). However, she will hide these concerns from the woman and her partner to avoid worrying them (these are her 'professional feeling rules'). The acting needed to manage her feelings and conceal her concerns is 'emotion work'. The feelings that the midwife then reveals to the woman and her partner is the 'displayed emotion', which in this situation might be the midwife assuming a reassuring and encouraging manner. When you begin to consider that this will be only one of many other emotions that the midwife may be feeling (for example, she may be concerned about whether her children got to school safely, annoyed with the behaviour of a colleague, happy that she will be on holiday next week), the complexity of her emotion work becomes clear.

Figure 9.1 A conceptual model of emotion work in midwifery

Source: Designed by B. Hunter, 2015.

**Box 9.6   Reflective Activity: Exploring felt emotion, feeling
rules, emotion work, displayed emotion**

In pairs:

- Look at the model in Figure 9.1. Take it in turns to tell a story about supporting a
  woman in labour where 'felt emotion', 'feeling rules', 'emotion work' and 'displayed emotion' were key elements of the experience.
- How might the model be useful in helping you to unpick the complexities of the
  emotion work that you do every day?
- How might you use this model when reflecting with colleagues?
- What are the issues to consider when thinking about pressures in our private lives
  that might impact on our emotions at work?

Emotions and intrapartum care: evidence from midwives

In this section we use midwives' own words to describe the emotional demands of providing
intrapartum care and how they manage these emotions. We draw on unpublished data from
Nicky's study of how midwives support women who are experiencing labour pain (Leap,
1996) and Billie's study of the emotion work of midwives (Hunter, 2002). There are several
key themes which crop up time and time again in midwives' stories: the emotional demands
of 'being there'; witnessing pain; body work and intimacy; self-expectations; the woman's
expectations; and the reactions of the birth partner.

The emotional demands of 'presence'

As we have seen in earlier chapters, women greatly value the authentic and attentive 'presence' of the midwife 'being there' for them. But this can take an emotional toll on midwives:

> You almost have to be like a chameleon and change constantly, and that in itself is quite
> wearing, tiring. I find the fact that you're constantly adapting, it wears you out, doesn't
> it? When you go home, and the children need you, you think, I haven't got anything left
> to give, I've spent everything I've got and I'm just like a wrung out sponge sometimes.
> (Midwife, Hunter, 2002, unpublished data)

A long labour can be particularly challenging for the midwife, and even more so when the
woman is in pain. These midwives discuss how the midwife's feelings may affect the care
that women receive:

Jackie: It is very draining looking after somebody in pain for hours and hours.
Sue: It's fine if it's a normal labour and it's all going ahead, but it's when it starts to
deviate away and you know that it's going to be a really drawn out thing and oh!
When they do decide to have an epidural, you often just think – thank God for
that! So that's more your feelings than theirs.
Voices: Yes exactly.

Linda: I've got to admit – not coercing them to have an epidural – but strongly suggesting that they do.
Carol: That's true, it is, it is true.
Sue: Because you can't stand their suffering.

(Hunter, 2002, unpublished data)

Witnessing pain

As this midwife says, there is a notable silence around how midwives feel about women's pain in labour:

> I still have my own agenda in the context of pain. When I translate a woman's pain into a feeling that she's being helpless, it triggers off a real irritation in me.
>   And if the woman's pain somehow makes me feel helpless, I sort of take it on as helplessness towards her. . . . There are some women and a particular kind of pain that triggers that off in me. We don't talk about any of the personal responses that women's pain evokes in us and I think that dialogue's incredibly important. I've learnt a hell of a lot from what other midwives have to say about, you know, what responses women's pain evokes.

(Midwife, Leap, 1996, p.51)

Supporting women who are experiencing pain can be emotionally challenging for some midwives even when the woman herself may be managing well. It may be that some midwives are not always able to cope with the uncomfortable personal feelings that witnessing pain creates. As the midwife above says: 'So that's more **your** feelings than theirs' (Hunter 2002, unpublished data). In some cases, these uncomfortable feelings may then lead to midwives encouraging pharmacological pain relief, but more for their own benefit than the woman's:

> Among a lot of midwives and doctors, they need women not to – not exactly not to have the pain, but **not to show** that they're having the pain. So that's where the 'Room 11's nicely sedated' comes in. It's about the midwife needing not to have to deal with someone else's pain, someone else's expression of pain.

(Midwife, Leap, 1996, p.42)

This self-protection is hinted at in the focus group discussions with midwives below and harks back to the early study by Menzies (1970), which suggested that hospital staff developed coping strategies to 'defend' themselves against anxiety:

Carol: I get quite upset when I see people in an awful lot of pain, when women are screaming, crying and saying, 'Oh help me.'
Linda: They're more or less pleading with you.
Carol: Yes, I do find that very difficult.
Sue: Sometimes they look at you as if they're like an animal caught in a trap – petrified.
Billie: How does that make you feel?
Jackie: It's the expectation that you can solve their pain instantly.
Linda: And if you can't you've let them down. Especially if you know them, they think you are going to work miracles right away.
Sue: I think we are rescued a bit by epidurals.

(Hunter, 2002, unpublished data)

It is also the case that supporting someone in pain is physically as well as emotionally demanding, as this midwife comments:

> Some midwives give Pethidine because they don't like the fuss and the noise and the agitation and the fact the woman won't settle down. I think that sometimes the midwife isn't coping with the pain either. They think the woman isn't and actually **they're** not. Because it's a lot more work for a midwife to be interacting with somebody. If someone's agitated and making a lot of noise and being demanding, then you have to be with her all of the time, you can't go and have cups of tea, or whatever.
>
> (Midwife, Leap, 1996, pp.41–42)

Midwives who have experience of supporting women who choose not to use pharmacological pain relief describe how they have learnt to cope with their own anxieties and develop trust in the process of labour and the woman's capacity to cope:

> I don't feel uncomfortable with watching people in labour when they're experiencing pain and making the sounds of normal labour. I mean, they're obviously having severe contractions, but looking at them as a whole I can see that they're actually doing what they need to do. I feel perfectly comfortable with just sitting back and being there with them. I don't feel the need to rush in and offer Pethidine or Entonox or anything.
>
> (Midwife, Leap, 1996, p.50)

This midwife reflects on how the feelings that she is left with may differ from those of the woman, who will probably have 'moved on' to her post-birth feelings:

> Afterwards, I'm still emotionally and physically wrecked and they've moved on completely. It's like, through a fog they can remember the time they were pleading for an epidural but they've moved on. So that's been significant for me just in terms of women's ability to recover or move on or have a different agenda in a very short space of time. And that's given me enormous confidence to . . . just be there . . . and not see pain as long term damage.
>
> (Midwife, Leap, 1996, p.54)

Box 9.7 Reflective Activity: Enhancing self-awareness

In pairs:
- The midwives who offered the reflections above showed a level of self-awareness that is not always easy to share with colleagues. How do their reflections resonate with you?
- How easy is it for you to share these emotional experiences?

The intimate sounds of childbirth

Undoubtedly, the noises a woman makes in labour can provoke strong emotions in all of us, particularly if she is distressed. Also, when a woman is powering on in a straightforward labour, the sounds she makes can be similar to those we associate with sexual activity. In hospital settings, such noises can feel very challenging, particularly if you are not in the same room:

> You can come out of a room where you were with someone who was making a lot of noise and they say, 'What's going on in there?' like it's something abnormal. 'Can't you do something about that?' And you say, 'She's fine, I think she's nearly there'. And they say, 'God, I hope she has that baby soon, she's making a dreadful racket.' And that's with normal noise, just the grunting and groaning.
>
> (Midwife, Leap, 1996, p.42)

Box 9.8   Reflective Activity: The intimate sounds of labour

In pairs:
- Think back to the first time you supported a woman in labour and discuss how you felt about the noises a woman makes when labouring and giving birth. How might these noises affect the woman's birth supporters as well as those involved in her care?
- Compare notes about the noises a woman who is well supported and not frightened might make at different stages in labour. Practise making the noises out loud and discuss how they make your feel.

The reactions of the birth partner

The reactions of the woman's birth partner can also feel like another emotional responsibility:

> It does make a difference if the birth partner starts to lose it. Because as long as I can instil trust that all is going fine and the partner can pick that up they can instil that too. . . . But when the partner is all falling to pieces and the woman is saying, 'I can't do it, I can't do it', then it starts to get to me sometimes because I think, 'I should have an answer to all this!' [laughter].
>
> (Midwife, Leap, 1996, p.50)

Box 9.9   Research Briefing: Midwives' emotions and intrapartum care

There has been little research specifically on this subject. The evidence that does exist has frequently been collected as part of broader studies, for example the study of uncertainty and decision making by midwives in labour conducted by Page and Mander (2014) and an early study by Niven (1994) of factors influencing women's experiences of pain in labour. The emotional aspects of providing intrapartum care are certainly worthy of more investigation.

Niven, C. (1994). Coping with labour pain: the midwife's role. In S. Robinson and A. Thompson (eds), *Research and Childbirth*. London: Chapman and Hall.

This study identifies the important role that midwives play in helping women to cope with labour pain and how a 'trusting relationship' between caregivers and women can influence a woman's experience of labour. Niven (p.116) makes the important point that supporting women with childbirth pain 'may cause distress to some midwives. They may feel rather helpless and inadequate. Such feelings will benefit neither midwife nor labouring woman'.

Page, M. and Mander, R. (2014). Intrapartum uncertainty: a feature of normal birth, as experienced by midwives in Scotland. *Midwifery, 30*, 28–35.

This study looked at how midwives experienced the uncertainties of intrapartum care and how this affected their decision making. Despite the fact that there are always many 'grey areas' in childbirth, some midwives felt a sense of personal and professional failure when they were unable to predict the unpredictable. They were also concerned about missing something important, and this underlying 'finger of fear' made them 'cautious in their approach' and 'zealous in their care' (Page and Mander, 2014, p.31). However, other midwives experienced the unknown-ness of labour as exciting and a source of curiosity. These different emotional responses reflect the midwives' accounts in the previous section.

Why do emotions matter?

So why does all of this matter? We think that there are three key reasons, which we shall explore in turn:

1   How midwives manage the emotional challenges of supporting women in labour will affect the way they care for women and how women experience this care.
2   How midwives cope with the emotional demands of their profession will affect their own wellbeing and job satisfaction.
3   How midwives cope with their felt emotions will affect their working relationships.

It is interesting to reflect on these three key reasons. At first glance, they seem obvious and self-evident. However, the psychological and emotional experiences of midwives (and indeed healthcare workers in general) have been poorly articulated and their importance has rarely been taken into account in discussions of quality of care, patient safety and user experiences. It is only very recently, prompted by the immense workforce challenges presented by the Covid-19 pandemic, that the psychological wellbeing of the workforce has begun to receive proper attention (Greenberg *et al.*, 2020; Hunter *et al.*, 2020; O'Connell *et al.*, 2020).

Emotions matter: evidence from women

Clearly midwives' emotions matter to women. As we explored in Chapter 1, universally, women tell us that the emotional components of the care they receive in labour are all important. Ellen Hodnett (2002) provides strong evidence for this. In a conclusion that should be writ large above the entrance to every labour ward or birth centre door, Hodnett states:

> The influences of pain, pain relief and intrapartum medical interventions on subsequent satisfaction are neither as obvious, as direct nor as powerful as the influences of the **attitude and behaviours of the caregivers**.
>
> (Hodnett, 2002, p.160)

In many ways, this is all we need to know. Labour and birth are the part of the whole childbirth journey that women are most apprehensive about, and how well they are supported emotionally can greatly enhance or damage the experience. Numerous studies provide examples of the caring and uncaring behaviours of midwives and the effect that this has on women. Developing a trusting relationship is vital for a woman to feel listened to, cared for and 'anchored' during her labour.

Conversely, when women feel invisible, ignored or 'processed' through the system, they are, understandably, unlikely to feel safe or trust their caregivers:

> But I felt as if she always came just 2 minutes too late. . . . I felt as if half of her was still in the other room.
>
> (Berg *et al.*, 1996, p.13)

> She didn't spend much time with me, coming in and out . . . she seemed quite distracted, like her mind wasn't really in the room.
>
> (Anderson, 2000, p.102)

In recent years, there has been an upsurge in focusing attention on unsupportive healthcare practices in Western countries. In the UK this has been prompted by high-level enquiries that have generated heated discussion and debate. How is it that some individuals become uncaring? Presumably, they all went into healthcare work initially wanting to provide the best quality care – so what has happened to them on the way?

The previous discussions about emotion management may provide some explanations. Hochschild's (1983) research into emotional labour identified the 'distancing' strategies that individuals use to protect themselves when their work feels emotionally and physically overwhelming. These strategies have also been identified in studies of emotion management in health and maternity care (Bone, 2009; Deery, 2005, 2009; Hunter, 2005, 2009; Smith, 1992).

Put simply, if midwives feel overwhelmed and unsupported, they are likely to withdraw emotionally by distancing themselves and 'going into robot' (Hochschild, 1983, p.129). This is also described as 'compassion fatigue'. It may also explain why some midwives describe using epidurals as a source of rescue for the midwife: their emotional 'reserve tank' has simply run out. This lack of caring usually manifests in the midwife being emotionally withdrawn and distant – 'her mind wasn't really in the room' (Anderson, 2000, p.102), rather than overt unkindness.

However, as we discussed in Chapter 1, global evidence also shows that women around the world can sometimes experience maternity care that is actually abusive or disrespectful (Bowser and Hill, 2010). Disrespectful care is not only damaging on an individual level; it is also likely to be an important contributor to global maternal and infant mortality and morbidity. Put simply, if women fear that they will not be treated with respect and kindness, they will not access healthcare facilities and providers.

The importance of respectful maternity care is increasingly recognised worldwide and addressed in a number of policies and reports, for example, the ICM Respect Toolkit and the White Ribbon Alliance Respectful Maternity Care Charter, which you will find on the respective ICM and White Ribbon Alliance websites, along with many useful Respectful Maternity Care Resources. We suggest that you search for these policies, reports and toolkits on the Internet and create a resource list to share with colleagues.

Emotions matter: midwives' wellbeing and job satisfaction

The danger for midwives of feeling emotionally overwhelmed and unsupported is that they may become stressed to the point where they become mentally or physically unwell and/or experience burnout. This can result in taking sick leave or even in midwives leaving the profession. A number of recent studies have investigated stress and burnout in midwifery and drawn attention to the challenges these negative experiences present for personal and professional sustainability, including staff retention (Creedy *et al.*, 2017; Fenwick *et al.*, 2018a; Harvie *et al.*, 2019; Hunter *et al.*, 2019). Worryingly, it is often the newest entrants to the profession whose psychological wellbeing is at most risk (Cull *et al.*, 2020).

These studies all point to systemic issues that commonly underpin midwives' negative work experiences, for example: chronic workforce shortages and work overload, poor quality management and leadership, lack of workplace autonomy. Importantly, for many midwives it is not being able to give high-quality care to women and their babies that is a major source of stress and job dissatisfaction. One recently qualified midwife in the study by Cull *et al.* (2020 p.4) summarised the feelings of many participants when she said: 'The feeling of failure when you've physically exhausted yourself and couldn't possibly do any more is demoralising. Above everything, not giving women and babies the care they deserve is the worst aspect.'

The review paper by Cramer and Hunter (2019) provides a comprehensive overview of what we currently know about the relationship between working conditions and midwives' wellbeing. The authors set out factors that could be 'modifiable' as well as those that are 'non-modifiable'. Importantly, where midwives have the opportunity to work in continuity of care schemes, which provide much greater opportunities to develop meaningful relationships with women and have workplace autonomy, levels of stress and burnout are considerably lower (Dawson *et al.*, 2018; Dixon *et al.*, 2017; Fenwick *et al.*, 2018b). This also applies to newly qualified midwives: when they are supported to work in continuity of care models, they are able to develop trusting relationships with women and with colleagues, which in turn enables them to develop confidence in their practice and job satisfaction (Evans *et al.*, 2020; Cummins *et al.*, 2015).

Box 9.10   Reflective Activity: Working conditions and emotional wellbeing

In preparation for this activity read the following review:

Cramer, E. and Hunter, B. (2019). Relationships between working conditions and emotional wellbeing in midwives. *Women and Birth, 32(6)*, 521–532.

In pairs or small groups:
- Consider *Figure 4* in the article by Cramer and Hunter (2019): *Summary of risk indicators identified in the review*. The authors suggest that some of these risk indicators can be modified (e.g. level of autonomy, model of care), whilst others are an inevitable part of the work (e.g. emergencies, bereavement).
- Think of the most recent clinical setting you've worked in and discuss how this figure relates to your own experiences. Do you agree with the distinction made between modifiable and non-modifiable factors?
- How could this figure provide a useful way to identify possible changes to improve emotional wellbeing in your working environment?
- Make a list of all the people who would need to be involved in order to make such changes sustainable.
- Conduct a search to identify an example of a maternity service that made changes to improve the emotional wellbeing of staff. Prepare a list of dot points identifying the factors that contributed to the success of the initiative/s to share with the wider group.

Clearly there are fundamental systems issues affecting midwives' emotional wellbeing which need tackling, rather than problems being personalised and directed back to individuals to resolve. It is essential, however, that midwives' occupational and associated emotional support needs are acknowledged and attended to within the workplace and that all midwives receive the support they need from within the health system. Such an approach and understanding is what Pat Brodie has referred to as 'midwifing the midwives' (Brodie, 2013).

Informal support to promote midwives' wellbeing

The importance of informal social support from colleagues is demonstrated in many studies. For example, Rosemary Mander (2001) vividly describes the value of this collegial support in her study of how midwives were affected by the death of a mother whom they had cared for. Midwives spoke of the importance of feeling that their colleagues were there for them. This support might never be called on but knowing that colleagues were willing to chat or be telephoned was an important source of comfort. Conversely, the negative impact of no collegial support was profoundly distressing, accentuating the pain already being felt.

Whilst Mander's study focuses on the extremely distressing situation of a maternal death, the importance of collegial support for nurturing emotional wellbeing appears time and time again in other studies of midwives' everyday work. Recent studies of stress and burnout in midwifery all identify the importance of positive teamworking and support from colleagues for emotional wellbeing (Cull *et al.*, 2020; Creedy *et al.*, 2017; Fenwick *et al.*, 2018a;

Harvie *et al.*, 2019; Hunter *et al.*, 2019). Denis Walsh draws on theories of 'social capital' to explain why social support is so important, drawing on observations in his ethnographic study of a midwife-led birth centre (Walsh, 2006a, 2006b, 2007).

Organisational support to promote midwives' emotional wellbeing

As well as informal peer support at work, it is also important that midwives are supported formally, as part of the care for employees which should be provided by the organisation where they work. It is increasingly being recognised that institutions have a responsibility to care for their workforce, if only because a cared-for workforce is much more likely to provide good-quality, safe care for patients and clients (Hall *et al.*, 2016; House of Commons, 2013). This has led to workplace initiatives such as Schwartz Rounds (facilitated meetings which provide an opportunity for staff to reflect on the emotional aspects of their work). Formal support can also take the form of structured staff counselling and clinical supervision sessions.

Support needs to be both reactive, responding to immediate emotional stresses and challenges, and proactive, building emotional support into the fabric of the everyday workplace. A number of recent reports and studies have drawn attention to the importance of this proactive organisational support for wellbeing, with an emphasis on workplace kindness and tolerance.

Professor Michael West has been particularly influential in calling for a new leadership approach based on compassion. His UK Kings Fund report *The Courage of Compassion* (West *et al.*, 2020) pulls together the research evidence which shows that, in order to minimise workplace stress and ensure staff wellbeing and motivation, people have three core needs that need addressing (the 'ABC Framework of Nurses' and Midwives' Core Needs'). All of these needs must be attended to in order for staff to flourish and thrive:

- *autonomy* – the need to have control over your work life, and to be able to act in accordance with your personal values;
- *belonging* – the need to feel that you belong and are connected to colleagues, and are valued and cared for by them;
- *contribution*– the need to feel that you are effective in what you do at work and are able to do what matters.

Michael West and colleagues caution that many healthcare workers across the world are so used to working in situations where there is chronic excessive workload, that it has become normalised – we just don't see it and the impact it has. Of course, addressing staff shortages requires long-term organisational solutions. There are no quick fixes, but focusing on these three core needs may offer employers and employees a way to create a more supportive work environment at least in the short term.

Emotions matter: the effect on working relationships

Finally, emotions also matter because they affect working relationships. The opposite is also true: working relationships generate emotions, and these work emotions permeate our non-working lives. As this emotional interplay is a characteristic of any workplace, not just maternity care, there is a wealth of literature available; see, for example, Fineman (2000) and

Waldron (2012). We recommend that you explore this material further, as it offers much that is relevant to maternity care work.

When working relationships are experienced negatively, this may be because there is a lack of interpersonal connection and mutual support. Staff can, at times, feel invisible and undervalued, mere cogs in the wheel of the organisation. At its worst, the workplace can be rife with disrespect and bullying behaviour. Healthcare organisations are particularly well known for being hierarchical and full of unwritten rules and sanctions. In such settings, it is easy for staff to feel undermined and it is very difficult to defend oneself or raise concerns about poor practice. Such situations were at the root of much of the poor care exposed in the Francis Report (House of Commons, 2013) and are often exemplified in the negative experiences of whistle-blowers.

Clearly, however, the workplace can also be a source of emotional fulfilment. Where working relationships are experienced positively, there is usually mutual support (practical and emotional) and a strong sense of trust and reciprocity. In the UK WHELM study (Cull *et al.*, 2020; Hunter *et al.*, 2019), the most commonly reported source of satisfaction was relationships with colleagues and feeling part of a team. Midwives described working in a strong team as a protective factor against stress: 'If I am working with a good team I don't mind how hard the work is' (Cull *et al.*, 2020, p.5).

Positive working relationships are usually characterised by emotional awareness and emotional intelligence (Waldron, 2012). Work colleagues 'suss out' how others are feeling and alter their behaviour accordingly. They may offer practical support or a listening ear, steer a situation away from difficult topics or celebrate each other's successes. It is easy to see how such a positive workplace will bring benefits, not only for its staff, but also for those receiving care from those staff.

Box 9.11   Reflective Activity: Identifying personal sources of support

Working in pairs:

- Take time individually to draw a mind map identifying yourself in the centre and all the sources of support that you can draw on. In whatever way you choose, portray the nature of the support (formal, informal, professional or personal) and the importance of each type of support in your working life.
- Share your mind map with one other person and discuss whether this represents the ideal picture in terms of enabling your wellbeing, job satisfaction, collegial relationships and your ability to offer the best possible care and support to pregnant women and new mothers.

Thinking about workplace culture

Christine Catling and colleagues have developed a Midwifery Workplace Culture Instrument which can facilitate insights into the quality of relationships and emotional support in the workplace (Catling *et al.*, 2020). In the following activity, we have adapted the instrument so that it focuses on positive statements, providing a constructive way to explore your workplace culture with colleagues.

Box 9.12   Reflective Activity: Thinking about workplace culture

At the start of this activity each participant needs to have access to a hard copy sheet of the ten Positive Statements extracted from the Australian Midwifery Workplace Culture Survey (see below).

Working in pairs:
Take a few minutes to complete the survey on your own, thinking of your most recent experiences of a maternity workplace. (You are only going to share this information in confidence with your partner, not the whole group).

Take 10 minutes to share how you each filled in the survey and discuss the issues it raised for you both, sharing experiences and ideas.

Still in your pair, take 5 minutes to choose the three statements in the survey that you think are most important in terms of promoting a positive workplace culture. You will be sharing the three items you chose with the whole group. This will stimulate a facilitated group discussion.

Table 9.1 Survey: Midwifery Workplace Culture

Statement	Strongly disagree	Disagree	Disagree somewhat	Agree somewhat	Agree	Strongly agree
1 I feel respected by my co-workers						
2 I feel good about working in this maternity unit						
3 I am able to influence the way things are done in the workplace						
4 When things get difficult, I can rely on my colleagues						
5 I feel I work in a place with a positive culture						
6 The people I work with are friendly						
7 When we are short staffed, we are given adequate support						
8 My philosophy of care is shared by the midwives in my workplace						
9 Our workplace culture celebrates when midwives achieve success (e.g. completes a course, uses innovation to improve practice)						
10 There are positive role models where I work						

Caring for ourselves: the key to resilience

Resilience – the ability to respond positively to adversity – has become an increasingly popular concept, with many healthcare employers offering resilience workshops and training to their staff. A scoping review of the midwifery resilience literature provides a useful overview of the evidence which informs this training (Wright *et al.*, 2017). Resilience-building sessions may offer some useful personal insights and coping strategies for individuals. However, we caution against taking an overly individualised approach to resilience, which can result in midwives feeling personally responsible for adverse work situations. From our experiences, when building resilience within a workforce group or team, what is really needed for long-term sustainable improvements is systemic change at a wider, organisational level.

In a study of resilience in midwifery by Billie and her colleague Lucie Warren, receiving and providing social support within a community of midwifery colleagues was identified as a key strategy for building resilience (Hunter and Warren, 2013, 2014, 2015). We have profiled this work in Box 9.13.

Box 9.13   Research Briefing: How can midwives be more resilient?

Hunter, B. and Warren L. (2014) Midwives' experiences of workplace resilience. *Midwifery*, *30*, 926–934.

Funded by the Royal College of Midwives UK, the *Investigating Resilience in Midwifery* study was a preliminary investigation into the experiences of 11 UK midwives with 15 or more years' experience, who all self-identified as resilient or 'able to bounce back after a difficult day at work'. Rich data were collected via a closed online discussion group over a one-month period, thematically analysed and then discussed with an expert panel to enhance data interpretation and refine modelling of the concept. The research provides important new insights into midwives' resilient responses to workplace adversity.

Key messages

- Midwifery is known to be demanding work that may lead to high levels of stress, low morale, sickness and attrition. But some midwives continue to enjoy their work despite the challenges. These individuals are said to demonstrate *resilience*.
- The study identified key challenges in the workplace, and three key resilient responses to these challenges: day-to-day reactive strategies of managing and coping; developing self-awareness; and proactive strategies of building resilience.
- Managing and coping strategies focused on trying to control whatever was possible and accepting what could not be controlled. Midwives described using reflection, positive mood changers such as music and exercise, social support and trying to keep a good work–life balance.
- The participants identified 'critical moments' in careers when midwives could be particularly vulnerable to workplace adversity. These occurred when midwives were newly qualified, when they had experienced a particularly difficult clinical situation or when they were 'under investigation'.

- The midwives thought that it was possible to develop personal resilience over time and also to support others to build their resilience. Ways of doing this included accessing support, developing self-awareness and learning self-protection. Midwives described how they built up their resilience by learning how to take care of themselves emotionally (for example, by increasing their self-awareness of potential triggers) and by supporting and empowering others (especially less experienced colleagues).
- A strong sense of professional identity and love of midwifery were seen as important for building resilience.
- Understanding more about resilience may help midwives and student midwives to cope with workplace challenges. However, this should not mean that the onus of responsibility falls on individual midwives at the expense of addressing wider environmental and organisational issues.

There are a number of practical ways to take care of yourself emotionally and develop professional resilience. As a starter, we suggest that you look at the Resilient Repertoire, which can be found in a book chapter: 'Caring for ourselves: the key to resilience' (Hunter and Warren, 2015). This Repertoire was derived from the study identified in Box 9.13 (Hunter and Warren, 2014). There is also growing evidence to support the use of more formal techniques, such as mindfulness to promote relaxation, reduce stress and anxiety, and enhance self-compassion (Foureur *et al.*, 2013; Warriner *et al.*, 2016). Related resources can be found on a number of websites and in I-learn modules (for example, explore the All4Maternity and Royal College of Midwives websites). We recommend investigating these and seeing what might work for you.

Finally, it is very important to be alert to the extreme responses to stress that may occur, within ourselves and our colleagues, which can be seriously debilitating. These can lead to compassion fatigue, secondary (or vicarious) traumatic stress and/or possibly post-traumatic stress disorder (PTSD). Quite often there is an event that triggers a response – for example, attending a traumatic birth or when there is loss and grief – which becomes the final straw (Wright *et al.*, 2017). The accumulation of chronic stress responses can tip over into panic attacks, insomnia and phobias. If you think that you or a colleague are at risk of, or suffering from, PTSD it is vital to seek skilled support without delay.

'Midwifing the midwife': global issues

The significance of emotional wellbeing for midwives across the world has been illustrated vividly in an important joint WHO/ICM/White Ribbon Alliance report 'Midwives voices, midwives realities' (WHO, 2016) and a related paper (Filby *et al.*, 2016). The authors explored why poor-quality maternity care can occur, from the perspective of midwives. They conducted a survey of 2,470 midwives from 93 countries, alongside a systematic review of the literature. Their analysis suggests that, particularly in low- and middle-income countries, midwives experience a multitude of social, cultural, economic and professional barriers to providing good care to women. These barriers are interlinked and are identified as stemming from gender inequality. It was recognised that they can lead to emotional burnout and moral distress, which in turn results in poor-quality care (WHO, 2016; Filby *et al.*, 2016).

The importance of emotional and practical support for midwives globally, so that they can provide safe, supportive care, is highlighted in Pat Brodie's (2013) commentary 'Midwifing the midwives'.

Box 9.14   Research Briefing: 'Midwifing the midwives'

Brodie, P. (2013). 'Midwifing the midwives': addressing the empowerment, safety of, and respect for, the world's midwives. *Midwifery, 29*, 1075–1076. doi:http://dx.doi.org/10.1016/j.midw.2013.06.012i.

Key messages

Retention and motivation are key strategies in global efforts to build and develop a sustainable midwifery workforce. Many midwives are working in unsafe, isolated and poorly equipped environments, with daily challenges that lead to disempowerment and demoralisation. Support that strengthens capacity and sustainability is essential for promoting 'emotional resilience' and the 'restoration of courage' for many of these midwives. Mentoring, peer support, networking and supportive supervision within the organisation or workplace can all play a role in effectively 'midwifing the midwives'.

Box 9.15   Reflective Activity: Supporting each other

The International Confederation of Midwives (ICM) has a 'Twinning' project to facilitate collaborative relationships among midwives' associations. You will find information on the ICM website.

- Explore your nearest local or national midwifery professional organisation's involvement in this initiative and ways in which you and your colleagues might be able to contribute.
- Explore other ways of being involved in support activities, for example:
  - attending local meetings of your professional organisation or other midwifery related interest and support groups;
  - mentoring or 'buddying' with a student or newly graduated midwife in your local area.

Conclusion

We finish with some recommendations for further reading around the issues that we have discussed in this chapter. And finally, in the postscript, midwifery lecturer Rachel Smith offers a message to students, one that applies to all of us in our efforts to support women for labour and birth:

'You can make a difference for every woman who crosses your path.'

Box 9.16   Recommended Resources for thinking about emotions in the workplace

Ballatt, J. and Campling, P. (2011). *Intelligent Kindness: Reforming the Culture of Healthcare.* London: Royal College of Psychiatrists RCPsych Publications.

This book takes as its focus the central importance of 'kindness' in healthcare, both kindness towards others and self-kindness, and how these are inextricably bound together – a deceptively simple idea that is ignored at peril!

Bunting M. (2020) *Labours of Love: The Crisis of Care*. London: Granta.

Based on Madeleine Bunting's research as a journalist and on her personal experiences, this stimulating book explores the 'crisis of care' in UK society. She argues that the welfare state has been dismantled by the pursuit of consumerism and economic growth, and that the network of care relationships that we all rely on is at breaking point. Although the focus is on care throughout the lifecycle, there is much in this book of relevance to maternity care.

Byrom, S. and Downe, S. (eds). (2015) *The Roar against the Silence. Why Kindness, Compassion and Respect Matter in Maternity Care*. UK: Pinter & Martin.

This book is a rich source of evidence about the importance of kindness and compassion in maternity care. The 32 chapters have been written by some of the leading thinkers in this area from across the world, including midwives, students, childbearing women, doctors, doulas, childbirth activists and lawyers. The authors say, 'Our intention is to shift the debate and practice of maternity care from being based in **fear** to being based in **love** (**caritas,** the basis of the word "caring")'. This is strongly recommended reading.

Hunter, B. and Deery, R. (eds). (2009) *Emotions in Midwifery and Reproduction*. Basingstoke: Palgrave Macmillan.

A useful and thought-provoking reader that brings together some of the key researchers into emotions in maternity care and wider reproductive healthcare (for example, infertility and pregnancy loss). The book includes an international perspective and has a strong emphasis on clinical relevance.

Youngson, R. (2012). *Time to Care: How to Love Your Patients and Your Job*. New Zealand: Rebelheart Publishers.

A personal and very readable account of Robin Youngson's transition from being an exhausted and detached doctor to an advocate for compassionate healthcare. It draws on literature related to positive psychology and neuroscience to suggest practical strategies for keeping alive one's love of the job. See also http://heartsinhealthcare.com.

Other useful texts

Fineman, S. (2000). *Emotion in Organizations*. London: SAGE Publications.
Gilbert, P. (2010). *The Compassionate Mind*. London: Constable.
Mander, R. (2001). *Supportive Care and Midwifery*. Oxford: Blackwell Science.
Waldron, V.R. (2012). *Communicating Emotion at Work*. Cambridge: Polity Press.

Online resources

Schwartz Rounds – see Point of Care Foundation. Schwartz Rounds are meetings that provide an opportunity for staff from all disciplines across the organisation to reflect on the emotional aspects of their work. www.pointofcarefoundation.org.uk/Schwartz-Rounds.
Hearts in Healthcare – The Movement for Human-centred Healthcare. http://heartsinhealthcare.com.
White Ribbon Alliance – Campaign for Respectful Maternity Care.
All4Maternity – various resources available online, including a Nurture Zone and learning modules such as Selfcare and Resilience in Midwifery. www.All4Maternity.com.
Royal College of Midwives – i-learn modules, including Building Resilient Practitioners and Promoting Compassionate and Supportive workplaces. www.ilearn.rcm.org.uk.

Postscript

'You can make a difference for every woman who crosses your path': an interview with midwifery lecturer Rachel Smith, April 2015

I acknowledge that it's hard for students. They have to fit into the culture of maternity care in order to survive. Because it's such a conveyor belt system the student is trying to be two people, trying to fit, sitting out at the desk making contributions to conversations or talking about things they don't really care about; the other part of the student really wants to be in the room with the woman. They see themselves as being judged if they do that, not a team player.

I say to the students:
You have stepped into a woman's life at the most vulnerable time of her life, uninvited, into a situation where 60 or 70 years later, she will remember everything you said to her, everything you did, how you made her feel. So it's about understanding your privileged position. You may not agree with that woman's life choices or whatever but there will be a whole back story that you don't know when you step in. Always remember you are the privileged one.

You don't have a choice as a midwife to have a bad day at work. That doesn't happen. If you're not a morning person don't do shift work. You have to turn up every day, ready to make a difference in a woman's life. Your cat might have died, you might have had a fight with your partner or whatever, but all of that does not come to work; you have to be ready to let everything go and focus on that woman, be there for her.

In the system, the only time you get to see other midwives practising is as a student. You'll see practices you abhor and practices you aspire to. This is your chance. Make the most of it because in midwifery we shut the door once we're qualified; hence there are midwives whose practice has barely changed in over 20 years. As a student you have a lot to offer the midwives through engaging with them about their practice. You can do that without being too challenging or being seen to be judging. So you might ask questions like, 'That was really interesting the way you put your hands like that. Can you explain to me why you do that because I've noticed others who don't do that?'

Being a student is a wonderful opportunity to sit in the corner of the room if the woman doesn't need direct support from you and listen and watch and learn the patterns of labour, the different patterns that women present with. Make connections with the noises women make at different times. And the behaviours: toe curling in transition, beads of sweat on the upper lip when fully, all those sorts of things. If you watch enough you'll learn the signs.

When labour is complicated, remember that, essentially, this is a normal life event – the birth of a baby. Try to work with the woman so that you keep that in focus in her mind. It so easily becomes a production with all the machines so it's really hard to do, but it could be as simple as holding the woman's hand and finding something positive to say, like, 'You've grown your baby really well up to now, sure the baby's going to be early but you've given her/him a good start. Let's work on making it as uncomplicated as possible.' It's the birth of her baby and if you can make just one thing positive – so that, for example, the woman might say afterwards, 'There were 20 people in the room but the midwife took my hand and told me I was doing great, that I was strong and that my baby was coming soon.' We all have to try to keep it as normal as it can be in a situation where there's not much normal to be had.

You can make a difference for every woman who crosses your path.

References

Allan, H.T. (2009). *Managing Intimacy and Emotions in Advanced Fertility Care*. Cumbria: M & K Publishing.

Anderson, T. (2000). Feeling safe enough to let go: the relationship between a woman and her midwife during the second stage of labour. In M. Kirkham (ed.), *The Midwife–Mother Relationship* (pp.92–119). London: Macmillan.

Berg, M., Lundgren, I., Hermansson, E. and Wahlberg, V. (1996). Women's experience of the encounter with the midwife during childbirth. *Midwifery*, *12*, 11–15.

Bolton, S.C. (2000). Who cares? Offering emotion work as a 'gift' in the nursing labour process. *Journal of Advanced Nursing*, *32(3)*, 580–586.

Bone, D. (2009). Epidurals not emotions: the care deficit in US maternity care. Chapter 3 in B. Hunter and R. Deery (eds), *Emotions in Midwifery and Reproduction* (pp.56–72). Basingstoke: Palgrave Macmillan.

Bowser, D. and Hill, K. (2010). *Exploring Evidence for Disrespect and Abuse in Facility-Based Childbirth: Report of a Landscape Analysis. USAID – Traction Project*. Retrieved from Cambridge, MA: Harvard School of Public Health University Research Co., LLC.

Brodie, P. (2013). 'Midwifing the midwives': addressing the empowerment, safety of, and respect for, the world's midwives. *Midwifery*, *29*, 1075–1076.

Catling, C., Rossiter, C. and McIntyre, E. (2020). Developing the Australian Midwifery Workplace Culture Instrument. *International Journal of Nursing Practice*, *26* (e12794).

Cramer, E. and Hunter, B. (2019). Relationships between working conditions and emotional wellbeing in midwives. *Women and Birth*, *32(6)*, 521–532.

Creedy, D. K., Sidebotham, M., Gamble J., Pallant J. and Fenwick, J. (2017). Prevalence of burnout, depression, anxiety and stress in Australian midwives: a cross-sectional survey. *BMC Pregnancy & Childbirth*, *17(13)*, 1–8.

Cull, J., Hunter, B., Henley, J., Fenwick, J., and Sidebotham, M. (2020). 'Overwhelmed and out of my depth': responses from early career midwives in the United Kingdom to the Work Health and Emotional Lives of Midwives Study *Women and Birth*, *23(6)*, e549–e557.

Cummins, A.M., Denney-Wilson, E. and Homer, C.S.E. (2015). The experiences of new graduate midwives working in midwifery continuity of care models in Australia. *Midwifery*, *31(4)*, 438–444.

Dawson. K., Newton, M., Forster, D. and Mclachlan, H. (2018). Comparing caseload and non-caseload midwives' burnout levels and professional attitudes: a national, cross- sectional survey of Australian midwives working in the public maternity system *Midwifery*, *63*, 60–67.

Deery, R. (2005). An action research study exploring midwives' support needs and the effect of group clinical supervision, *Midwifery*, *21(2)*: 161–176.

Deery, R. (2009). Community midwifery 'performances' and the presentation of self. In B. Hunter and R. Deery (eds), *Emotions in Midwifery and Reproduction* (pp.73–89). Basingstoke: Palgrave Macmillan.

Dempsey, R. (2020). *Beyond the Birth Plan: Getting Real about Pain and Power*. Fairfield, Victoria, Australia: Boathouse Press.

de Vries, R. (2004). *A Pleasing Birth: Midwives and Maternity Care in the Netherlands*. Philadelphia, PA: Temple University Press.

Dixon, L., Guilliland, K., Pallant, J., Sidebotham, M., Fenwick, J., McAra-Couper, J. and Gilkison, A. (2017). The emotional wellbeing of New Zealand midwives: comparing responses for midwives in caseloading and shift work settings. *New Zealand College of Midwives Journal*, *53*, 5–14.

Evans, J., Taylor, J., Browne, J., Sally Ferguson, S., Atchan, M., Penny Maher, P., . . . Davis, D. (2020). The future in their hands: graduating student midwives' plans, job satisfaction and the desire to work in midwifery continuity of care. *Women and Birth*, *33*, e59–e66.

Fenwick, J., Lubomski, A., Creedy, D.K. and Sidebotham, M. (2018a). Personal, professional and workplace factors that contribute to burnout in Australian midwives. *Journal of Advanced Nursing*, *74(4)*, 852–863.

Fenwick, J., Sidebotham, M., Gamble, J. and Creedy, D.K. (2018b). The emotional and professional wellbeing of Australian midwives: a comparison of those providing continuity of midwifery care and those not providing continuity. *Women and Birth, 31*, 38–43.

Filby, A., McConville, F. and Portela, A. (2016). What prevents quality midwifery care? A systematic mapping of barriers in low and middle income countries from the provider perspective. *PLoS ONE, 11(5)*, e0153391.

Fineman, S. (2000). *Emotion in Organizations*. London: SAGE Publications.

Foureur, M., Besley, K., Burton, G., Yu, N. and Crisp, J. (2013). Enhancing the resilience of nurses and midwives: pilot of a mindfulness based program for increased health, sense of coherence and decreased depression, anxiety and stress. *Contemporary Nurse, 45(1)*, 114–125.

Gilbert, P. (2010). *The Compassionate Mind*. London: Constable.

Greenberg, N., Docherty, M., Gnanapragasam, S. and Wessely, S. (2020). Managing mental health challenges faced by healthcare workers during Covid-19 pandemic. *British Medical Journal, 368*, m1211.

Hall, L.H., Johnson, J., Watt, I., Tsipa, A. and O'Connor, D.B. (2016). Healthcare staff wellbeing, burnout, and patient safety: a systematic review. *PLoS ONE, 11(7)*, e0159015.

Halperin, O., Goldblatt, H., Noble, A., Raz, I., Zvulunov, I. and Liebergall Wischnitzer, M. (2011). Stressful childbirth situations: a qualitative study of midwives. *Journal of Midwifery & Women's Health, 56(4)*, 388–394.

Harvie, K., Sidebotham, M. and Fenwick, J. (2019). Australian midwives' intentions to leave the profession and the reasons why. *Women and Birth, 32*, e584–e593.

Hochschild, A.R. (1983). *The Managed Heart: Commercialization of Human Feeling*. Berkeley, CA: University of California Press.

Hodnett, E.D. (2002). Pain and women's satisfaction with the experience of childbirth: a systematic review. *American Journal of Obstetrics and Gynaecology, 186(5)*, S160–S172.

House of Commons (2013). Report of the Mid Staffordshire NHS Foundation Trust public inquiry chaired by Robert Francis QC. London: The Stationery Office.

Hunter, B. (2002). Emotion work in midwifery: an ethnographic study of the emotional work undertaken by a sample of student and qualified midwives in Wales. Unpublished Ph.D. University of Wales, Swansea.

Hunter, B. (2002, unpublished data). Emotion work in midwifery: an ethnographic study of the emotional work undertaken by a sample of student and qualified midwives in Wales. Unpublished PhD, University of Wales, Swansea.

Hunter, B. (2004). Conflicting ideologies as a source of emotion work in midwifery. *Midwifery, 20*, 261–272.

Hunter, B. (2005). Emotion work and boundary maintenance in hospital based midwifery. *Midwifery, 21*, 253–266.

Hunter, B. (2006). The importance of reciprocity in relationships between community-based midwives and mothers. *Midwifery, 22*, 308–322.

Hunter, B. (2009). Mixed messages: midwives' experiences of managing emotion. In B. Hunter and R. Deery (eds), *Emotions in Midwifery and Reproduction* (pp.175–179). Basingstoke: Palgrave Macmillan.

Hunter, B. (2010). Mapping the emotional terrain of midwifery: what can we see and what lies ahead? *International Journal of Work Organisation and Emotion, 3(3)*, 253–259.

Hunter, B. (2015, unpublished data). Identifying the experiences of receiving and providing support in labour.

Hunter, B. and Deery, R. (eds). (2009). *Emotions in Midwifery and Reproduction*. Basingstoke: Palgrave Macmillan.

Hunter, B., Fenwick, J., Sidebotham, M. and Henley, J. (2019). Midwives in the United Kingdom: levels of burnout, depression, anxiety and stress and associated predictors *Midwifery, 79*, 102526.

Hunter, B., Renfrew, M.J. and Downe, S. (2020). Supporting the emotional wellbeing of midwives in a pandemic. London. https://www.rcm.org.uk/media/4095/rcm-supporting-the-emotional-wellbeing-of-midwives-during-a-pandemic-v1-submitted-to-rcm_mrd.pdf.

Hunter, B. and Segrott, J. (2014). Renegotiating interprofessional boundaries in maternity care: implementing a clinical pathway for normal labour. *Sociology of Health & Illness, 36(5)*, 719–737.

Hunter, B. and Warren, L. (2013). Investigating resilience in midwifery. Final report. Cardiff: Cardiff University.

Hunter, B. and Warren L. (2014) Midwives' experiences of workplace resilience. *Midwifery, 30*, 926–934.

Hunter, B. and Warren, L. (2015). Caring for ourselves: the key to resilience. In S. Byrom and S. Downe (eds), *The Roar against the Silence. Why Kindness, Compassion and Respect Matter in Maternity Care*. London: Pinter & Martin.

James, N. (1992). Care = organisation + physical labour + emotional labour. *Sociology of Health & Illness, 14(4)*, 489–509.

Kenworthy, D. and Kirkham, M. (2011). *Midwives Coping with Loss and Grief*. London: Radcliffe Publishing.

Leap, N. (1996). A midwifery perspective on pain in labour. Unpublished MSc dissertation, South Bank University, London. Available on request from nickyleap@me.com.

Mander, R. (2001). *Supportive Care and Midwifery*. London: Blackwell Science.

Mander, R. (2006). *Loss and Bereavement in Childbearing*. London: Routledge.

Mander, R. and Murphy-Lawless, J. (2013). *The Politics of Maternity*. Abingdon: Routledge.

Menzies, I.E.P. (1970). *The Functioning of Social Systems as a Defence against Anxiety*. London: The Tavistock Institute of Human Relations.

Mollart, L., Skinner, V.M., Newing, C. and Foureur, M. (2013). Factors that may influence midwives work-related stress and burnout. *Women and Birth, 26(1)*, 26–32.

Montgomery, E. (2013). Feeling safe: a metasynthesis of the maternity care needs of women who were sexually abused in childhood. *Birth, 40(2)*, 88–95.

Niven, C. (1994). Coping with labour pain: the midwife's role. In S. Robinson and A. Thompson (eds), *Research & Childbirth*. London: Chapman & Hall.

O'Connell, M.A., Crowther, S., Ravaldi, C. and Homer, C. (2020). Midwives in a pandemic: a call for solidarity and compassion. *Women and Birth, 33*, 205–206.

Page, M. and Mander, R. (2014). Intrapartum uncertainty: a feature of normal birth, as experienced by midwives in Scotland. *Midwifery, 30*, 28–35.

Pezaro, S., Clyne, W., Turner, A., Fulton, E.A. and Gerada, C. (2015). 'Midwives overboard!' Inside their hearts are breaking, their makeup may be flaking but their smile still stays on. *Women and Birth, 29*, 59–66.

Revans, R.W. (1964). *Standards for Morale: Cause and Effect in Hospitals*. Oxford: The Nuffield University Hospitals Trust, Oxford University Press.

Sheen, K., Spiby, H. and Slade, P. (2015). Exposure to traumatic perinatal experiences and posttraumatic stress symptoms in midwives: prevalence and association with burnout. *International Journal of Nursing Studies, 52(2)*, 578–587.

Slade, P., Sheen, K., Collinge, S., Butters, J. and Spiby, H. (2018). A programme for the prevention of post-traumatic stress disorder in midwifery (POPPY): indications of effectiveness from a feasibility study. *European Journal of Psychotraumatology, 9(1)*, 1518069.

Smith, P. (1992). *The Emotional Labour of Nursing*. London: Macmillan.

Waldron, V.R. (2012). *Communicating Emotion at Work*. Cambridge: Polity Press.

Walsh, D. (2006a). Birth centres, community and social capital. *MIDIRS Midwifery Digest, 16(1)*, 7–15.

Walsh, D. (2006b). 'Nesting' and 'matrescence' as distinctive features of a free-standing birth centre in the UK. *Midwifery, 22(3)*, 289–239.

Walsh, D. (2007). *Improving Maternity Services. Small is Beautiful – Lessons from a Birth Centre*. Oxford: Radcliffe Publishing.

Warriner, S., Hunter, L. and Dymond, M. (2016). Mindfulness in maternity: evaluation of a course for midwives. *British Journal of Midwifery, 24(3)*, 188–195.

West, M., Bailey, S. and Williams, E. (2020). *The Courage of Compassion*. London: The Kings Fund.

WHO. (2016). Midwives voices, midwives realities. Findings from a global consultation on providing quality midwifery care. Geneva: World Health Organization.

Wright, E., Matthai, M.T. and Warren, N. (2017). Methods for alleviating stress and increasing resilience in the midwifery community: a scoping review of the literature *Journal of Midwifery & Women's Health, 62*, 737–745.

Youngson, R. (2012). *Time to Care: How to Love Your Patients and Your Job*. New Zealand: Rebelheart Publishers.

Epilogue

A support person offers a continuous, uninterrupted presence and it is this commitment that brings its own reward for those who are curious about how birth happens and observant of the intimacies of the process. It is also a great adventure, full of possibilities and unexpected discoveries.

Most of all, enjoy your work for what it offers: magic moments of rare beauty, excitement and never-ending wonderment.

(Andrea Robertson, *The Midwife Companion: The Art of Support During Birth*, Sydney: Birth International, 2007, p.ix)

List of Reflective Activities, Student Assignments and Assessments

Chapter 1: What do we mean by 'support' in labour?

Exploring local implementation of one-to-one support in labour
Talking to women about support in labour
Advice about supporting women in labour – YouTube
Creating environments that enable companions to provide support
Exploring the potential effect of our values and attitudes when supporting women in labour
The roles of the doula and the midwife in community-based continuity of care
Being in the room with women in labour
Continuous support in labour and safety
'Break the silence' – thinking about respectful maternity care

Chapter 2: Approaches to pain in labour

Stories of women's experiences of pain in childbirth
Factors that might influence the way pain in labour is approached and experienced by women
Being alongside a woman in labour and reading her experiences
Women's responses to pain in labour – cultural considerations
Discussing evidence about pain management
Explaining the rationale for 'working with pain'

Chapter 3: Addressing fear and anxiety about labour and birth

Recognising symptoms, risk factors, consequences and treatments of fear of childbirth and PTSD
What are women's worst fears?
Paternal anxiety in labour – what might be the consequences?
Picking up on the cues when women are fearful
Identifying resources in the community for women who fear childbirth
Exploring our own fears
Conversations about reality TV shows and representations of birth
'The things that count cannot be counted' – microbiology, epigenetics and birth
Professional attitudes to planned caesarean or vaginal birth
Practising 'The Midwifery Wave'
Encouraging words when talking to a pregnant woman about labour
Scenario-based workstation (OSCE): addressing a pregnant woman's anxiety

Chapter 4: Supporting women preparing for labour and birth

Enabling 'Active Birth' and 'non-disturbance' in labour
Thinking about birth plans and choice
Discussing Internet information sources with a pregnant woman
Identifying women's individual needs for support in labour
Learning from women through VBAC blogs
Identifying values in childbirth education
Group facilitation – honouring women's expertise
Demystifying physiology
Using birth photos in groups
Simulating labour behaviour and sounds
Explaining 'mindfulness' approaches in labour
Discussing hypnobirthing and calm birthing with women and their birth companions
Talking to women about choice of birthplace
Encouraging conversations with pregnant women and their partners: some examples to practise

Chapter 5: Communication and thoughtful encouragement

First impressions and communication with pregnant women and their families
Suggestibility and the effect of tone and emphasis in communication
Exploring the role of persuasion in practice
Discussing homeopathy – contested opinions
A journey metaphor for childbirth
Metaphor promoting meaning in *The Squire*
Language, communication and power dynamics
The 'delivery' word
The words we use for contractions
The problem with 'normal'
Enhancing communication through midwifery continuity of care
When personal values get in the way of rapport
Communication and thoughtful encouragement: a student assignment

Chapter 6: Supporting women for normal birth

Concerted efforts to define, measure and promote normal birth
Why normal birth matters
'Midwifery muttering'
'I just want to talk. And I want you to listen'
Confronting the stereotyping of labouring women
'Looking after Auntie'
Supporting partners to provide labour support
When midwives need to step in with support
Interactions with birth support people
Changing the culture to promote home birth
Conversations with women contemplating 'freebirthing'
Supporting women in birth centres
Thinking about how birth unit design affects supportive care in labour
Facilitating normal birth in practice

Chapter 7: Supporting women in labour: practicalities

Supportive strategies in labour – identifying individual competency and learning needs
Supporting women who want to use complementary therapies in labour
Supporting women who have prepared for labour using self-hypnosis techniques
Supporting women in early labour
Behavioural clues
Positions for labour and birth
Facilitating active birth and privacy
Water to promote comfort in labour and birth
'Cluefulness' and the Coping with Labor Algorithm ©
'She believed in me when I didn't believe in myself'
'You can do it' – supporting women in transition
Supporting women for 'the first embrace'

Chapter 8: Supporting women with complex needs in labour

A midwifery model of care for women at high risk of complications
Promoting normal birth around technology
Creating a sense of calm in the birth room
Epidural dilemmas – a student midwife's story
Supporting women faced with induction
Talking through what to expect in theatre
Planned caesarean birth – exploring choices
Support for a breech birth – Tanya's story
'Pilots through stormy seas' – Carol's story
Supporting women around the loss of a baby

Chapter 9: Emotions and labour support

Identifying our emotions when caring for a woman in labour
Acknowledging emotional work in maternity care
Discussing emotions in midwifery
Exploring felt emotion, feeling rules, emotion work, displayed emotion
Enhancing self-awareness
The intimate sounds of labour
Working conditions and emotional wellbeing
Identifying personal sources of support
Thinking about workplace culture
Supporting each other

Index

Printed in the United States
by Baker & Taylor Publisher Services